AJPH
A PUBLICATION OF THE
AMERICAN PUBLIC HEALTH ASSOCIATION

AMERICAN JOURNAL of PUBLIC HEALTH
AUGUST 2025
Issue 8

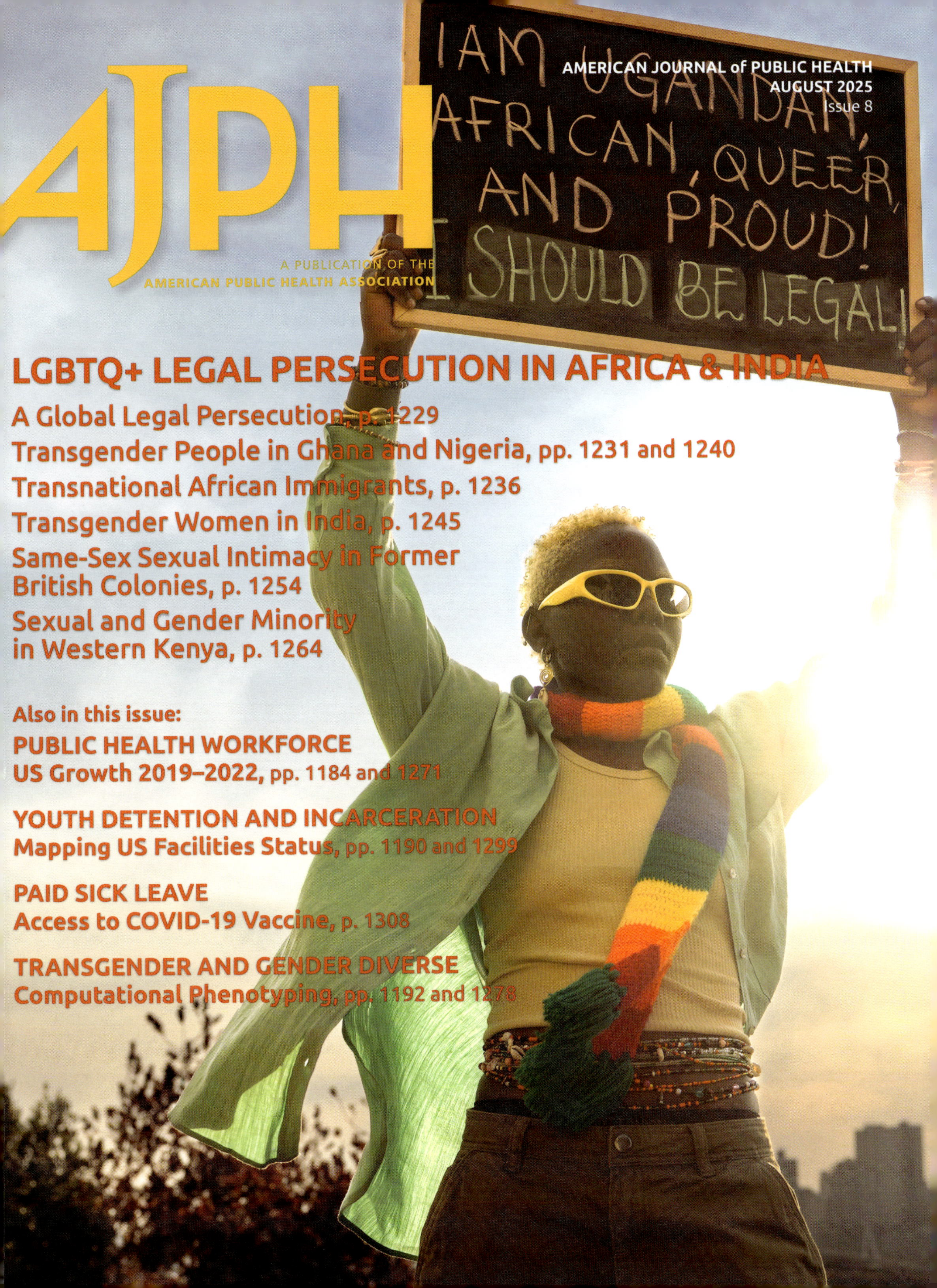

LGBTQ+ LEGAL PERSECUTION IN AFRICA & INDIA

A Global Legal Persecution, p. 1229
Transgender People in Ghana and Nigeria, pp. 1231 and 1240
Transnational African Immigrants, p. 1236
Transgender Women in India, p. 1245
Same-Sex Sexual Intimacy in Former British Colonies, p. 1254
Sexual and Gender Minority in Western Kenya, p. 1264

Also in this issue:

PUBLIC HEALTH WORKFORCE
US Growth 2019–2022, pp. 1184 and 1271

YOUTH DETENTION AND INCARCERATION
Mapping US Facilities Status, pp. 1190 and 1299

PAID SICK LEAVE
Access to COVID-19 Vaccine, p. 1308

TRANSGENDER AND GENDER DIVERSE
Computational Phenotyping, pp. 1192 and 1278

APHA
AMERICAN PUBLIC HEALTH ASSOCIATION
For science. For action. For health.

AJPH®, published monthly, is the official Journal of the American Public Health Association®, 800 I St NW, Washington, DC 20001-3710; (202) 777- APHA; TDD (202) 777-2500. APHA is a nongovernmental professional society founded in 1872, representing all disciplines and specialties in public health.

The *American Journal of Public Health*® (*AJPH*) (print ISSN: 0090-0036; electronic ISSN: 1541- 0048), first published in 1911, is the official journal of the American Public Health Association® (APHA). The oldest and largest organization of public health professionals in the world, APHA represents approximately 30 000 members from more than 50 occupations of public health.

Submissions: Visit www.editorialmanager.com/ajph or ajph.edmgr.com for online manuscript preparation and submission guidelines. Contributions of original unpublished research, social science analyses, scholarly essays, critical commentaries, departments, and letters to the editor are welcome. Questions? Write ajph.submissions@apha.org or call APHA at (202) 777-2469.

Print plus online subscriptions: Institutional price (print copy with online access for a single institution and all authorized users, regardless of geographic location) varies by size of organization and ranges from $993–$1445 for US organizations, and $1073–$1526 for international organizations (air delivery); multiple campuses not permitted without special arrangement. Details of the tiered pricing system at https://subscriptionoffice.com/pages/apha-landing-page. To order, write apha.subscriptions@apha.org.

Online-only subscriptions: Institutional price for one institution and its authorized users (regardless of geographic location) is $878–$1307. To order, write apha.subscriptions@apha.org. For academic consortia or multisite corporate subscriptions, contact apha.subscriptions@apha.org.

Print-only subscriptions: Institutional price is US $701, $782 international.

Back print issues: A limited number of print issues are for sale. Single copies are US $65, $75 international (air delivery). Shipping included; prepay only. To order, write apha.subscriptions@apha.org.

Reprints: For prices and ordering information on 50 or more reprints, check the Reprints section at www.ajph.org. To order smaller quantities of reprints (rush delivery), use the "Purchase Article" link on the article site itself.

Electronic access: Online articles more than 10 years old are available free for personal use at www.ajph.org. Recent articles are available through pay-per-view: single PDF article for $24, single issue access for 24 hours for $33, or entire site access for 24 hours for $38.

Postal information: Periodicals postage paid at Washington, DC, and additional mailing offices. Postmaster: Send address changes to American Journal of Public Health, 800 I St NW, Washington, DC 20001-3710.

Address changes: Send to AJPH, Membership Department (members) or AJPH Subscriptions (subscribers), APHA, 800 I St NW, Washington, DC 20001-3710. Or write to membership.mail@apha.org (members) or apha.subscriptions@apha.org (subscribers).

Advertising: For pricing and other information, see www.ajph.org. Please write to brian.selzer@apha.org or call (202) 777-2470 for other advertising opportunities. Ask about special exhibit packages and sponsorships. Acceptance of advertising by the *Journal* does not imply endorsement of products.

Indexes: Publications that index or abstract articles from *AJPH* include the following: Ageline, Assia (Applied Social Science Index and Abstracts), Biological Abstracts, Chemical Abstracts, CINAHL, Criminal Justice Abstracts, EMBASE, EMCare, Environmental Abstracts, e-psyche, ERIC, ETOH (Alcohol and Alcohol Problems Science Database), Excerpta Medica, Food Science and Technology, General Science Index, Grateful Med, Hospital Literature Index, Human Resources Abstracts, International Pharmaceutical Abstracts (IPA), Medline, Physical Education Index, Pollution Abstracts, Psychological Abstracts, PsychINFO, Safety Science Abstracts, Sage Family Studies Abstracts, Sage Human Resources Abstracts, Science Citation Index, SCOPUS, SIIC Data Bases, Social Work Research and Abstracts, and Statistical Reference Index (SRI)/LexisNexis.

AJPH

A PUBLICATION OF THE
AMERICAN PUBLIC HEALTH ASSOCIATION

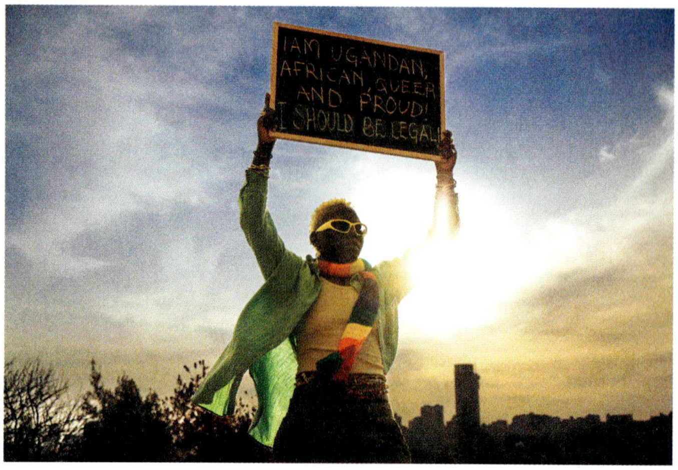

COVER: DeLovie Kwagala (papa De), self-described, as the first openly nonbinary Queer photographer from Uganda, human rights activist, and photojournalist. DeLovie is in exile from Uganda for safety reasons.

Cover concept and selection by Aleisha Kropf. Photo by Brent Stirton/Getty Images. Printed with permission.

APHA
AMERICAN PUBLIC HEALTH ASSOCIATION
For science. For action. For health.

Promoting public health research, policy, practice, and education is the *AJPH* mission. As we widen our scope to embrace global issues, we also sharpen our focus to support the needs of public health practitioners. We invite contributions of original unpublished research, opinion and commentary, and letters to the editor.

The *Journal* is printed on acid-free recycled paper.

OPEN ACCESS ONLINE ONLY PODCAST DATA SUPPLEMENT AVAILABLE

EDITOR'S CHOICE

1182 US Schools and Programs, Don't Forget Federal Grants Expire in 2027
J. P. Leider and P. Erwin

OPINIONS, IDEAS, & PRACTICE

EDITORIALS

1184 Fleeting Fixes, Fractured Systems: Confronting the Continuing Crisis of the Public Health Workforce
B. C. Castrucci

1187 The AIDS Drug Assistance Program Is a Model for Chronic Disease Treatment Support
J. C. Dombrowski, A. Thompson, and J. Feinberg

1190 Centering Youth and Family Needs in Juvenile Justice Reform Efforts
L. Helmcamp

1192 Now, More Than Ever, We Need Institutional Commitments to Transgender Health Research
D. M. Tordoff, N. K. Tran, J. Obedin-Maliver, and M. R. Lunn

PERSPECTIVES

1196 Legal Recognition of Same-Sex Marriage in Asia Is an Opportunity to Improve LGBTQ+ Physical and Mental Health
Y. T. Suen

1200 The Impact of Anti-LGBTQ+ Legislation on Mental Health and Substance Use and HIV Prevention and Care Among Gay and Bisexual Men in Kenya
G. W. Harper, E. O. Odhiambo, L. Jadwin-Cakmak, F. O. Okuta, K. Bauman, K. O. Olango, D. M. Moore, E. Gumbe, T. Aloo, and S. A. Hussen

1206 Tobacco Company Efforts to Persuade Consumers to Fight the Proposed Federal Menthol Cigarette and Flavored Cigar Bans in the United States
O. Ganz, A. C. Villanti, A. Altunbilek, A. Johnson, J. Garmon, O. A. Wackowski, and K. L. Sterling

1211 Designating Cartels as Terrorist Organizations: The Wrong Path to Addressing the Illicit Fentanyl Crisis
J. Wolthuis and D. G. Aaron

RADICAL HOPE

1215 The Power of Community in Promoting Water Safety in Rural Madagascar
S. Brown

1217 Tackling Wicked Problems: The Power of Community Among the Unhoused
K. Marnfeldt, L. Xie, and A. Zhang

EDITOR'S CORNER

1220 The Escalating War on Immigrants Is a Public Health Crisis
L. N. Borrell and F. Kapadia

NOTES FROM THE FIELD

1222 Time Scarcity, Health Behaviors, and Unconditional Cash in Los Angeles
A. Castro, M. Philips, I. Kim, S. West, and B-K. E. Kim

1226 Breaking Barriers: Advancing Employment Opportunities for Black Women
C. Tucker, T. L. Foust, N. Baldwin, and T. Moore

GLOBAL LGBTQ+ PUBLIC HEALTH IN THE FACE OF LEGAL PERSECUTION

1229 Global LGBTQ+ Public Health in the Face of Legal Persecution
S. Landers and B. E. Coston

1231 Barriers to Gender-Affirming Care, Health Care Services, and Experiences of Health Care Provider Bias Among Transgender People in Nigeria
A. Ogunbajo, T. Oke, C. Fitch, A. Restar, A. Barney, O. Oginni, and D. Hickson

1236 The Effects of LGBTQ+ Persecution on Transnational African Immigrants
K. Ibe-Lamberts and D. Onyeise

1240 The Public Health Implications of Ghana's Anti-LGBTQ+ Bill: A Lesson From Nigeria
E. P. Akadinma and S. Hillier

RESEARCH & ANALYSIS

GLOBAL LGBTQ+ PUBLIC HEALTH IN THE FACE OF LEGAL PERSECUTION

1245 Transgender Women in India: A Syndemic and Intersectional Framework Addressing HIV Care Gaps
W. Lodge II, S. Rawat, A. Dange, M. Agénor, V. R. Anand, D. Operario, M. J. Mimiaga, and K. B. Biello

1254 Strategic Litigation, Public Health, and the Decriminalization of Same-Sex Sexual Intimacy: Lessons From Legal Challenges Across Former British Colonies
S. Wallach, J. Ratevosian, T. Smith, K. Duval, S. Baral, and C. Beyrer

1264 US Right-Wing, Pro-Family Movements in East Africa: Furthering Legislation That Fuels Health Inequities Among Sexual and Gender Minority Persons Assigned Female Sex at Birth in Western Kenya
H. M. Tucker, A. Mbanda, R. Odhiambo, and G. W. Harper

POLICY

1271 Sustainability of the Growth of the Local Public Health Workforce During the COVID-19 Pandemic, 2019–2022
K. Patel, T. C. McCall, M. Cunningham, C. Garofalini, J. Lee, and A. A. Alford

METHODS

1278 Identification of Transgender and Gender-Diverse Individuals in the All of Us Research Program, 2017–2022
F. Shi, X. Yang, R. Cai, J. Zhang, S. E. Harrison, S. Qiao, S. G. Frary, and X. Li

OPEN-THEMED RESEARCH

1288 Trends in AIDS Drug Assistance Program Support for People With HIV, by Age, Sex, Race, and US Region, 2008–2021
K. A. McManus, A. Killelea, T. Horn, A. Steen, B. Sun, J. Keim-Malpass, A. Hamp, A. Strumpf, and E. T. R. McQuade

1299 Youth Detention and Incarceration Facilities in the United States (2010 to February 2023): Mapping Closure Intents and Implementation
E. J. Johnson, H. Pluckebaum, K. D. Martin, B. Danielson, B. Majercin, S. A. Capestany, and V. H. Lyons

1308 Access to Paid Sick Leave and COVID-19 Vaccination Status Among Employed Adults Aged 18–64 Years in the United States, 2021–2022
E. W. Lundstrom, A. Asfaw, and R. Tsai

1312 Expiration of the Expanded Child Tax Credit and Energy Insecurity in US Households With Children, 2021–2022
C. Yama, J. M. Rook, L. E. Wisk, R. Dudovitz, D. Hernández, D. P. Eisenman, and K. M. Leifheit

1322 Preventing Real-World Pediatric Vehicular Heatstroke Events With Technology
J. Maheshwari, E. Sartin, G. Chingas, and K. B. Arbogast

BACKMATTER

LETTERS & RESPONSES

1327 Collecting Data Is Just the First Step: The Importance of Training Providers for Patient Encounters
S. Chang and M. Kano

1328 Tamí-Maury and Millett Respond
I. Tamí-Maury and M. L. E. Millett

ERRATA

1330 Erratum In: “Intersectional HIV Stigma Among Black Women: Regional Differences and Implications From the Black Women First Initiative”

OTHER DEPARTMENTS

1336 Subscription Form

US Schools and Programs, Don't Forget Federal Grants Expire in 2027

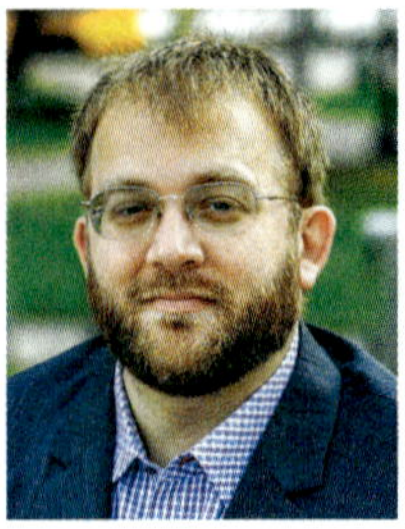
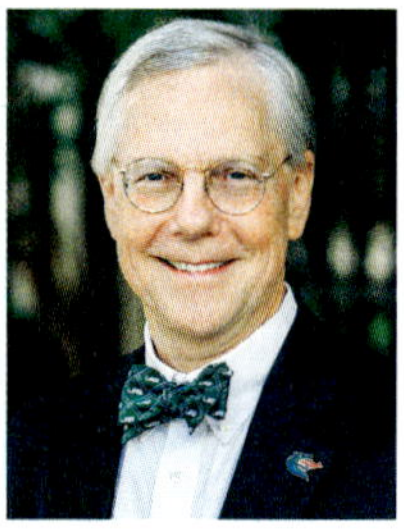

Jonathon P. Leider, PhD
School of Public Health, University of Minnesota, Minneapolis
Paul Erwin, MD, DrPH
School of Public Health, University of Alabama, Birmingham

AJPH August 2025, Vol. 115, No. 8

For all the clear and present threats of the here and now, leaders in public health academia also need to keep one eye toward 2027. It is a year when we will experience a shrinking pool of students because of demographic shifts, a year when undergraduate and graduate education will be threatened, and a year when nearly all remaining pandemic era federal grants will expire. Absent a recession—which very likely would result in an increase in post-secondary applications that could counter the demographic changes—enrollment in undergraduate and graduate education is expected to decline nationwide, and public health programs may well experience the same.

The demographic cliff has been well described for more than a decade: in or around 2025, the number of those aged 18 years is expected to peak, after which fewer students will be around to attend college. For this we have the Great Recession of 2008 to thank, when birth rates plummeted. In addition, macroeconomic shifts and a previously strong labor market have diminished the perceived value of postsecondary education. The relative increases in proportion and absolute numbers of Asian, Hispanic/Latino, and Black/African American students are not expected to offset the decrease in White students seeking postsecondary education. Although a future recession or other macroeconomic shifts could alter this trajectory, the current outlook warrants serious consideration.

As the demographic cliff approaches, so too does a federal funding cliff: one-time funds tied to pandemic recovery and COVID-19 response are set to expire in 2027. Moreover, the current presidential administration has shown a clear interest in decreasing or eliminating pandemic era funds (witness the recent $12 billion cut to the Center for Disease Control and Prevention's Epidemiology and Laboratory Capacity Program), even when those funds support ongoing public health activities not associated with COVID-19 response. Tens of billions more in funding will expire, much of which would have gone to colleges and universities across the United States directly or indirectly through grants and contracts from state and local entities.

Academic public health must acknowledge these potential realities and

Continued on page 1183...

HISTORY CORNER

22 YEARS AGO

Culturally Appropriate Interventions Targeting Men Who Have Sex With Men

Modern terminology and biomedical models of homosexuality were developed in the 19th century, and became the object of study for pioneers such as Hirschfeld and Westermarck. The pervasive assumption that these "scientific" concepts of sexuality apply universally is not only incorrect, it also impedes appreciation of the relative differences within and between cultures with respect to same-sex behavioral phenomena. As Carrier writes, "Additional anthropological research on human sexual behavior is urgently needed in different culture areas of the world . . . to counteract the myopia of many who continue to view it only through the screen of Western behavior, beliefs, and social and clinical labels." . . . The concept of the berdache, or two-spirit, individuals in Native American cultures provides some of the best-documented examples of gender-defined patterns for MSM. These patterns refer to the assumption of some or all of the conventional roles and responsibilities of the opposite gender, or of a combined or distinctive third gender role. . . . Human sexuality cannot be definitively fixed or located in a static taxonomy, and ongoing cultural change must also be accounted for. Failure to appreciate this level of historical complexity undermines not only the cultural competencies of public health personnel, but also the effectiveness of public health education, research, and service.

From *AJPH*, June 2003, pp. 867–870

address them head on. Redefining the value proposition of a public health degree in the current political and funding environment is critical. Current students are already asking, "Should I remain in public health? Will I have immediate and long-term career opportunities?" Although we can answer with our belief that science will ultimately prevail over the present chaos—repeating the useful American Public Health Association phrase "Science is evidence, not opinion"—the budgetary assault on higher education in general, and public health specifically, makes it difficult for students to accept this as a value proposition, especially because the average master of public health graduate leaves school with almost $50 000 in debt on average.

Will schools of public health compete for a shrinking pool of students, seek to expand it through online programs or international recruitment (if still permissible), or create new pathways from the natural and social sciences? In support of those who want to chart the problem, a new dashboard (https://z.umn.edu/county2025) helps to compare graduation trends in public health and overall with local demographic data. Although some areas are seeing stability or growth, the national decline is, indeed, mirrored in local contexts.

Everyone likes a good metaphor for the moment. In times of uncertainty, the idea of a roller coaster gets bandied about with some frequency, and with good reason: the gravity pressing you down, the apex and weightlessness, the freefall that follows, and the horrific fear of falling out and getting run over. For this time, though, it may be that the whirling teacups or carnival spider are more apt: incongruent, unpredictable motion with no clear end that just might make you throw up seems a reasonable fit. To say that the state of academic public health is uncertain does some injustice to the notion of certainty. Billions of dollars have been cut, schools are experiencing nationwide revenue freezes, and indirect cuts have been threatened. As we divine the appropriate metaphor for the moment, we need to also keep our eyes toward the future. More cuts are sure to come, and more challenges will present themselves. The tumult of early 2025 showed that we cannot predict the future, but the field can try to prepare for it. AJPH

DOI: https://doi.org/10.2105/AJPH.2025.308204

ORCID iDs:
Jonathon P. Leider https://orcid.org/0000-0001-9905-476X
Paul Erwin https://orcid.org/0000-0002-0580-4855

HISTORY CORNER

24 YEARS AGO

Lesbian and Gay Health Research in South Africa

In this commentary, we describe our difficulties in obtaining research ethics committee (or institutional review board) approval for research into human rights abuses of gay men and lesbians in the South African Defence Force by health professionals during the apartheid era. We use this case study to raise concerns that institutional heterosexism and a reluctance to explore professional abuses of power continue to shape health research in South Africa. . . . Apartheid provided the ideologic framework for decades of South African health research that allowed racism, sexism, and heterosexism to masquerade as "scientific objectivity." Despite democratic transition, the enactment of a wide-ranging bill of rights (which includes protection against discrimination on the basis of sexual orientation), and the findings of the Truth and Reconciliation Commission, these hegemonic ideologies have yet to be fundamentally challenged in many institutions in South Africa. . . . Researchers and research institutions have an important role to play in building a culture of human rights in South Africa and elsewhere. This can be achieved, however, only through inclusion and through ensuring that all research domains, including lesbian and gay health, are supported as valid topics for scientific inquiry.

From *AJPH*, June 2001, p. 867

Fleeting Fixes, Fractured Systems: Confronting the Continuing Crisis of the Public Health Workforce

Brian C. Castrucci, DrPH, MA

ABOUT THE AUTHOR

Brian C. Castrucci is with the de Beaumont Foundation, Bethesda, MD.

See also Patel et al., p. 1271.

In their article "Sustainability of the Growth of the Local Public Health Workforce During the COVID-19 Pandemic, 2019–2022" (p. 1271), Patel et al. document a 19% increase in staffing across local governmental public health departments between 2019 and 2022. At first glance, this suggests a long-overdue reversal of years of chronic underinvestment. Yet beneath the surface of this apparent resurgence lies a more troubling reality—one that warrants scrutiny, not celebration.

TEMPORARY GAINS, ENDURING GAPS

Although total staffing levels increased during the pandemic, this growth was overwhelmingly concentrated in temporary, contractual, and seasonal positions. In contrast, full-time employment, the foundational pillar of a stable and enduring public health workforce, rose by only 7%. These modest gains were underwritten by short-term federal investments, including the CARES Act and the American Rescue Plan. Now, as these appropriations expire, the positions they funded are rapidly disappearing, taking with them any illusion of lasting progress.

Even if the pandemic-era workforce gains were permanent, they would fall far short of what is required. According to the Staffing Up report by the de Beaumont Foundation and the Public Health National Center for Innovations, the local public health workforce must expand by 80% to ensure the delivery of foundational public health services to all communities.[1] A short-lived 19% increase—heavily concentrated in temporary and contractual roles—barely registers against that benchmark. What appeared to be a turning point was, in truth, a familiar cycle: a fleeting surge that left the system's structural deficiencies untouched.

RURAL AMERICA LEFT BEHIND—AGAIN

Patel et al. also reveal profound inequities in how pandemic-era investments were allocated. Although medium and large health departments absorbed most of the new staffing, small and rural jurisdictions—those most urgently identified in the Staffing Up report as underresourced[1]—were largely bypassed. This is not simply a failure of implementation; it is a failure of equity. Rural communities, which already experience higher rates of preventable disease, disability, and premature death, were once again left with the fewest resources. Yet during the largest public health crisis in a century, they received the smallest share of workforce investment.[2] When funding mechanisms reward complexity and scale rather than demonstrated need, they do more than miss the mark—they reinforce the very disparities public health is charged with addressing. Equity is not a slogan. It is a structural obligation—and it must be funded accordingly.

In the United States, public health funding has long followed a predictable and perilous pattern: crisis prompts investment, and stability invites retreat. Funding typically flows in response to discrete threats—Ebola, opioids, Zika, COVID-19—while the essential infrastructure that enables prevention, detection, and response remains chronically underfunded. The Centers for Disease Control and Prevention's (CDC's) Public Health Infrastructure Grant (PHIG) represented an important departure from this model: a rare, flexible investment aimed at bolstering core capabilities across jurisdictions, regardless of disease or emergency.[3] Yet despite its innovation, the PHIG remains a grant—time-limited by statute and vulnerable to shifting political priorities. It is, at best, a down payment on the infrastructure the nation requires. And history offers a sobering reminder: aspirations for continued funding cannot substitute for permanent, structural investment. This is not recovery. It is a mirage evaporating fast—revealing a nation more exposed than ever and a system still unfit for the threats ahead.

Academic research provides critical insight, but it often reflects conditions

AJPH August 2025, Vol. 115, No. 8

that have already begun to shift by the time findings are published. This is not a critique of Patel et al.'s contribution, but a reflection of the volatility and velocity of the current policy landscape. In COVID-19's aftermath, few could have anticipated the scale and ferocity of the political backlash against public health: sweeping legislative rollbacks of public health authority, sustained harassment of health officials, and—perhaps most consequentially—the Trump administration's proposal to cut more than $12 billion from the budgets of the CDC and the Health Resources and Services Administration.[4] These proposed reductions, now the subject of ongoing legal challenges, threaten to dismantle the very infrastructure the pandemic exposed as dangerously fragile.

These are not routine budgetary corrections—they are deliberate efforts to erode an already strained public health infrastructure. The narrow policy window that enabled flexible investments like the PHIG has closed, and the prevailing political environment is now actively working to undercut their longevity. In this climate, long-term planning becomes fiction. Health departments cannot meaningfully build capacity when their very survival depends on transient political will.

ASSAULTING THE PUBLIC HEALTH WORKFORCE

The erosion of public health infrastructure has been paralleled by a profound psychological toll on the workforce itself. According to the Public Health Workforce Interests and Needs Survey (PH WINS), 44% of state and local public health employees reported symptoms consistent with posttraumatic stress disorder during the COVID-19 response.[5] The pandemic pushed health departments to their operational and emotional limits. Staff were pulled from core responsibilities, essential non-COVID-19 services were suspended,[6] and frontline professionals faced relentless harassment, political interference, and public vilification.[7] They continued their work even as the scaffolding beneath them gave way. Now, amid renewed funding threats and mounting political hostility, the message is unmistakable: their service was circumstantial, their labor expendable.

This is not merely a technical crisis—it is a crisis of values. When school budgets are slashed, families rightly worry about their children's education. When police departments face cuts, communities fear for their safety. But when public health departments are dismantled, the response is silence. There is no public outcry, no widespread alarm, no collective recognition of what has been lost. That absence speaks volumes—not about the importance of public health, but about the failure to make its value visible and understood.

The public health literature has long articulated a coherent and evidence-based blueprint for reform. Across decades of scholarship and policy analysis, the calls have remained consistent: sustained and flexible funding,[8] modernization of data systems,[9] and strategic investments in workforce development, including loan repayment programs.[10] These priorities are neither new nor contested. Yet despite their clarity and the growing urgency of the moment, the response has been intermittent and inadequate. This is not a failure of knowledge—it is a failure of political and fiscal resolve. That failure, in part, stems from a deeper problem: public health has never successfully made its value visible. Policymakers rarely fund what the public does not understand.

VISIBILITY IS SURVIVAL: MAKING PUBLIC HEALTH SEEN AND VALUED

Public health has long suffered from a deficit not of impact, but of visibility. When schools hire more teachers, parents expect smaller class sizes. When police departments expand, residents anticipate increased patrols. But when a health department brings on an epidemiologist or an environmental health officer, the public often sees no immediate, tangible benefit. The outcomes are diffuse, the value abstract—and that obscurity has become a critical vulnerability.

Without the ability to articulate its contributions in ways that resonate with the public, public health remains politically vulnerable and chronically underfunded. The field must move beyond technical vernacular and lead with outcomes the public can see and feel: cleaner air, safer food, healthier children, longer lives. A national communications strategy is no longer optional. It is essential.

Public health must trade ambiguity for clarity, invisibility for resonance. It must abandon the assumption that its value is self-evident and instead demonstrate it—relentlessly, creatively, and in terms that matter to the communities it serves.

The responsibility for safeguarding public health cannot rest solely with the federal government. State and local governments must recognize public health for what it is: essential civic infrastructure, no less vital than police departments, fire services, or public libraries. A system built on the hope of periodic federal investments is not a system built to last. It is one perpetually at risk for collapse. Public health departments must be sustained by predictable, locally anchored investments that reflect their foundational role in community well-being. If public health truly matters, it must be reflected not in rhetoric, but in appropriations.

The pandemic delivered a temporary surge of investment. But attention is not infrastructure, resources are not systems, and growth without permanence is not progress.

Today, as funding recedes and political resistance hardens—even as H5N1 and mpox persist and measles, once considered eliminated, returns with force—the public health system is contracting once again. Without sustained and equitable investment in the workforce and infrastructure that protect the nation's health, the consequence will not simply be a loss of personnel. It will be a loss of capacity—the very ability to anticipate, respond to, and contain future crises.

Readiness cannot be improvised. It cannot be summoned when the sirens start. It must be constructed—deliberately, durably, and with unwavering resolve. If that foundation erodes, it is the public who will bear the full cost. AJPH

CORRESPONDENCE

Correspondence should be sent to Brian C. Castrucci, 7501 Wisconsin Ave #1310e, Bethesda, MD 20814 (e-mail: castrucci@debeaumont.org). Reprints can be ordered at http://www.ajph.org by clicking the "Reprints" link.

PUBLICATION INFORMATION

Full Citation: Castrucci BC. Fleeting fixes, fractured systems: confronting the continuing crisis of the public health workforce. *Am J Public Health*. 2025;115(8):1184–1186.

Acceptance Date: April 29, 2025.

DOI: https://doi.org/10.2105/AJPH.2025.308184

CONFLICTS OF INTEREST

The author has no conflicts of interest to report.

REFERENCES

1. de Beaumont Foundation and Public Health National Center for Innovations. Staffing Up: workforce levels needed to provide basic public health services for all Americans. 2021. Available at: https://debeaumont.org. Accessed April 20, 2025.
2. Coates A, Zahnd W, Burgin C. Toward a sustainable and diversified rural health workforce. National Rural Health Association. February 2022. Available at: https://www.ruralhealth.us/getmedia/f7b57994-8fb2-47b0-a6e0-12ee74591314/NRHA-Toward-a-Sustainable-Rural-Health-Workforce-Policy-Brief-2022.pdf. Accessed April 21, 2025.
3. Centers for Disease Control and Prevention. Public Health Infrastructure Grant. 2024. Available at: www.cdc.gov/infrastructure-phig/about/index.html. Accessed April 20, 2025.
4. Goldman M, Moreno S. Trump admin cancels over $12B in health care grants. *Axios*. March 27, 2025. Available at: https://www.axios.com/2025/03/27/trump-admin-cancels-state-health-care-grants. Accessed April 20, 2025.
5. de Beaumont Foundation and Association of State and Territorial Health Officials. Public Health Workforce Interests and Needs Survey (PH WINS) 2021: stress and burnout. 2022. Available at: https://debeaumont.org/phwins/2021-findings/stress-and-burnout. Accessed April 20, 2025.
6. McCullough JM, Robins M. The opportunity cost of COVID for public health practice. *J Public Health Manag Pract*. 2023;29(suppl 1):S64–S72. https://doi.org/10.1097/phh.0000000000001656
7. Fraser MR. Harassment of health officials: a significant threat to the public's health. *Am J Public Health*. 2022;112(5):728–730. https://doi.org/10.2105/AJPH.2022.306797
8. DeSalvo K, Parekh A, Hoagland GW, et al. Developing a financing system to support public health infrastructure. *Am J Public Health*. 2019; 109(10):1358–1361. https://doi.org/10.2105/AJPH.2019.305214
9. Milliken L. Modernizing public health: the critical role of technology and workforce training. National Network of Public Health Institutes. October 31, 2024. Available at: https://nnphi.org/modernizing-public-health-the-critical-role-of-technology-and-workforce-training. Accessed April 21, 2025.
10. Association of Schools and Programs of Public Health (ASPPH). ASPPH signs on to letter to fund public health workforce loan repayment. March 28, 2024. Available at: https://aspph.org/aspph-signs-on-to-letter-to-fund-public-health-workforce-loan-repayment. Accessed April 21, 2025.

The AIDS Drug Assistance Program Is a Model for Chronic Disease Treatment Support

Julia C. Dombrowski, MD, MPH, Adam Thompson, MPH, and Judith Feinberg, MD

ABOUT THE AUTHORS

Julia C. Dombrowski is with the Department of Medicine at University of Washington, Seattle. Adam Thompson is a patient advocate who lives in Willingboro, NJ. Judith Feinberg is with the Department of Behavioral Medicine and Psychiatry and the Department of Medicine, Division of Infectious Diseases, West Virgina University, Morgantown.

See also McManus et al., p. 1288.

By virtually any definition, the AIDS Drug Assistance Program (ADAP) stands out as an effective US government program. It emerged from collective advocacy by and for people with AIDS who could not afford life-saving medication, was created through bipartisan cooperation, and is cost-effective.[1] Initially established in 1987 as a one-year emergency measure to cover the cost of newly available but prohibitively expensive antiretroviral medication, ADAP was later incorporated into the 1990 Ryan White HIV/AIDS Program (RWHAP).[2] The RWHAP is a federally funded program that provides health care and support services for low-income people with HIV (PWH). For nearly 40 years, ADAP has played a critical role in providing prescription drugs for uninsured and underinsured PWH.

ADAP and the broader RWHAP legislation have had sustained political support across party lines. The Ryan White CARE Act (Ryan White Comprehensive AIDS Resources Emergency Act; Pub L No. 101–381; 1990) was introduced with bipartisan sponsorship from Senator Orrin Hatch (R, UT), Senator Edward Kennedy (D, MA), and Representative Henry Waxman (D, CA). In 2004, President George W. Bush launched an initiative to supplement ADAPs in 10 states with ADAP waiting lists, underscoring the need to avert delays in HIV treatment initiation. Because RWHAP authorization formally expired in 2013, each subsequent Congress has funded the program through the annual appropriations process. A key reason for enduring support of the program is the substantial flexibility that ADAP grants the states, allowing it to adapt to changes in HIV treatment and insurance availability while addressing local needs.

In this issue of *AJPH*, McManus et al. (p. 1288) present a longitudinal analysis of ADAP from 2008 to 2021. Using data from public ADAP reports, the Ryan White Compass Dashboard, and Centers for Disease Control and Prevention–funded HIV surveillance, McManus et al. enumerate and describe the characteristics of PWH who received ADAP services, estimate the proportion of PWH supported by ADAP, and describe utilization trends over time. Because ADAP eligibility data vary by state and are not available, the investigators estimated utilization among the total population of PWH. Perhaps their most important finding is also the most straightforward: as of 2021, 22.3% of PWH rely on ADAP services, a substantial proportion for a safety net program. Utilization increased from 14.0% in 2008 and had its biggest increase in 2014 to 2015 during the implementation of the Affordable Care Act (Patient Protection and Affordable Care Act, Pub L No. 111–148, 124 Stat. 855 [March 2010]). Since then, ADAP funding has largely transitioned from direct payment for antiretrovirals to purchasing or subsidizing insurance.[3]

Although many Southern states did not expand Medicaid, ADAP coverage in the South nearly doubled—from 12.7% of PWH in 2008 to 23.2% in 2021—likely driven by the availability of Affordable Care Act marketplace insurance plans. By contrast, ADAP utilization decreased in states that expanded Medicaid, as people on Medicaid have fewer ADAP needs. Remarkably, the large expansion in ADAP utilization nationwide occurred despite flat federal funding, probably reflecting increased contributions from manufacturer rebates, the 340B pharmacy program (a federal program that allows eligible providers to purchase outpatient drugs at discounted prices), and the program's shift toward paying for insurance premiums. The expansion of services without an increase in federal spending demonstrates the flexibility of ADAP, which is a potential model for expanding medication access for people with other complex chronic diseases.

Differences in health outomes by race, ethnicity, geography, and socioeconomic status are a persistent feature of the country's HIV epidemic.[4] The article of McManus et al. comes at a critical moment, when funding for HIV research and prevention programs is being eliminated.[5] Funding for research explicitly focused on health disparities has been foremost among the cuts, and the National Institutes of Health has labeled equity objectives as "nonscientific" in termination letters sent to researchers.[6] Nonetheless, health disparities are very real. The RWHAP is a safety net that supports PWH who have the fewest resources and the greatest unmet needs. McManus et al. demonstrate why we must remain focused on improving health outcomes in communities that continue to be disproportionately affected by HIV. Although the difference in ADAP coverage between Black PWH and White PWH narrowed over the study period, it still persisted in 2021: 25.2% of Black PWH received services compared with 28.4% of White PWH.

The success of ADAP may reflect the flexibility granted to states in designing their programs—facilitating adapation to the local context and creative service expansion. However, this flexibility also leads to uneven outcomes, with some state models more successful than others despite ostensibly offering similar services. Notably, the federal data source McManus et al. used for their analysis of differences in utilization by race[7] is no longer available online at the time of this writing (the most recent copy on a web archive is from January 2025[8]), making it more difficult going forward to monitor differences at the national level.

Sustaining funding for ADAP is critical. As of May 2025, ADAP funding has not yet been cut, but the future of the program is uncertain, largely because ADAP depends on annual congressional appropriations. However, ADAP does exactly what it is supposed to do—prevent people in the United States from dying of AIDS—a goal as important today as it was when the program began. Two of us are privileged to provide medical care for people with HIV and routinely witness the phenomenal recovery to health after individuals seek care for advanced HIV disease, and one of us has lived experience as a RWHAP client relying on ADAP to cover the costs of medication that would have otherwise been inaccessible. We are fortunate to live in a country where death from AIDS is now rare. The dramatic decline in AIDS deaths in the United States should be a national point of pride. It is a triumph of our science, advocacy, medical care, social services, and communities. We should not forget this achievement, even as we strive to do better: to rectify disparities, improve quality of life for PWH, and, ultimately, end the epidemic—a goal made possible by unflagging medical research.

The central goal of the current presidential administration's Make America Healthy Again initiative is to end the chronic disease epidemic in the United States.[9,10] ADAP and the RWHAP offer a proven model for the treatment of chronic diseases, as HIV is itself a complex chronic disease, and PWH are disproportionately diagnosed with associated chronic diseases, such as diabetes, cardiovascular disease, mental health disorders, and cancer. The RWHAP has evolved from its initial focus on providing access to expensive HIV medication to supporting a comprehensive system of care for PWH. Consistent with the Make America Healthy Again initiative,[9] RWHAP services support a whole person–centered approach, including facilitating access to transportation to medical appointments, food and housing, and addressing "the root causes of why Americans are getting sick."[9] Approaches modeled on ADAP and the RWHAP could be applied successfully to the care of Americans with, for example, diabetes and cardiovascular disease.

In the United States, approximately one in five PWH rely on ADAP, which represents a substantial portion of the larger population receiving RWHAP services.[2] As McManus and collegues have demonstrated, both the need for ADAP services and the urgency to address disparities in access to treatment are growing. Sustaining funding for ADAP and restoring data transparency are critical to ending the HIV epidemic in the United States. The conditions that led to ADAP's creation remain today: medication costs still exceed what many people can afford, especially in states that have not expanded Medicaid. We have the opportunity to not only preserve this essential program but do even better in the future. AJPH

CORRESPONDENCE

Correspondence should be sent to Julia C. Dombrowski, MD, MPH, 325 9th Ave, Box 359777, Seattle, WA 98104 (e-mail: jdombrow@uw.edu) Reprints can be ordered at http://www.ajph.org by clicking the "Reprints" link.

PUBLICATION INFORMATION

Full Citation: Dombrowski JC, Thompson A, Feinberg J. The AIDS Drug Assistance Program is a model for chronic disease treatment support. *Am J Public Health*. 2025;115(8):1187–1189.
Acceptance Date: May 1, 2025.
DOI: https://doi.org/10.2105/AJPH.2025.308189
ORCID iD:
Julia C. Dombrowski https://orcid.org/0000-0003-1907-9428

CONTRIBUTORS

J. C. Dombrowski drafted the editorial. A. Thompson and J. Feinberg revised the article for important intellectual content. All authors conceptualized the work and approved the final version of the editorial to be published.

CONFLICTS OF INTEREST

J. C. Dombrowski has conducted research unrelated to this work with materials donated by Hologic and Mayne Pharmaceuticals. A. Thompson and J. Feinberg have no conflicts of interest to report.

REFERENCES

1. Goyal R, Luca D, Klein PW, et al. Cost-effectiveness of HRSA's Ryan White HIV/AIDS Program? *J Acquir Immune Defic Syndr*. 2021;86(2):174–181. https://doi.org/10.1097/QAI.0000000000002547
2. Kaiser Family Foundation. The Ryan White HIV/AIDS Program: the basics. November 3, 2022. Available at: https://www.kff.org/hivaids/fact-sheet/the-ryan-white-hivaids-program-the-basics. Accessed May 14, 2025.
3. McManus KA, Strumpf A, Killelea A, Horn T, Hamp A, Keim-Malpass J. Economic benefits of the United States' AIDS Drug Assistance Program: a systematic review of cost analyses to guide research and policy priorities. *Prev Med Rep*. 2022;29:101969. https://doi.org/10.1016/j.pmedr.2022.101969
4. Sullivan PS, Satcher Johnson A, Pembleton ES, et al. Epidemiology of HIV in the USA: epidemic burden, inequities, contexts, and responses. *Lancet*. 2021;397(10279):1095–1106. https://doi.org/10.1016/S0140-6736(21)00395-0
5. Basilio H. Trump team guts AIDS-eradication programme and slashes HIV research grants. March 31, 2025. Available at: https://www.nature.com/articles/d41586-025-00969-5. Accessed May 14, 2025.
6. Kozlov M, Mallapaty S. Exclusive: NIH to terminate hundreds of active research grants. *Nature*. 2025;639(8054):281–282. https://doi.org/10.1038/d41586-025-00703-1
7. Health Resources and Services Administration. Dashboards. Available at: https://data.hrsa.gov/data/dashboards. Accessed April 7, 2025.
8. Health Resources and Services Administration. Ryan White HIV/AIDS program compass dashboard. Archived January 31, 2025. Available at: https://web.archive.org/web/20250131022358/https://data.hrsa.gov/topics/hiv-aids/compass-dashboard. Accessed April 7, 2025.
9. White House. Establishing the president's Make America Healthy Again Commission. February 13, 2025. Available at: https://www.whitehouse.gov/presidential-actions/2025/02/establishing-the-presidents-make-america-healthy-again-commission. Accessed April 7, 2025.
10. US Department of Health and Human Services. Fact sheet: HHS' transformation to make America healthy again. April 2, 2025. Available at: https://www.hhs.gov/press-room/hhs-restructuring-doge-fact-sheet.html. Accessed April 7, 2025.

Centering Youth and Family Needs in Juvenile Justice Reform Efforts

Leslie Helmcamp, MPAff

ABOUT THE AUTHOR

Leslie Helmcamp is with Strengthening Chicago's Youth at Ann & Robert H. Lurie Children's Hospital, Chicago, IL.

See also Johnson et al., p. 1299.

State and local communities have made progress in reducing youth violent crime and incarceration, but more work remains, particularly to reduce racial and ethnic inequities. Since 2000, youth violent crime has declined 68%, while the number of youths incarcerated has dropped by 75%.[1,2] Declines in the use of secure confinement for youths are attributable in part to a drop in youth crime, the emergence of community-based alternatives to divert youths away from incarceration, and a recognition by system partners and advocates that punitive measures to address youth delinquency do not reduce crime. Despite the positive move away from incarceration, reform efforts to close youth prison and jail facilities must do more to reduce disparities in the justice system, while also addressing the best interest of young people and their families.

The continued operation of youth jails and prisons has devastating health and financial costs for youths, families, and the broader community. Each year, states and localities waste taxpayer dollars on ineffective and costly jails and prisons, with average daily costs across the United States reaching $588 per day per youth in 2020, despite ongoing evidence of high recidivism rates for detained youths.[3] Roughly 70% of previously detained youths are rearrested within two years.[4] And in one longitudinal study conducted by Gatti et al., youths placed in a juvenile correctional institution were 38 times more likely to have adult records compared with other justice-involved youths who were not incarcerated.[5]

As juvenile justice systems consider closing youth prisons, policymakers must design program alternatives that seek to repair harm and keep youths connected with their families and communities. A new analysis demonstrates that prison closures alone do not necessarily lead to declines in confinement for most incarcerated youths. In "Youth Detention and Incarceration Facilities in the United States (2010 to February 2023): Mapping Closure Intents and Implementation," Johnson et al. (p. 1299) explore the stated reasons for youth detention and prison closures, with cost and declining numbers being the driving factors influencing attempts to close these facilities. Although the study found that most efforts to close youth prisons and jails were successful, with 62% (73 out of 118 facilities) closing, these closures did not greatly reduce the use of confinement as nearly all the facilities that closed (89%) transferred youths to another facility. In the remaining facilities, some youths were provided services in the community or released to family members while the remaining youths were transferred to other facilities.

The economics of incarceration should not mandate that when prisons become too expensive to operate, youths are transferred farther from their families and communities to other equally ineffective and harmful facilities. As Johnson et al. point out, these practices disproportionately affect Black and brown youths compared with their share of the overall population, and despite evidence that youths of color are more likely to be arrested for similar offenses compared with their White peers. Ensuring that prison closure considerations recognize youth developmental needs and rightfully acknowledge the harms that are rooted in American chattel slavery and Native American boarding schools will allow for a system that more effectively repairs harm, while also addressing the underlying causes of youth delinquency.

Developmental and age-appropriate responses to youth delinquency are essential for reducing future offending. Because young people are still developing, they are capable of learning new behaviors and developing new skills as they grow.[6] The cognitive, emotional, and social support a young person needs for healthy development requires a different justice system approach.

Using punitive measures such as detention and incarceration to address youth misbehavior is in direct conflict with what we know about adolescent brain development. Current research on the developing brain shows that children and adolescents differ from adults in their ability to assess risk, respond to peer influences, and make decisions. Because the brain continues

AJPH August 2025, Vol. 115, No. 8

to develop into a person's mid-20s, youths have a greater ability to change and improve their behavior.[7] However, exposure to toxic stress, trauma, and abuse can alter a child's brain development and can have harmful long-term consequences if left unaddressed.[8] Detaining a young person exposes them to harsh conditions during confinement, including increased exposure to harmful peer influences and isolation from families, schools, and communities. Furthermore, youths who are incarcerated suffer from poorer health outcomes into adulthood.[9] A 2017 study found that youths who had been detained at any point during the previous 12 months had 126% more emergency department visits and 479% more hospital night stays in the previous year compared with youths without justice system involvement.[10]

Although there is no one-size-fits-all approach to address youth delinquency, many state and local governments have adopted responses that prioritize community-based alternatives over incarceration. Keeping youths in their communities has produced positive results, reducing their likelihood of offending again.[11] Milwaukee, Wisconsin's Wraparound Milwaukee program and Redeploy Illinois both offer community-based programming for youths with felony convictions that focuses on positive youth development, employment, and education. Importantly, these programs prioritize addressing youths' unmet needs, which contribute to involvement in the justice system.[12] Other approaches, including peer mentoring, workforce development programs, and programs that prioritize family engagement, have been shown to reduce future delinquency.[13] As these programs and approaches are deployed in new areas, implementation and outcome research should accompany them to ensure fidelity, continued positive outcomes, and reduced costs. AJPH

CORRESPONDENCE

Correspondence should be sent to Leslie Helmcamp, 225 E. Chicago Ave, Box 33, Chicago, IL 60611 (e-mail: lhelmcamp@luriechildrens.org). Reprints can be ordered at http://www.ajph.org by clicking the "Reprints" link.

PUBLICATION INFORMATION

Full Citation: Helmcamp L. Centering youth and family needs in juvenile justice reform efforts. *Am J Public Health*. 2025;115(8):1190–1191.

Acceptance Date: May 14, 2025.

DOI: https://doi.org/10.2105/AJPH.2025.308200

ORCID iD:

Leslie Helmcamp https://orcid.org/0009-0008-7023-751X

CONFLICTS OF INTEREST

The author has no conflicts of interest to disclose.

REFERENCES

1. Office of Juvenile Justice and Delinquency Prevention. *Juvenile Residential Facility Census*. Washington, DC: US Census Bureau, 2022.
2. Bureau of Justice Statistics. Rate of violent victimizations, 1993–2020. NCVS Dashboard (N-DASH). Available at: https://ncvs.bjs.ojp.gov/Home. Accessed April 4, 2025.
3. Justice Policy Institute. Sticker Shock 2020: the cost of youth incarceration. 2020. Available at: Sticker_Shock_2020.pdf. Accessed April 3, 2025.
4. Petrosino A, Turpin-Petrosino C, Guckenburg S. Formal system processing of juveniles: effects on delinquency. *Campbell Syst Rev*. 2010;6(1):1–88. https://doi.org/10.4073/csr.2010.1
5. Gatti U, Tremblay RE, Vitaro F. Iatrogenic effect of juvenile justice. *J Child Psychol Psychiatry*. 2009;50(8):991–998. https://doi.org/10.1111/j.1469-7610.2008.02057.x
6. Neir E, Nelson EE, James Blair R, Pine DS, Ernst M. Neural substrates of choice selection in adults and adolescents: development of the ventrolateral prefrontal and anterior cingulate cortices. *Neuropsychologia*. 2007;45(6):1270–1279. https://doi.org/10.1016/j.neuropsychologia.2006.10.004
7. Giedd JN, Blumenthal J, Jeffries NO, et al. Brain development during childhood and adolescence: a longitudinal MRI study. *Nat Neurosci*. 1999;2(10):861–863. https://doi.org/10.1038/13158
8. Center on the Developing Child, Harvard University. In brief: the science of early childhood development. 2007. Available at: https://developingchild.harvard.edu/resources/inbriefs/inbrief-science-of-ecd/. Accessed March 30, 2025.
9. Barnert E, Dudovitz R, Nelson BB, et al. How does incarcerating young people affect their adult health outcomes? *Pediatrics*. 2017;139(2):2016–2624. https://doi.org/10.1542/peds.2016-2624
10. Winkelman TNA, Genao I, Wildeman C, Wang EA. Emergency department and hospital use among adolescents with justice system involvement. *Pediatrics*. 2017;140(5):2017–1144. https://doi.org/10.1542/peds.2017-1144
11. The Pew Charitable Trusts. Re-examining juvenile incarceration: high cost, poor outcomes spark shift to alternatives. April 20, 2015. Available at: http://www.pewtrusts.org/en/research-and-analysis/issue-briefs/2015/04/reexamining-juvenile-incarceration. Accessed March 30, 2025.
12. Gebler E, Buck L, Goyal-Carkeek R, Kissi J. New Medicaid opportunities to support youth leaving incarceration: building community well-being and advancing prevention efforts. Center for Health Care Strategies. 2024. Available at: https://www.chcs.org/resource/new-medicaid-opportunities-to-support-youth-leaving-incarceration-building-community-well-being-and-advancing-prevention-efforts/. Accessed April 4, 2025.
13. Mendel R. Effective alternatives to youth incarceration. The Sentencing Project. 2023. Available at: https://www.sentencingproject.org/reports/effective-alternatives-to-youth-incarceration. Accessed April 3, 2025.

Now, More Than Ever, We Need Institutional Commitments to Transgender Health Research

Diana M. Tordoff, PhD, MPH, Nguyen K. Tran, PhD, MPH, Juno Obedin-Maliver, MD, MPH, MAS, and Mitchell R. Lunn, MD, MAS

ABOUT THE AUTHORS

Diana M. Tordoff, Nguyen K. Tran, and Juno Obedin-Maliver are with the Department of Obstetrics and Gynecology, Stanford University School of Medicine, Palo Alto, CA. Mitchell R. Lunn is with the Division of Nephrology, Department of Medicine, Stanford University School of Medicine. All authors are affiliated with the PRIDE Study/PRIDEnet, Stanford University School of Medicine.

AJPH August 2025, Vol. 115, No. 8

See also Shi et al., p. 1278.

Twenty-five years ago, Viviane Namaste wrote, "Erasure is the defining condition of trans people."[1(p53)] Transgender and gender diverse (henceforth "trans") people's health has suffered as a result of erasure: the systematic exclusion from institutional realms.[1] Institutional erasure produces informational erasure, so trans people, their families, and health care providers must make health decisions based on limited data, clinical guidance, and evidenced-based interventions.[2]

FROM ERASURE TO INCLUSION IN RESEARCH

Historically, trans people have been excluded from population-based research, clinical trials, and public health surveillance. The past decade has produced a surge in both research studies and publications focused on trans health, reflecting strengthened institutional commitments to this field (Figure 1). Between 2014 and 2017, several key changes accelerated the institutional capacity to conduct trans health research through funding and data availability. The Behavioral Risk Factor Surveillance System (BRFSS), the first federal study to collect data on trans identities, and the US Transgender Survey,[3] with the largest sample of trans participants recruited at the time, facilitated access to large national samples of trans adults for the first time. Concurrently, the National Institutes of Health (NIH) designated sexual and gender minority people as a health disparities population for research in 2016 and issued its first trans-specific funding announcement the following year; these actions created explicit trans health research funding avenues. Alongside other shifts in institutional support, this contributed to a sixfold increase in the annual number of research publications about trans populations between 2014 and 2024.

ALL OF US AS A TOOL FOR TRANS HEALTH EQUITY

Among these efforts, the All of Us Research Program played an important role in actively including trans people in biomedical research by collecting data on self-reported gender identity and sex assigned at birth—often regarded as the gold standard for identifying trans individuals.[4] Launched in 2015 under the Barack Obama presidential administration, the All of Us Research Program's primary goal is to enroll 1 million adults (with 80% from communities that are underrepresented in biomedical research, e.g., ethnoracial minority people, sexual and gender minority people, people living in rural areas, people living in poverty) to accelerate biomedical research and improve health outcomes for historically marginalized and underrepresented communities.[5]

All of Us aims to achieve this by partnering with a broad network of community organizations and health care providers to collect diverse data and materials, including health questionnaire responses, electronic health records (EHRs), physical measurements, digital health metrics, and biospecimens for genomic and other assays. Integration into a single data repository would enable linkage of self-reported gender identity to objective health measures. This structure would facilitate knowledge generation across many health outcomes for trans people throughout their lifespans, including in the areas of cancer, cardiovascular disease, diabetes, and reproductive health, which are understudied owing to the systemic exclusion of trans people from research and institutional data collection efforts.[6]

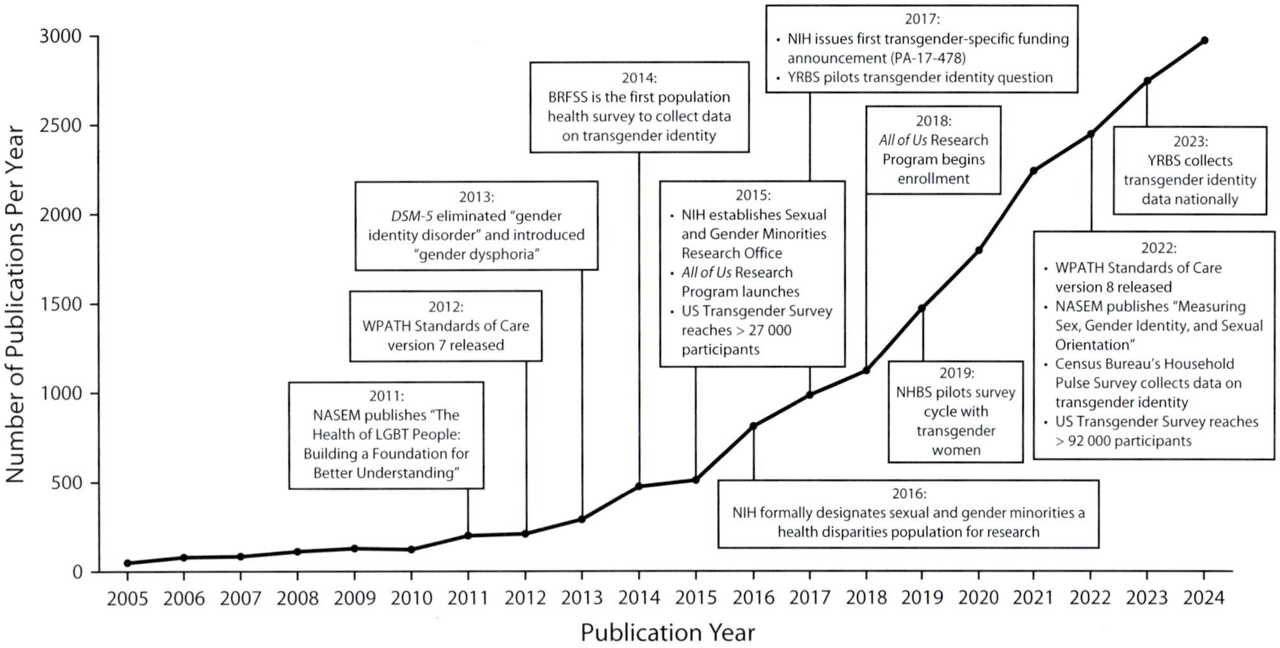

FIGURE 1— Milestones of Institutional Supports for Transgender Health Research and Annual Number of PubMed Publications Including Transgender or Gender Diverse Terms in the Title or Abstract: 2005–2024

Note. BRFSS = Behavioral Risk Factor Surveillance System; *DSM-5* = *The Diagnostic and Statistical Manual of Mental Disorders, Fifth Edition*; LGBT = lesbian, gay, bisexual, transgender; NASEM = National Academies of Sciences, Engineering, and Medicine; NHBS = National HIV Behavioral Surveillance; NIH = National Institutes of Health; WPATH = World Professional Association for Transgender Health; YRBS = Youth Risk Behavior Survey. The figure presents the results of our PubMed search conducted April 3, 2025, using the following search syntax: "Transgender"[Tiab] or "Transsexual"[Tiab] or "Gender-Diverse"[Tiab] or "Gender Diverse"[Tiab] or "Gender-Expansive"[Tiab] or" Gender Expansive"[Tiab] or "Nonbinary People"[Tiab] or "Non-Binary People"[Tiab].

In this issue of *AJPH*, Shi et al. (p. 1278) present an algorithm they developed using All of Us survey responses and EHR data to identify trans participants. The authors found that nearly all (95.6%) trans individuals were identified by survey questions alone and that EHR-based algorithms identified only 8.2% of participants. This may be in part because many trans participants did not authorize EHR data sharing with All of Us. Overall, approximately a third of the cohort is missing EHR data, and trans participants are less likely to have linked EHR records than are cisgender heterosexual participants.[6] These results underscore the importance of asking patients and participants about their gender identity.

Self-report has long been considered the most reliable method for assessing identity-related measures. However, few studies, clinical programs, or surveillance systems use validated and recommended methods for measuring gender identity. EHR algorithms to identify trans patients were developed to fill this methodological gap, but they have limitations.[7] EHR algorithms use a combination of gender dysphoria diagnosis codes, trans-specific medical intervention codes, and natural language processing of free text clinical notes. These algorithms systematically fail to identify trans people who do not experience dysphoria, do not desire or have access to gender-affirming interventions, or choose not to disclose their trans status.[8] Although most gender identity measurement literature emphasizes the importance of self-report, Shi et al. highlight that survey-only approaches may exclude individuals who are less comfortable disclosing trans identity. In All of Us, however, this composed only 4.4% of trans participants; survey-only methods disproportionately excluded transfeminine individuals, those aged 65 years or older, and heterosexual people.

NEW THREATS TO TRANS HEALTH RESEARCH

On January 20, 2025, Donald Trump's presidential administration issued Executive Order 14168 ("Defending Women From Gender Ideology Extremism and Restoring Biological Truth to the Federal Government"). Among other rhetorical devices in this order, "women" are equated to "females," and "men" are equated to "males," with the goal of erasing trans and intersex people's existence. On January 28, 2025, the Trump administration issued Executive Order 14187 ("Protecting Children From Chemical and Surgical Mutilation") to withhold funding from institutions that provide gender-affirming medical care to youths younger than 19 years. Despite ongoing legal challenges, these orders have had a significant impact on the day-to-day lives of trans communities, including limiting access to identity documents and health care and removing antidiscrimination protections. They also have had an unprecedented impact on government communication and funding for trans health and health research, amounting to abandoning trans people and their health.

Amid wide-scale attempts to dismantle federally funded scientific infrastructure and the independence of universities more broadly, trans health research and health care are being disproportionately targeted.[9] Government agencies have been directed to remove all references to the following terms: "gender, transgender, pregnant person, pregnant people, LGBT, transsexual, nonbinary, nonbinary, assigned male at birth, assigned female at birth, biologically male, biologically female."[10(p620)]

By January 31, 2025, vital federally funded surveys (e.g., BRFSS, Youth Risk Behavior Surveillance System) had been removed from the Centers for Disease Control and Prevention website, which was also scrubbed of all mentions of trans identities and stripped of variables related to trans identity in publicly available data sets. As of April 2025, more than 200 NIH grants for research on trans health have been terminated, accounting for 24% of all terminated NIH grants.[11] These terminations frequently contain language dismissing research based on gender identity as "unscientific" and having "no return on investment."

At the same time, the Trump administration directed the NIH to study "regret and detransition" among trans individuals.[12] These topics were already being researched, with multiple studies reporting very low rates of regret (< 1% to 2%).[13]

Beyond being politically and ideologically motivated, redirecting funding to focus on regret and detransition ignores the critical gaps in our understanding of trans health and is unlikely to improve the health or the quality of clinical care for the vast majority of trans people. Collectively, these attacks are dismantling the carefully built, critical infrastructure to support high-quality, high-impact trans health research.

After a 10-year commitment to bolstering trans health research, All of Us was directed to scour all mentions of trans health, and sexual and gender minority health more broadly, from their public-facing online presence. The public-facing data browser no longer displays summary data for gender identity or sex assigned at birth, which were collected in the core survey administered to all participants. Importantly, as of this writing in May 2025, these variables are still accessible to researchers and have not yet been removed from the All of Us data. Thus, the large (n = 4781) and diverse (43.2% ethnoracial minority, 35.1% 45 years and older, 67.6% sexual minority) data set of trans participants identified by Shi et al. remains accessible as a rich resource for trans health research.

DEFENDING RESEARCH AMID ERASURE

Institutional commitments are necessary to ensure the continuation of high-quality trans-inclusive and trans-specific research (especially longitudinal, population-based studies and clinical trials). This is critical to combat the current administration's active erasure of the existence, health, and health care needs of trans people. Notwithstanding federal policies, individual institutions must stand up to support trans health rather than capitulating to the Trump administration's demands that infringe on freedom of speech and scientific inquiry. This can include providing bridge funding for researchers affected by the recent politicized grant terminations, joining lawsuits that challenge the legality of NIH terminations,[14] developing internal trans health funding mechanisms, collecting comprehensive gender identity data in EHR systems, hiring trans scholars, and cultivating expertise to support all investigators in designing trans-inclusive studies.

The successes of the US Transgender Survey (with more than 27 000 participants in 2015 and more than 92 000 participants in 2022)[3] and the PRIDE (Population Research in Identity and Disparities for Equality) study (with a longitudinal cohort that has enrolled more than 33 000 sexual and gender minority participants)[15] demonstrate the potential of nongovernmental and community-driven trans health research initiatives. Even these research programs require institutions to stand up against the recent attempts at erasure to support, defend, and fund the current generation of scientists and health care providers fiercely dedicated to trans health research and justice. AJPH

CORRESPONDENCE

Correspondence should be sent to Diana M. Tordoff, 453 Quarry Rd, Palo Alto, CA 94304 (e-mail: dtordoff@stanford.edu). Reprints can be ordered at https://www.ajph.org by clicking the "Reprints" link.

PUBLICATION INFORMATION

Full Citation: Tordoff DM, Tran NK, Obedin-Maliver J, Lunn MR. Now, more than ever, we need institutional commitments to transgender health research. *Am J Public Health.* 2025;115(8):1192–1195.

Acceptance Date: May 8, 2025.

DOI: https://doi.org/10.2105/AJPH.2025.308195

ORCID iDs:
Diana M. Tordoff https://orcid.org/0000-0002-9238-9927

Nguyen K. Tran https://orcid.org/0000-0002-5093-4499

Mitchell R. Lunn https://orcid.org/0000-0002-0068-0814

CONTRIBUTORS

D. M. Tordoff conceptualized, drafted, and revised the editorial. N. K. Tran, J. Obedin-Maliver, and M. R. Lunn critically reviewed and revised the editorial.

ACKNOWLEDGMENTS

All authors are affiliated with PRIDEnet, which served as a national community engagement partner for the All of Us Research Program from 2017 to 2025 via the National Institutes of Health (NIH), Office of the Director (award OT2OD025276). This award was prematurely terminated by the NIH on March 14, 2025, which said, "Research programs based on gender identity are often unscientific, have little identifiable return on investment, and do nothing to enhance the health of many Americans. Many such studies ignore, rather than seriously examine, biological realities. It is the policy of NIH not to prioritize these research programs." D. M. Tordoff is currently funded by the National Institute of Allergy and Infectious Disease, NIH (award K01AI182507).

Note. The contents of this editorial are solely the responsibility of the authors and do not necessarily represent the official views of the NIH.

CONFLICTS OF INTEREST

J. Obedin-Maliver has received consultation fees from Ibis Reproductive Health, Hims and Hers Health Inc., Folx Health Inc., Sage Therapeutics and Upstream Inc. on topics unrelated to this work. M. R. Lunn received consultation fees from Hims and Hers Health Inc., Folx Health Inc., Otsuka Pharmaceutical Development and Commercialization, Inc., and the American Dental Association on topics unrelated to this work. D. M. Tordoff and N. K. Tran have no conflicts of interest to disclose.

REFERENCES

1. Namaste VK. *Invisible Lives: The Erasure of Transsexual and Transgendered People.* Chicago, IL: University of Chicago Press; 2000.
2. Bauer GR, Hammond R, Travers R, Kaay M, Hohenadel KM, Boyce M. "I don't think this is theoretical; this is our lives": how erasure impacts health care for transgender people. *J Assoc Nurses AIDS Care.* 2009;20(5):348–361. https://doi.org/10.1016/j.jana.2009.07.004
3. James SE, Herman JL, Durso LE, Heng-Lehtinen R. Early insights: a report of the 2022 US Transgender Survey. February 2024. Available at: https://transequality.org/sites/default/files/2024-02/2022%20USTS%20Early%20Insights%20Report_FINAL.pdf. Accessed April 8, 2025.
4. All of Us Research Program Investigators. The "All of Us" research program. *N Engl J Med.* 2019;381(7):668–676. https://doi.org/10.1056/NEJMsr1809937
5. Mapes BM, Foster CS, Kusnoor SV; All of Us Research Program Investigators, et al. Diversity and inclusion for the All of Us research program: a scoping review. *PLoS One.* 2020;15(7):e0234962. https://doi.org/10.1371/journal.pone.0234962
6. Tran NK, Lunn MR, Schulkey CE, et al. Prevalence of 12 common health conditions in sexual and gender minority participants in the All of Us research program. *JAMA Netw Open.* 2023;6(7):e2324969. https://doi.org/10.1001/jamanetworkopen.2023.24969
7. Streed CG, King D, Grasso C, et al. Validation of an administrative algorithm for transgender and gender diverse persons against self-report data in electronic health records. *J Am Med Inform Assoc.* 2023;30(6):1047–1055. https://doi.org/10.1093/jamia/ocad039
8. Lett E, Everhart A. Considerations for transgender population health research based on US national surveys. *Ann Epidemiol.* 2022;65:65–71. https://doi.org/10.1016/j.annepidem.2021.10.009
9. McFarling UL. Day by day, how Trump is roiling science and health. *STAT.* April 24, 2025. Available at: https://www.statnews.com/2025/04/24/trump-100-days-timeline-science-health-nih-cdc-fda-hhs. Accessed April 28, 2025.
10. Krieger N, Gruskin S. Gender removal by fiat: impacts of new Trump administration edicts. *Lancet.* 2025;405(10479):620. https://doi.org/10.1016/S0140-6736(25)00243-0
11. Kozlov M, Ryan C. How Trump 2.0 is slashing NIH-backed research—in charts. *Nature.* 2025;640(8060):863–865. https://doi.org/10.1038/d41586-025-01099-8
12. Kozlov M. Exclusive: Trump White House directs NIH to study "regret" after transgender people transition. *Nature.* [Epub ahead of print April 3, 2025]. https://doi.org/10.1038/d41586-025-01029-8
13. Bustos VP, Bustos SS, Mascaro A, et al. Regret after gender-affirmation surgery: a systematic review and meta-analysis of prevalence. *Plast Reconstr Surg Glob Open.* 2021;9(3):e3477. https://doi.org/10.1097/GOX.0000000000003477
14. American Civil Liberties Union. Researchers challenge NIH's politically driven grant cancellations. April 2, 2025. Available at: https://www.aclu.org/press-releases/researchers-challenge-nihs-politically-driven-grant-cancellations. Accessed April 18, 2025.
15. Obedin-Maliver J, Hunt C, Flentje A, et al. Engaging sexual and gender minority (SGM) communities for health research: building and sustaining PRIDEnet. *J Community Engagem Scholarsh.* 2024;16(2):9. https://doi.org/10.54656/jces.v16i2.484

Legal Recognition of Same-Sex Marriage in Asia Is an Opportunity to Improve LGBTQ+ Physical and Mental Health

Yiu Tung Suen, DPhil, MSc

ABOUT THE AUTHOR

Yiu Tung Suen is with the Gender Studies Programme and (by courtesy) the Jockey Club School of Public Health and Primary Care at the Chinese University of Hong Kong.

AJPH August 2025, Vol. 115, No. 8

Asia is home to millions of sexual and gender minority people, who may or may not use the term "LGBTQ+" (lesbian, gay, bisexual, transgender, and queer) to identify themselves. It is a diverse region in terms of cultural, social, and political histories, including periods of colonization with long-lasting impact on contemporary understandings of diverse genders and sexualities.

It has been argued that being LGBTQ+, as it is now defined, was associated with a relatively high level of tolerance or even acceptance in earlier Asian historical periods, during which very different cultural and religious lenses were used to understand and interpret gender identities and sexualities, and before Asia increasingly opened up to the world and adopted Western religious and medical viewpoints.

Currently, the legal landscape for sexual and gender minorities in Asia is very diverse.[1] Same-sex sexual acts are punishable by death in places like Iran, Iraq, and Pakistan. Same-sex sexual acts (for both men and women) are criminalized in Malaysia and Indonesia. Changes in legal recognition of gender can be observed in Pakistan, India, and Nepal, albeit with legal uncertainties over how they are applied.

Recently, there has been rapid development in terms of legal recognition of same-sex relationships in the region. Legislation legalizing same-sex marriage became effective in Taiwan in 2019, and Nepal registered its first same-sex marriage in 2023. In 2024, the Thai House of Representatives and the Thai Senate approved a same-sex marriage bill by an overwhelming majority, and the bill came into effect in January 2025. There are also other jurisdictions in Asia that are actively debating same-sex marriage, or at least certain forms of legal recognition of same-sex relationships. The official recognition of same-sex partnership in Japan started in 2015, when the municipal government of Shibuya began allowing same-sex couples to register their partnership at the ward office, followed by other municipal bodies that issued guidelines on and acknowledgments of such partnerships. In a judicial review case in 2023, Hong Kong's Court of Final Appeal ordered the city's government to set up an "alternative framework" to legally recognize the rights of same-sex couples, although it fell short of a demand for full marriage equality.

LGBTQ+ people face physical and mental health disparities compared with their non-LGBTQ+ counterparts. Minority stress theory argues that minority group members, including LGBTQ+ people, experience additional minority stressors (including distal and proximal stressors) in society as a result of stigmatized social status, in addition to experiencing general stressors that the dominant social group members face in society.[2] The minority stress that LGBTQ+ people face results in adverse mental health as well as physical health outcomes.[3] Research in different parts of the world has shown that legal recognition of same-sex relationships has implications for LGBTQ+ individuals, same-sex couples, and economies and societies as a whole.[4] In particular, it has been argued that legal recognition of same-sex marriage can have health implications for LGBTQ+ people.

An established research literature sheds light on the ways in which legal recognition of same-sex marriage can improve LGBTQ+ physical and mental health.[5] First, it helps to reduce the structural, interpersonal, and intrapersonal stigma faced by same-sex couples (whether or not they enter into same-sex marriage), their family members, and LGBTQ+ individuals, thereby alleviating some of the minority stress that LGBTQ+ people experience in society.[6] Studies have found that public acceptance increases in the longer run after recognition of same-sex marriage (despite the emergence of backlash in some instances).[7] Other studies found increased interpersonal validation, such as perceptions of being viewed as a "real" couple and the increased social inclusion[8] that same-sex couples experience after legalization of same-sex marriage. Research has consistently found that LGBTQ+ people who live in places with legal recognition of same-sex marriage report significantly less depression and anxiety, and better psychological well-being. For example, according to a national cross-sectional online survey of 1824 lesbian, gay, and bisexual participants in the United States during the period in which same-sex couples had equal marriage rights in some but not all states, sexual minorities who resided in states with equal marriage rights reported less identity concealment, vigilance, and isolation than their peers in states without equal marriage rights.[9] The protective effect of same-sex marriage on mental health has been found to be particularly significant among younger sexual minority individuals. Second, legalization of same-sex marriage provides same-sex households with rights to key financial and legal benefits and access to health care, health insurance, and survivor protections, which previously excluded recognition of same-sex households.[10] Altogether, these findings suggest that legalization of same-sex marriage provides LGBTQ+ people with a society in which they experience greater self-worth, and a more socially and a legally supportive environment with a sense of greater security, stability, and safety. It can be described as a social legitimization process.

It is important to acknowledge the complex and variable health outcomes associated with legalization of same-sex relationships among LGBTQ+ people.[11] For example, research has shown that whether and how same-sex marriage rights may improve health outcomes and access vary according to age, gender, race, ethnicity, and socioeconomic status. Studies also found that, despite legalization of same-sex relationships, sexual minority stigma persisted. Some same-sex couples also reported feeling hurt and betrayed when familial reactions to their legalized status were negative or when reactions among family members were divided. Research to date also has several limitations[11]; for example, it disproportionately represents samples from the United States and White populations, and rarely examines differences by sexual or gender identity or other demographic characteristics.

These findings that legal recognition of same-sex marriage has health benefits for LGBTQ+ individuals are worth considering for policymakers and governments around the world. The debates about same-sex marriage in Asia have often been emotive. Oftentimes the public debate has been about cultural values and "cultural compatibility," and whether or not it is compatible with "Asian traditions" (although it is important to note that sometimes such "traditions" may be invented to suit the opposition's argument).[12] At other times, economic considerations have been on some governments' mind for legalizing same-sex marriage. For example, in Thailand, it has been claimed that the possibility of attracting more international tourists, and therefore generating greater income, is one consideration in the government's thinking about same-sex marriage legalization.[13] However, so far, there has been little discussion of how legal recognition of same-sex marriage can have implications for public health in Asia.

LGBTQ+ physical and mental health in Asia is affected by a mix of factors, such as lack of legal protection, lack of social recognition (especially in terms of family acceptance), and lack of access to LGBTQ+ friendly health care providers, among others.[14] It is important to highlight that intersecting identities (e.g., race, ethnicity, socioeconomic status) affect the health outcomes of LGBTQ+ individuals in Asia.[15] Socioeconomic factors compound the health disparities faced by LGBTQ+ individuals in different Asian countries. In such a vast region of diverse cultural, economic, geographic, and social landscapes, research has found that LGBTQ+ people who are residing in rural areas, are unemployed, and have lower educational and income levels face even more adverse mental and physical health outcomes.

In particular, the lack of legal protection has been found to affect health behaviors. For example, in Asia, it was found that a change of human rights for sexual minorities, from a score of 0.0 to 1.0 (as measured by the Sexual Orientation and Gender Identity Human Rights Index), was correlated with a decrease in unprotected anal intercourse of 25.5% ($P = .075$), increases in recent HIV testing of 42.9% ($P = .011$), increases in HIV knowledge of 29.5% ($P = .032$), and exposure to HIV prevention services of 37.9% ($P = .119$).[16] These findings provide clear empirical evidence that increased rights for LGBTQ+ people in Asia benefits their health, in line with findings from other parts of the world.

Of course, this is not to say that legal recognition of same-sex marriage is a panacea for all LGBTQ+ health issues in Asia, nor does it suggest that improvements in LGBTQ+ health after legal recognition of same-sex marriage will come overnight. Indeed, the process of legal recognition of same-sex marriage itself will be full of struggles in Asia.

If legal recognition of same-sex relationships is to improve LGBTQ+ health in Asia, it has to be accompanied by social and cultural changes, particularly social acceptance of families of origin, and attitudinal changes of health care providers. The impact of legal recognition of same-sex marriage on transgender health may be less certain, considering the additional legal and social challenges they face, such as issues related to the lack of protection against gender identity–based discrimination, the lack of a legal gender recognition system, and systematic barriers to access health care. Also, varying levels of social acceptance, traditional values, and legal frameworks across Asian societies may mean that the potential health benefits of the legalization of same-sex marriage may be highly uneven—it is not difficult to imagine there might be backlash in some Asian societies that are less accepting of LGBTQ+ people.

The process leading up to legal recognition of same-sex relationships in Asia will be long. It needs to be remembered that the way in which legal recognition of same-sex relationships develops also has implications for LGBTQ+ health. In Taiwan, the first in Asia to legalize same-sex marriage, a controversial referendum took place in 2018 before eventual legalization in 2019. According to a study survey, it was found that the suicide ideation rate among nonheterosexual people in Taiwan was lower in wave 1 (23 months before the same-sex marriage referendums) than in wave 2 (one week after the referendums).[17] The study's authors commented that "The suicidal ideation rate significantly increased in nonheterosexual participants experiencing the same-sex marriage referendums in Taiwan. Whether civil rights of sexual minority individuals can be determined through referendums should be evaluated."[17] Another study also found that the suicide rates among LGBTQ+ adults during the referendum were higher than those found in previous studies prior to the referendum.[18] Therefore, the process of legalizing same-sex relationships in Asia needs careful consideration. Whether it is to be through legislature or courts in different jurisdictions, legal development of same-sex marriage in Asia needs to be accompanied by thoughtful, well-facilitated, and well-informed social debates to combat misunderstanding and disinformation, which can unnecessarily create fear among the general public, thus adversely affecting the health of LGBTQ+ people.

Same-sex marriage as an opportunity to improve LGBTQ+ physical and mental health in Asia deserves public, policy, and government attention. It is hoped that this editorial can further ignite debates in this direction in Asia. AJPH

CORRESPONDENCE

Correspondence should be sent to Yiu Tung Suen, Room 250, 2nd Floor, Sino Building, Gender Studies Programme, The Chinese University of Hong Kong, Hong Kong SAR (e-mail: suenyiutung@cuhk.edu.hk). Reprints can be ordered at https://www.ajph.org by clicking the "Reprints" link.

PUBLICATION INFORMATION

Full Citation: Suen YT. Legal recognition of same-sex marriage in Asia is an opportunity to improve LGBTQ+ physical and mental health. *Am J Public Health*. 2025;115(8):1196–1199.

Acceptance Date: February 26, 2025.

DOI: https://doi.org/10.2105/AJPH.2025.308102

ORCID iD:

Yiu Tung Suen https://orcid.org/0000-0001-9113-1169

ACKNOWLEDGMENTS

The writing of the article was enabled by funding support from the General Research Fund of the University Grants Committee in Hong Kong (14604221).

CONFLICTS OF INTEREST

The author has no conflicts of interest to report.

REFERENCES

1. Lau H. Courts, the law, and LGBT rights in Asia. *Oxford Research Encyclopedia of Politics (2020), UNC Legal Studies Research Paper*. March 2020. Available at: https://papers.ssrn.com/abstract=3573177. Accessed September 19, 2024.
2. Meyer IH. Prejudice, social stress, and mental health in lesbian, gay, and bisexual populations: conceptual issues and research evidence. *Psychol Sex Orientat Gend Divers*. 2013;1(S):3–26. https://doi.org/10.1037/2329-0382.1.S.3
3. Lick DJ, Durso LE, Johnson KL. Minority stress and physical health among sexual minorities. *Perspect Psychol Sci*. 2013;8(5):521–548. https://doi.org/10.1177/1745691613497965
4. Badgett MVL, Waaldijk K, Rodgers Y van der M. The relationship between LGBT inclusion and economic development: macro-level evidence. *World Dev*. 2019;120:1–14. https://doi.org/10.1016/j.worlddev.2019.03.011
5. Buffie WC. Public health implications of same-sex marriage. *Am J Public Health*. 2011;101(6):986–990. https://doi.org/10.2105/AJPH.2010.300112
6. Fingerhut AW, Riggle EDB, Rostosky SS. Same-sex marriage: the social and psychological implications of policy and debates. *J Soc Issues*. 2011;67(2):225–241. https://doi.org/10.1111/j.1540-4560.2011.01695.x
7. Lewis GB, Gossett CW. Changing public opinion on same-sex marriage: the case of California. *Polit Policy*. 2008;36(1):4–30. https://doi.org/10.1111/j.1747-1346.2007.00092.x
8. Gonzales G, Blewett LA. National and state-specific health insurance disparities for adults in same-sex relationships. *Am J Public Health*. 2014;104(2):e95–e104. https://doi.org/10.2105/AJPH.2013.301577
9. Riggle EDB, Rostosky SS, Horne SG. Marriage amendments and lesbian, gay, and bisexual individuals in the 2006 election. *Sex Res Social Policy*. 2009;6(1):80–89. https://doi.org/10.1525/srsp.2009.6.1.80
10. Carpenter CS, Eppink ST, Gonzales G, McKay T. Effects of access to legal same-sex marriage on marriage and health. *J Policy Anal Manage*. 2021;40(2):376–411. https://doi.org/10.1002/pam.22286
11. Drabble LA, Wootton AR, Veldhuis CB, et al. Perceived psychosocial impacts of legalized same-sex marriage: a scoping review of sexual minority adults' experiences. *PLoS One*. 2021;16(5):e0249125. https://doi.org/10.1371/journal.pone.0249125
12. Wan M. The invention of tradition: same-sex marriage and its discontents in Hong Kong. *Int J Const Law*. 2020;18(2):539–562. https://doi.org/10.1093/icon/moaa026
13. Sinsomboonthong T. On homosexual love and right to same-sex marriage: questioning the paradox of #LoveWins discourse. In: Mayer CH, Vanderheiden E, eds. *International Handbook of Love: Transcultural and Transdisciplinary Perspectives*. Cham, Switzerland: Springer International Publishing; 2021:405–421. https://doi.org/10.1007/978-3-030-45996-3_22
14. Suen YT, Chan RCH. A nationwide cross-sectional study of 15,611 lesbian, gay and bisexual people in China: disclosure of sexual orientation and experiences of negative treatment in health care. *Int J Equity Health*. 2020;19(1):46. https://doi.org/10.1186/s12939-020-1151-7

15. Tan KKH, Saw ATW. Prevalence and correlates of mental health difficulties amongst LGBTQ people in Southeast Asia: a systematic review. *J Gay Lesbian Ment Health.* 2023;27(4):401–420. https://doi.org/10.1080/19359705.2022.2089427
16. Anderson JE, Kanters S. Lack of sexual minorities' rights as a barrier to HIV prevention among men who have sex with men and transgender women in Asia: a systematic review. *LGBT Health.* 2015; 2(1):16–26. https://doi.org/10.1089/lgbt.2014.0024
17. Lin IH, Ko NY, Huang YT, Chen MH, Lu WH, Yen CF. Effect of same-sex marriage referendums on the suicidal ideation rate among nonheterosexual people in Taiwan. *Int J Environ Res Public Health.* 2019;16(18):3456. https://doi.org/10.3390/ijerph16183456
18. Wang Y, Chang S, Miao N. Suicide attempts among Taiwanese lesbian, gay, bisexual, and transgender adults during the 2018 Taiwan referendum on same-sex issues. *J Nurs Scholarsh.* 2022;54(3):388–395. https://doi.org/10.1111/jnu.12744

The Impact of Anti-LGBTQ+ Legislation on Mental Health and Substance Use and HIV Prevention and Care Among Gay and Bisexual Men in Kenya

Gary W. Harper, PhD, MS, MPH, Elijah Ochieng Odhiambo, Laura Jadwin-Cakmak, MPH, Felix Odhiambo Okuta, Kenneth Bauman, BA, Kennedy Otieno Olango, Darius M. Moore, MPH, Edwin Gumbe, Teddy Aloo, and Sophia A. Hussen, MD, MPH

AJPH August 2025, Vol. 115, No. 8

ABOUT THE AUTHORS

Gary W. Harper, Laura Jadwin-Cakmak, Kenneth Bauman, and Darius M. Moore are with the Department of Health Behavior and Health Equity, School of Public Health, University of Michigan, Ann Arbor. Elijah Ochieng Odhiambo is with the Salina Youth Initiative, Kisumu, Kenya. Felix Odhiambo Okuta is with the Impact Research and Development Organization, Kisumu, Kenya. Kennedy Otieno Olango is with the Mission for Advocacy and Advisory for Young Generation, Kisumu, Kenya. Edwin Gumbe is with Nafasi Innovations, Kisumu, Kenya. Teddy Aloo is with Nyanza Reproductive Health Society–Anza Mapema, Kisumu, Kenya. Sophia A. Hussen is with the Hubert Department of Global Health, Emory University Rollins School of Public Health, Atlanta, GA.

We present a conceptual model to provide insights into the radiating negative effects of anti-LGBTQ+ (lesbian, gay, bisexual, transgender, queer or questioning, and all subsects) legislation on health inequities related to mental health and substance use (MHSU) and HIV prevention and care among gay and bisexual men in Kenya. Our model is based on individual and shared indigenous knowledge of these phenomena gained from lived experiences and findings from multiple participatory action research projects centering the realities of Kenyan gay and bisexual men during the past 15 years.

We chose to write an editorial to allow our diverse voices to be expressed, privileging lived experiences and stories shared outside the confines of a traditional research project. We are Kenyan and US researchers, practitioners, community organizers, and activists. Among us are gay and bisexual men who are living with and at risk for HIV and individuals experiencing mental health concerns. We have different sexual orientations, gender identities, ethnic/racial categories, and ages. Our disciplinary backgrounds, educational levels, career positions, and socioeconomic statuses are diverse. Given power differentials in our partnership, those with more power strive to engage in a continual process of intersectional reflexivity that specifically recognizes and interrogates proximities to power.[1] This editorial represents our collective viewpoints and experiences.

Before presenting our model, we feel it is important to examine the roots of anti-LGBTQ+ belief systems and restrictions in Kenya and other regions of Africa. Early British colonizers criminalized same-sex behavior and other sexual acts they deemed to be unnatural to "set standards of behaviour to reform the colonized and protect the colonizers against moral lapses."[2(p7)] This created systems of surveillance and punishment designed to suppress same-sex behaviors and replace precolonial sexual and gender fluidity with puritanical Western heteronormativity and rigid adherence to the gender binary.[2–4]

As Kenya and other colonized regions of Africa adopted oppressive colonial laws and embraced Christianity and Islam, the unique histories of indigenous normative same-sex practices and marriages, gender fluidity, and indigenous spirituality in African tribes were slowly erased and replaced with an essentialized notion of one homogenous African value system.[2,3,5] This denies the existence of diverse tribal-specific precolonial expressions of gender and sexuality and positions LGBTQ+ people and practices as un-African.[2,6] Scholars and activists suggest that to gain liberation from anti-LGBTQ+ laws across Africa there needs to be a "demystification of homophobic pseudo-history"[5(p267)] and a rejection of the notion that a monolithic anti-LGBTQ+ African value system exists.

CONSEQUENCES OF LGBTQ+ CRIMINALIZATION

Criminalization of same-sex sexual behavior and pervasive cultural and religious anti-LGBTQ+ rhetoric in Kenya serve as sociostructural forms of oppression that promote violence against LGBTQ+ people and create barriers to education, housing, and health care.[7–9] Kenyan Penal Codes 162–165 criminalize consensual same-sex sexual behaviors. Despite organized efforts to overturn these colonial era laws beginning in 2016, Kenya's High Court ruled to uphold them in 2019.[10]

The most recent anti-LGBTQ+ bill introduced in Kenya, the Family Protection Bill of 2023, would ban same-sex marriage and impose a minimum 10-year sentence for various activities, including engaging in same-sex sexual activity, promoting or funding prohibited activities, and receiving or providing gender-affirming hormones or surgery. Although not enacted into law, the bill has stirred intense media attention and anti-LGBTQ+ public discourse. A recent qualitative study with leaders of community-based LGBTQ+ health organizations representing 19 Kenyan counties suggests that the recent introduction of anti-LGBTQ+ bills such as the Family Protection Bill of 2023 is linked to their inability to provide health services because of growing religious tensions, threats of physical attacks, and the withdrawal of local county government financial support.[11]

The subjugation of LGBTQ+ people as criminals, intertwined with residual colonial era beliefs that LGBTQ+ people and behaviors are un-African, creates a sinister syndemic of hatred and oppressive sociostructural forces. These serve to erode the health and well-being of LGBTQ+ people in Kenya directly through victimization and murder and indirectly through increased levels of distress, leading to negative physical and mental health outcomes.[7,9]

There have been several high-profile accounts of Kenyan LGBTQ+ people being tortured and murdered. In 2023, Edwin Chiloba, a gay university student and LGBTQ+ activist, was murdered and his body was stuffed into a metal box on the side of a road.[12] In 2022, Sheila Lumumba, a nonbinary lesbian person, was raped and murdered in their own home.[13] In 2021, Erica Chandra, a transgender woman, was murdered and her body was dumped in a ditch; Joash Mosoti, a gay man and LGBTQ+-health worker, was tortured and strangled to death in his apartment; and Chriton Atuhwera, an LGBTQ+ Ugandan activist, died after being firebombed at a Kenyan refugee camp.[14] We share the names of these victims of LGBTQ+ extreme violence to honor their lives and remember them as humans who were taken from this earth for simply being their authentic selves. These brutal acts of violence have been highly publicized through social media to pressure police to investigate and take action, but this has had the unintended consequence of leading some LGBTQ+ people to conceal their sexual orientation and gender identity and expression for fear they may also become victims.[8]

ANTI-LGBTQ+ LEGISLATION EFFECTS ON HEALTH

Our work and that of others in Kenya has demonstrated disproportionate challenges with MHSU and HIV prevention and treatment. We found that more than half (52%) of gay and bisexual men in Western Kenya reported clinically significant posttraumatic stress symptoms and that 28% reported clinically significant depressive symptoms.[7] Gay and bisexual men in the capital city of Nairobi reported similar rates (29.8%) of clinically significant depressive symptoms, with 39.2% reporting harmful substance use.[15] In a study of 1476 gay and bisexual men in Kisumu, Kenya; Nairobi; and coastal Kenya, 31% of participants reported clinically significant depressive symptoms and 51% reported harmful alcohol use.[16]

Gay and bisexual men make up an estimated 15% of people with HIV in Kenya.[17] The estimated HIV prevalence among the general population of Kenya is 4.3%; the prevalence among gay and bisexual men is estimated to be at least four times higher.[18] Only 52% of gay and bisexual men in Kenya know their HIV status, with 80% of those who know receiving treatment and only 74% of those on treatment virally suppressed.[19]

Preexposure prophylaxis (PrEP) has been included in Kenya's comprehensive HIV prevention strategy for gay and bisexual men and other men who have sex with men (GBMSM) since 2017. Despite high levels of interest in PrEP, adherence and continuation have been low. A cohort study of 172 PrEP-eligible GBMSM in Kenya demonstrated that only 14.6% had protective levels of PrEP at any follow-up visit,[20] and a large-scale service delivery project found that only 7% of 4848 GBMSM who initiated PrEP returned for their three-month follow-up.[21] Common barriers to PrEP uptake and adherence include misinformation, mistrust in medical providers and facilities, and stigma and discrimination.[20]

CONCEPTUAL MODEL COMPONENTS

Our model is grounded in intersectionality[22,23] and the minority stress model.[24] We use intersectionality as both a framework and an epistemological stance, whereby we privilege gay and bisexual men's lived knowledge and narratives of social phenomena and actively engage in an interrogation of power, centering the impact of interlocking systems of oppression and privilege when examining health inequities.[22,23]

In Meyer's conceptualization of the minority stress model,[25] he describes individual experiences of sociostructural LGBTQ+ violence and discrimination as distal minority stressors and internalized responses to these experiences as proximal minority stressors. These two stress processes combine synergistically with general life stressors (e.g., financial stress, political unrest) to negatively affect physical and mental health. Despite being developed in the United States, the minority stress model has proven effective for understanding the mental health of gay and bisexual men in Kenya.[7,9]

Anti-LGBTQ+ Legislation

At the top of our model is anti-LGBTQ+ legislation (Figure 1). Kenyan Penal Codes 162–165 are currently the most notable, but others may emerge, as the Family Protection Bill did. These are inconsistent with the current Kenyan constitution of 2010 and with other national health policies, including the most recent Kenya AIDS Strategic Framework.[11] In alignment with our foundation in intersectionality,[22,23] we view various forms of anti-LGBTQ+ legislation in Kenya as part of other interlocking systems of oppression that synergistically create sociostructural barriers to the health of gay and bisexual men and other LGBTQ+ Kenyans. Given the pervasive and endemic nature of these intersectional forms of oppression, it is difficult to determine direct causality. Still, we honor the lived knowledge and voices of gay and bisexual Kenyan men in both our studies and our team, who perceive that criminalization is a contributing factor to MHSU and HIV prevention and care challenges.

Proximal LGBTQ+ Stressors and Barriers

We propose that anti-LGBTQ+ legislation contributes to proximal stressors in the form of internalized antigay stigma, shame, fears of rejection, feelings of powerlessness, and concealment of one's gay or bisexual identity and behaviors. We have often heard from gay and bisexual men that concealment can be a survival mechanism and a way to gain a sense of control and escape anti-LGBTQ+ violence—but with the consequence of increasing negative perceptions of self, psychological distress, and mental health challenges. Concealment also leads to the social invisibility of resilient gay and bisexual men in positions of power. Some men said that such internal turmoil increased HIV-related risk behaviors and substance use and created barriers to seeking services for both MHSU challenges and HIV prevention and care.

Distal LGBTQ+ Stressors and Barriers

We propose that anti-LGBTQ+ legislation contributes to distal stressors in the form of antigay violence and attacks, discrimination across multiple settings (e.g., school, housing, health care), family and community rejection, stigmatizing social practices, and verbal and physical harassment. One form of violence related to anti-LGBTQ+ laws has been police officers using forced anal exams to obtain physical evidence of same-sex activity, although this was deemed unconstitutional in March 2018. More recently, perpetrators have posed as potential romantic partners on dating apps, luring a victim to a secret location, where he is beaten, sexually assaulted, or robbed. Sometimes he is blackmailed using screenshots from the app or pictures taken during the assault. The traumatic nature of this violence may increase MHSU challenges and lead some to avoid seeking health-related services.

Sociostructural Stressors and Barriers

Gay and bisexual men in Kenya must contend with other sociostructural stressors also experienced by non-LGBTQ+ Kenyans, including lack of stable housing, lack of education and job skills training, and limited access to health care. Unemployment and poverty are also common sociostructural barriers to achieving optimal health among most minoritized Kenyans. We have heard many stories about the economic marginalization of gay and bisexual men owing to limited job opportunities in the current economy, which is exacerbated by discrimination in the workplace and transportation services.

Care Services Avoidance

Kenyan gay and bisexual men struggle with a range of mental health challenges and problematic substance use in the form of store-bought alcohol, traditional home brew alcohol, and, to

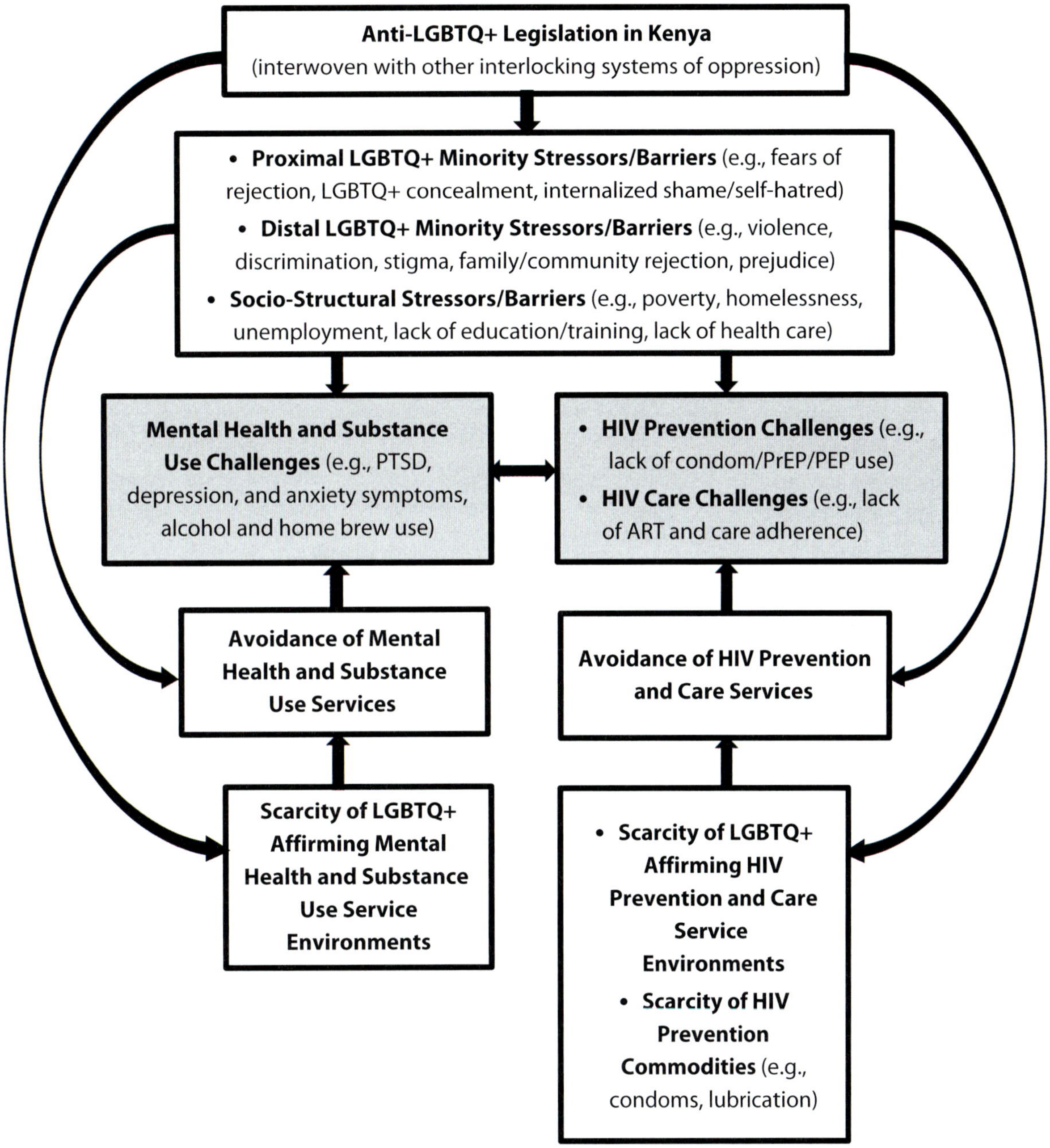

FIGURE 1— Multiple Influences of Anti-LGBTQ+ Legislation on Mental Health and Substance Use and HIV-Related Challenges Among Gay and Bisexual Men: Kenya

Note. ART = antiretroviral therapy; LGBTQ+ = lesbian, gay, bisexual, transgender, queer or questioning, and all subsects; PEP = postexposure prophylaxis; PrEP = preexposure prophylaxis; PTSD = posttraumatic stress disorder.

a lesser extent, marijuana. In our conceptual model, we propose that these health challenges are influenced by interactions among both proximal and distal LGBTQ+ minority stressors, as well as other sociostructural stressors and barriers. Team members and study participants have shared that the confluence of these stressors creates high levels of psychosocial distress, which can lead to significant levels of depression, anxiety, or posttraumatic stress symptoms—all followed by substance use to "self-medicate" and relieve discomfort. Avoidance of mental health services, because of proximal and distal LGBTQ+ minority stressors, such as fears of revealing one's sexual orientation to others or negative experiences of attempted "conversion therapy" by mental health providers, can lead to exacerbations of MHSU challenges.

In our model, we suggest a bidirectional relationship between MHSU challenges and HIV prevention and care challenges. Our previous work and team member experiences demonstrate that MHSU challenges can interfere with adherence to HIV prevention and care practices through cognitive or affective states that present barriers to health-promoting behaviors and may encourage participation in high-risk behaviors. Additionally, when a gay or bisexual man has challenges adhering to HIV prevention and care practices, he may experience frustration or disappointment, and even increase substance use to avoid feeling negative emotions.

HIV Prevention and Care Challenges

Disproportionately high rates of HIV among gay and bisexual men in Kenya persist despite the availability of HIV prevention strategies such as condom use, PrEP, and postexposure prophylaxis. For those living with HIV, adherence to medication and visits with health care providers can result in an undetectable viral load. Our model proposes that, similar to MHSU challenges, HIV-related health challenges are influenced by interactions among proximal and distal LGBTQ+ minority stressors, as well as other sociostructural stressors and barriers.[25] This confluence of stressors can burden gay and bisexual men with pervasive negativity, leading some to engage in non–condom-protected sex to feel a deeper human connection and euphoria that block negative affect. Others may cease health protective practices (e.g., PrEP, antiretroviral therapy) as they succumb to negative messaging and give up on life. Kenyan gay and bisexual men have shared their inability to access HIV prevention and care services and the barriers to using them consistently and correctly.

Avoidance of HIV prevention and care services can occur because of proximal and distal LGBTQ+ minority stressors, such as fears of revealing one's sexual orientation or HIV status to providers and other patients in clinics and anxiety that receiving HIV-related services will make it more difficult to deny their own gay or bisexual identity. Others have had negative experiences of discrimination and violence perpetrated by health care providers once the provider identified them as gay or bisexual. Avoiding HIV prevention services can lead to HIV seroconversions, and avoiding HIV care services can lead to serious health declines.

Service Environments and HIV Prevention

In addition to anti-LGBTQ+ legislation's direct effect on proximal, distal, and other sociostructural stressors and barriers, we view such legislation as limiting the number of LGBTQ+-affirming service environments that provide tailored MHSU and HIV-related services and offer free condoms and lubrication. Increases in anti-LGBTQ+ bills and political and religious rhetoric have already led to decreases in local government financial support for gay and bisexual men's health care, forcing service providers to reduce or eliminate services.[11] Health care facilities serving gay and bisexual men are often the last to receive condoms from the government and are not provided with lubrication because anal sex is a criminalized behavior. This scarcity of LGBTQ+-affirming service environments may lead gay and bisexual men to forego MHSU and HIV-related services if no such local facilities exist and they do not have the economic resources to travel to one. When MHSU and HIV prevention and care services are available but not located in an LGBTQ+ affirming service environment, many gay and bisexual men would rather not receive care than risk suffering stigma, discrimination, and even violence in health care settings.

CONCLUSIONS

With the use of our model, and through community-centered discussion, research, and action, we believe activists, practitioners, and sympathetic lawmakers can challenge anti-LGBTQ+ legislation in Kenya and defeat harsher and more extensive anti-LGBTQ+ proposed legislation, such as the Family Protection Bill of 2023. AJPH

CORRESPONDENCE

Correspondence should be sent to Gary W. Harper, PhD, MPH, 1415 Washington Heights, School of Public Health I, Ann Arbor, MI 48109 (gwharper@umich.edu). Reprints can be ordered at https://www.ajph.org by clicking the "Reprints" link.

PUBLICATION INFORMATION

Full Citation: Harper GW, Odhiambo EO, Jadwin-Cakmak L, et al. The impact of anti-LGBTQ+ legislation on mental health and substance use and HIV prevention and care among gay and bisexual men in Kenya. *Am J Public Health*. 2025;115(8):1200–1205.

Acceptance Date: February 24, 2025.

DOI: https://doi.org/10.2105/AJPH.2025.308097

ORCID iDs:

Gary W. Harper https://orcid.org/0000-0003-1011-1751

Laura Jadwin-Cakmak https://orcid.org/0000-0001-5744-9632

Sophia A. Hussen https://orcid.org/0000-0002-5726-1637

CONTRIBUTORS

G. W. Harper wrote the first draft of the editorial. All authors conceptualized and developed the model, offered feedback and recommendations on the writing, and approved the final draft.

ACKNOWLEDGMENTS

We wish to thank the many gay and bisexual men and other men who have sex with men in Kisumu County, Kenya, who have generously shared their life stories with us over the past 15 years. We also wish to thank the many LGBTQ+ (lesbian, gay, bisexual, transgender, queer or questioning, and all subsects) community-based organizations that provide safe havens and services for those in the community and give hope for health equity.

CONFLICTS OF INTEREST

We have no conflicts of interest to report.

REFERENCES

1. Esposito J, Evans-Winters V. *Introduction to Intersectional Qualitative Research.* Thousand Oaks, CA: Sage: 2022.
2. ReportOUT. The permanent shadow: colonialism, sexual orientation and gender identity in Zimbabwe and Kenya. 2023. Available at: https://www.ohchr.org/sites/default/files/documents/cfi-subm/2308/subm-colonialism-sexual-orientation-cso-reportout-input-2.pdf. Accessed April 19, 2025.
3. Murray SO, Roscoe W. *Boy-Wives and Female Husbands: Studies of African Homosexualities.* New York, NY: St. Martin's Press; 1998.
4. Zlozie B. Did Europe bring homophobia to Africa? 2021. Available at: https://www.aaihs.org/did-europe-bring-homophobia-to-africa. Accessed April 17, 2025.
5. Ibrahim AM. LGBT rights in Africa and the discursive role of international human rights law. *Afr Hum Rights Law J.* 2015;15(2):263–281. https://doi.org/10.17159/1996-2096/2015/v15n2a2
6. Buckle L. African sexuality and the legacy of imported homophobia. 2023. Available at: https://www.stonewall.org.uk/news/african-sexuality-and-legacy-imported-homophobia. Accessed April 17, 2025.
7. Harper GW, Crawford J, Lewis K, et al. Mental health challenges and needs among sexual and gender minority people in Western Kenya. *Int J Environ Res Public Health.* 2021;18(3):1311. https://doi.org/10.3390/ijerph18031311
8. Lewis KA, Jadwin-Cakmak L, Walimbwa J, et al. "You'll be chased away": sources, experiences, and effects of violence and stigma among gay and bisexual men in Kenya. *Int J Environ Res Public Health.* 2023;20(4):2825. https://doi.org/10.3390/ijerph20042825
9. Jauregui JC, Mwochi CR, Crawford J, et al. Experiences of violence and mental health concerns among sexual and gender minority adults in Western Kenya. *LGBT Health.* 2021;8(7):494–501. https://doi.org/10.1089/lgbt.2020.0495
10. Odula T, Kazziha K. Kenyan court upholds laws criminalizing same-sex relations. 2019. Available at: https://www.apnews.com/58b315e5dbcf4b9e97a2127b0634f6f7. Accessed April 16, 2025.
11. Walimbwa J, Macharia P, Wambua S, Lazarus L, Lorway R. Political homophobia and the effect on GBMSM programmes in Kenya: the significance of a community-led rapid agency assessment. *Glob Public Health.* 2023;18(1):2271989. https://doi.org/10.1080/17441692.2023.2271989
12. Ombuor R. Murder of gay activist triggers trauma for Kenya's LGBTIQ community. 2023. Available at: https://www.opendemocracy.net/en/5050/edwin-chiloba-murder-lgbtiq-kenya-africa. Accessed April 16, 2025.
13. Wepukhulu SK, Madegwa N. Sheila Lumumba: hopes for justice as man charged with lesbian's murder. July 20, 2022. Available at: https://www.opendemocracy.net/en/5050/sheila-lumumba-lesbian-murder-rape-kenyan-police. Accessed April 16, 2025.
14. National Gay and Lesbian Human Rights Commission. *Protect the Lives and Rights of LGBTIQ+ Persons in Kenya.* Nairobi, Kenya; 2022.
15. Doshi M, Macharia P, Mathenge J, et al. Beyond biomedical and comorbidity approaches: exploring associations between affinity group membership, health and health seeking behaviour among MSM/MSW in Nairobi, Kenya. *Glob Public Health.* 2020;15(7):968–984. https://doi.org/10.1080/17441692.2020.1739729
16. Korhonen CJ, Kimani M, Wahome E, et al. Depressive symptoms and problematic alcohol and other substance use in 1476 gay, bisexual, and other MSM at three research sites in Kenya. *AIDS.* 2018;32(11):1507–1515.
17. Moyer E, Igonya E. Queering the evidence: remaking homosexuality and HIV risk to "end AIDS" in Kenya. *Glob Public Health.* 2018;13(8):1007–1019. https://doi.org/10.1080/17441692.2018.1462841
18. US President's Emergency Plan for AIDS Relief. *Kenya: Country Operational Plan 2022 Strategic Direction Summary.* July 18, 2022. Available at: https://www.state.gov/wp-content/uploads/2022/09/Kenya-COP22-SDS-.pdf. Accessed April 19, 2025.
19. Musyoki H, Bhattacharjee P, Sabin K, et al. A decade and beyond: learnings from HIV programming with underserved and marginalized key populations in Kenya. *J Int AIDS Soc.* 2021;24(suppl 3):e25729. https://doi.org/10.1002/jia2.25729
20. Graham SM, Okall DO, Mehta SD, et al. Challenges with PrEP uptake and adherence among gay, bisexual, and other men who have sex with men in Kisumu, Kenya. *AIDS Behav.* 2023;27(4):1234–1247. https://doi.org/10.1007/s10461-022-03860-w
21. Were D, Musau A, Mutegi J, et al. Using a HIV prevention cascade for identifying missed opportunities in PrEP delivery in Kenya: results from a programmatic surveillance study. *J Int AIDS Soc.* 2020;23(suppl 3):e25537. https://doi.org/10.1002/jia2.25537
22. Bowleg L. The White racial frame of public health discourses about racialized health differences and "disparities": what it reveals about power and how it thwarts health equity. *Front Public Health.* 2023;11:1187307. https://doi.org/10.3389/fpubh.2023.1187307
23. Collins PH, Bilge S. *Intersectionality.* 2nd ed. Cambridge, UK: Polity Press; 2020.
24. Brooks VR. *Minority Stress and Lesbian Women.* Lexington, MA: Lexington Books; 1981.
25. Meyer IH. Prejudice, social stress, and mental health in lesbian, gay, and bisexual populations: conceptual issues and research evidence. *Psychol Bull.* 2003;129(5):674–697. https://doi.org/10.1037/0033-2909.129.5.674

Tobacco Company Efforts to Persuade Consumers to Fight the Proposed Federal Menthol Cigarette and Flavored Cigar Bans in the United States

Ollie Ganz, DrPH, MSPH, Andrea C. Villanti, PhD, MPH, Aila Altunbilek, MPH, BS, Amanda Johnson, MPH, BS, Jeannie Garmon, PhD, MPH, Olivia A. Wackowski, PhD, MPH, and Kymberle L. Sterling, DrPH

ABOUT THE AUTHORS

Ollie Ganz, Andrea C. Villanti, Olivia A. Wackowski, and Kymberle L. Sterling are with the Department of Health Behavior, Society, and Policy at the Rutgers School of Public Health in Piscataway, NJ, and the Rutgers Institute for Nicotine and Tobacco Studies at Rutgers Health in New Brunswick, NJ. Aila Altunbilek, Amanda Johnson, and Jeannie Garmon are with the Rutgers Institute for Nicotine and Tobacco Studies at Rutgers Health, New Brunswick.

AJPH August 2025, Vol. 115, No. 8

In April 2022, the US Food and Drug Administration (FDA) proposed product standards that would ban menthol cigarettes and flavored cigars. From May through August 2022, there were open dockets for both proposed rules where public comments could be submitted to the FDA.

HEALTH EQUITY VS TOBACCO COMPANY PROFITS

The proposed bans on menthol cigarettes and flavored cigars, which target the manufacturing and sales of these products, not purchasing or use by individuals, would have important implications for health equity, with modeling studies estimating that a ban on menthol cigarettes would save approximately 650 000 Black/African American lives in the United States over 40 years.[1] Indeed, most Black/African American adults who smoke cigarettes in the United States smoke menthols,[2] attributable in large part to decades of predatory tobacco company marketing.[3] Furthermore, the use of flavored cigars—cheap, mass-merchandise cigarillos (e.g., Swisher Sweets) in particular—is disproportionately high among young Black/African American individuals.[4]

Menthol cigarettes and flavored cigars comprise substantial proportions of the cigarette and cigar market share in the United States.[5,6] Cigarettes remain the dominant product in the tobacco marketplace (60% of tobacco sales),[7] followed by cigars (23% of tobacco sales); importantly, menthol cigarettes constitute 36% of the cigarette market,[8] and flavored cigars account for more than half (53%) of cigar sales in US convenience stores.[6] As a consequence, the proposed bans threaten tobacco companies' profits. As with many previous profit-threatening policies,[9] tobacco companies have engaged in numerous strategies to prevent the flavor bans from advancing, including meetings with top White House officials[10] and financial contributions to prominent leaders in the Black/African American community.[11] Companies have also engaged in concerted efforts to leverage their consumer base.

MARKETING TO ENCOURAGE CONSUMERS TO FIGHT THE BANS

We examined direct-to-consumer advertisements sent by tobacco companies encouraging consumers to fight the proposed federal menthol cigarette and flavored cigar bans. Specifically, we used Trinkets & Trash (an academic monitoring system; https://trinketsandtrash.org) and Mintel (a commercial market research company) to obtain a convenience sample of direct-to-consumer ads (i.e., direct mail and e-mail ads that customers sign up to receive) from tobacco companies referencing impending policies proposing to ban menthol cigarettes or flavored cigars from April 2022, when the proposed bans were announced, through December 2023. The Appendix (available as a supplement to the online version of this article at https://ajph.org)

contains additional information about the data sources used.

As part of a larger project,[12] the research team developed a coding guide to identify the themes and framing of arguments related to the proposed FDA menthol and flavored cigar bans. The initial coding guide was developed deductively based on the project's research questions and the research team's previous research and experience. The guide was refined through two rounds of pilot testing across different data sources to ensure the clarity of the codes and integrity of the process; several other codes were added inductively during pilot testing.

We identified a total of 18 relevant e-mail ads and double-coded them for company and brand characteristics, cues to action, key phrases, and arguments against the bans. We did not identify any direct mail ads. We imported data into StataMP version 18 and used frequencies to characterize the ads. See Figure A (available as a supplement to the online version of this article at https://ajph.org) for example ads. In addition to reviewing the ads, we also examined one of the website landing pages listed in most of the e-mails ("Own it. Voice it."; https://ownitvoiceit.com). Because the content relevant to the menthol and flavored cigar bans is no longer on the website, we could only view content via Wayback Machine, an Internet archive.[13] This limited the scope of our analysis. However, we were able to conduct a cursory review of the content of the website from the beginning of our study period (April 2022).

Most e-mail ads originated from cigarette brands (61.1%; n = 11), but more than a third were from cigar and smokeless tobacco brands (Table 1). Two thirds of the ads originated from

TABLE 1— Characteristics of E-Mails Sent to Consumers by Tobacco Companies Encouraging Them to Fight the Proposed Menthol and Flavored Cigar Bans, April 2022–December 2023

	No. (%)
Product type	
Cigarettes	11 (61.1)
Cigars	3 (16.7)
Snus or smokeless tobacco	3 (16.7)
Electronic cigarettes	1 (5.6)
Brand (product type indicated where not otherwise specified)	
Black & Mild (cigars)	1 (5.6)
Camel cigarettes	2 (11.1)
Camel Snus (smokeless tobacco)	1 (5.6)
Grizzly (smokeless tobacco)	2 (11.1)
Marlboro (cigarettes)	2 (11.1)
Natural American Spirit (cigarettes)	2 (11.1)
Newport (cigarettes)	4 (22.2)
Optimo (cigars)	1 (5.6)
Swisher Sweets (cigars)	1 (5.6)
Vuse (electronic cigarettes)	1 (5.6)
Winston (cigarettes)	1 (5.6)
Company	
Altria	3 (16.7)
Reynolds American Inc	12 (66.7)
Swisher International	3 (16.7)
ITG	2 (11.1)
Date of appearance	
2022	8 (44.4)
May	4 (22.2)
June	2 (11.1)
July	1 (5.6)
December	1 (5.6)
2023	10 (55.6)
July	8 (44.4)
October	2 (11.1)
Ban mentioned	
Menthol cigarette	9 (50.0)
Flavored cigar	3 (16.7)
Both	6 (33.3)
Website provided to protest ban	15 (83.3)
Explicit mention of speaking out against ban	18 (100.0)
Submitting a comment opposing ban mentioned	5 (27.8)
Key phrases	
Act now	2 (11.1)
Don't miss your chance	2 (11.1)
Don't stay silent	6 (33.3)
Speak your voice	9 (50.0)

Continued

TABLE 1— Continued

	No. (%)
Take a stand	1 (5.6)
Take action	6 (33.3)
Arguments against the ban	
Ban would do more harm than good	2 (11.1)
Ban is government overreach	9 (50.0)
Evidence doesn't support the ban	2 (11.1)
Ban would result in loss of tax revenue	2 (11.1)
Ban will cause businesses and jobs to suffer	4 (22.2)
Ban threatens adult choices	5 (27.8)
Ban will lead to illicit market	2 (11.1)
Ban will lead to increased criminalization	2 (11.1)

Note. The sample size was n = 18. Sources of e-mail ads: Trinkets & Trash (an academic monitoring system; https://trinketsandtrash.org) and Mintel (a commercial market research company).

Reynolds American Inc (66.7%; n = 12), which owns Newport, the most popular US menthol cigarette brand,[14] which also sent the most e-mails compared with other brands (cigarette; 22.2%; n = 4).

All e-mail ads explicitly mentioned speaking out against the ban and leveraged phrases encouraging customers to "speak your voice" (50%; n = 9), "don't stay silent" (33.3%; n = 6), and "take action" (33.3%; n = 6). Arguments featured in the ads noted that the bans are government overreach (50.0%; n = 9), threaten adult choice (27.8%; n = 5), and will cause businesses and jobs to suffer (22.2%; n = 4). Seven ads (38.9%) were sent during an open public FDA comment period for both proposed rules (May to August 2022), and eight were sent in July 2023 (44.4%), one month before the FDA had originally planned to issue the final rules (August 2023).

ADVOCACY WEBSITES FACILITATED CONSUMER OPPOSITION TO BANS

Most e-mails linked consumers to advocacy websites where they could take action against the bans (83%; n = 15). The most commonly linked website was "Own it. Voice it." (66.7%; n = 12), an advocacy website sponsored by RAI Service Company, a subsidiary of Reynolds American Inc, which is the parent company of brands such as Newport, Grizzly, and Vuse. The second most commonly linked website was "Citizens for Tobacco Rights" (https://tobaccorights.com; 16.7%; n = 3), which is operated on behalf of Philip Morris USA (maker of Marlboro cigarettes), US Smokeless Tobacco Company (maker of Copenhagen and Skoal), John Middleton Inc (maker of Black & Mild cigars), Helix Innovations (maker of on! oral nicotine pouches), and NJOY (electronic vapor products).

Our examination of the "Own it. Voice it." website from April 2022 demonstrates how the website encouraged consumers to act against the proposed bans and enabled them to generate and submit customized comments to the FDA dockets on menthol cigarettes and flavored cigars (Figure B, available as a supplement to the online version of this article at https://ajph.org). Consumers first selected the category with which they most identified: an adult menthol consumer, business owner, concerned citizen, or farmer. Then they were directed to select the anti-ban arguments that most concerned them. The list included both arguments featured in e-mail ads and unique arguments, including that the ban would "cause fractures in the criminal justice system" and have "negative impacts on farming and the agricultural industry." Users were also provided text boxes for open-ended comments.

CREATING A SENSE OF URGENCY TO FIGHT THE PROPOSED BANS

While previous evidence has shown tobacco companies using social media to encourage advocacy against tobacco-control policies,[15] our analyses document the use of tobacco companies' extensive direct-to-consumer databases to target customers and tobacco users with ads to persuade them to advocate against tobacco control policies. Direct-to-consumer marketing is a unique advertising channel for tobacco companies. It allows them to leverage their extensive direct mail database to facilitate carefully targeted messaging to consumers with minimal legal restrictions and in a manner that is largely out of public view.[16,17] The e-mails sent in July 2023, a month after the FDA announced its intentions to finalize the proposed rules, may have been a push to encourage customers to voice their opposition to the ban before the final regulations were published. The keywords and phrases such as "speak your voice," "take action," and "don't stay silent" create a sense of urgency and may be interpreted as directives to consumers to protest the ban. These types of messages also suggest that the proposed bans are an injustice that individuals must stand up to and resist. Previous studies of industry advocacy messages have also found that many of them encourage citizen advocacy[15] and contain pleas for action.[18]

Interestingly, anti-ban e-mails were not only sent from cigarette and cigar brands but also from brands of products that would not be directly impacted by the bans, including smokeless tobacco and e-cigarettes. Indeed, most of the anti-ban arguments featured in the e-mails and on the "Own it. Voice it." website were not product-specific but were more general arguments about tobacco control policies and regulations.[19] This was likely an attempt to appeal to a broader consumer base to generate more comments and, possibly, to confuse consumers into believing that the bans would affect a larger number of products. Furthermore, the e-cigarette and smokeless tobacco brands (e.g., Camel Snus) that sent e-mails are from companies that also sell menthol cigarettes and flavored cigars and therefore would benefit from consumers speaking out against the proposed bans.

HISTORY OF TOBACCO COMPANIES RALLYING CONSUMER OPPOSITION

The tobacco company–sponsored websites promoted in the e-mail ads have been used in the past to disseminate key messages articulating their opposition to various tobacco control policies, such as tobacco taxes, and to encourage and facilitate action among consumers to fight such policies.[18] Because the FDA comment period had ended when we conducted our evaluation of the website, we could not confirm how these comments were submitted to the docket; however, quick keyword searches available in the comment portals indicate that phrases from the "Own It. Voice It." website were present in a large number of comments in the menthol cigarette docket (e.g., n = 14 416 comments with "cause fractures in the criminal justice system").

Notably, our study relied on e-mails sent to a prespecified panel of consumers and likely underestimates the total number of e-mails sent. Furthermore, we were unable to identify the number or demographic characteristics of the individuals who received them, though previous research suggests that the prevalence of receiving tobacco coupons by e-mail or mail tends to higher among adults who smoke who are female, White, have lower education, and have more difficulty paying important bills, compared with adults who smoke who did not receive coupons.[20] Future research should consider the demographic characteristics of the recipients of these ads and examine the impact of their messages on consumer perceptions of the proposed bans.

PUBLIC HEALTH IMPLICATIONS

The proposed federal bans on menthol cigarettes and flavored cigars aim to restrict the manufacturing and distribution of the products by tobacco companies. However, tobacco company messaging about the proposed bans is meant to generate anger and fear among consumers, highlighting "loss of freedom" and "adult choice," without reference to the health harms incurred by tobacco products or the potential health benefits of reductions in cigarette and cigar smoking. Tobacco company anti-ban messages using freedom and choice themes obfuscate key points: tobacco products are highly addictive—initiation typically starts before adulthood[21]—and tobacco company profits come at the expense of public health, particularly among marginalized communities (e.g., Black/African Americans, youths) that have been targeted with menthol cigarette and flavored cigar advertising.

Messages about "freedom" and "choice" remain pervasive in tobacco company communications and were also employed by conservative nonprofit groups seeking to influence the 2024 presidential election.[22] To counter this, public health advocates should educate consumers about the purpose and public health benefits of the bans, the role of menthol cigarettes and flavored cigars in appealing to young people and making quitting smoking more difficult, and the history of targeted marketing of these products toward historically minoritized communities. These efforts should be tailored and culturally relevant for the people and communities experiencing disproportionate health harms from menthol cigarette and flavored cigar use, including Black/African Americans, sexual minority individuals, and young people.[2] This may improve policy support and build the political will needed to counteract industry antiregulation efforts, which is especially needed at this time since the FDA withdrew the proposed rules banning menthol cigarettes and flavored cigars in January 2025.[23]

The public health community can benefit from awareness of tobacco company tactics used to oppose public health policies in the era of electronic communication and direct-to-consumer advertising. Understanding the history of tobacco company efforts to oppose public health policies and the methods by which tobacco companies provide incomplete and sometimes misleading information to encourage their consumer base to actively oppose policies may inform regulators tasked with making sense of thousands of public comments. These insights may also apply to researchers and practitioners whose work focuses on other public health issues, such as alcohol, food, and gun violence, where corporate influences on public policies have negative impacts on public health.[24] AJPH

CORRESPONDENCE

Correspondence should be sent to Ollie Ganz, Rutgers Institute for Nicotine and Tobacco Studies, 303 George St, Suite 500, New Brunswick, NJ 08901 (e-mail: og96@sph.rutgers.edu). Reprints can be ordered at https://www.ajph.org by clicking the "Reprints" link.

PUBLICATION INFORMATION

Full Citation: Ganz O, Villanti AC, Altunbilek A, et al. Tobacco company efforts to persuade consumers to fight the proposed federal menthol cigarette and flavored cigar bans in the United States. *Am J Public Health*. 2025;115(8):1206–1210.

Acceptance Date: March 12, 2025.

DOI: https://doi.org/10.2105/AJPH.2025.308116

ORCID iDs:

Ollie Ganz https://orcid.org/0000-0002-7933-8463

Andrea C. Villanti https://orcid.org/0000-0003-3104-966X

Amanda Johnson https://orcid.org/0009-0006-4498-1420

Jeannie Garmon https://orcid.org/0009-0007-8177-7063

CONTRIBUTORS

All authors contributed to the conceptualization and design of the study, and were involved in the interpretation of data, writing of the original draft, and revision of the final draft. A. Altunbilek, A. Johnson, and J. Garmon coded the advertisements, and O. Ganz analyzed the data.

ACKNOWLEDGMENTS

This work was supported in part by the National Institute on Minority Health and Health Disparities (NIMHD) of the National Institutes of Health under award R01MD018728.

Note. This content is solely the responsibility of the authors and does not necessarily represent the official views of NIMHD.

CONFLICTS OF INTEREST

The authors report no conflicts of interest.

REFERENCES

1. Issabakhsh M, Meza R, Li Y, Yuan Z, Sanchez-Romero LM, Levy DT. Public health impact of a US menthol cigarette ban on the non-Hispanic Black population: a simulation study. *Tob Control*. 2023;33(1):126–130. https://doi.org/10.1136/tobaccocontrol-2022-057298
2. Goodwin RD, Ganz O, Weinberger AH, Smith PH, Wyka K, Delnevo CD. Menthol cigarette use among adults who smoke cigarettes, 2008–2020: rapid growth and widening inequities in the United States. *Nicotine Tob Res*. 2023;25(4):692–698. https://doi.org/10.1093/ntr/ntac214
3. Gardiner PS. The African Americanization of menthol cigarette use in the United States. *Nicotine Tob Res*. 2004;6(suppl 1):S55–S65. https://doi.org/10.1080/14622200310001649478
4. Watkins SL, Pieper F, Chaffee BW, Yerger VB, Ling PM, Max W. Flavored tobacco product use among young adults by race and ethnicity: evidence from the Population Assessment of Tobacco and Health Study. *J Adolesc Health*. 2022;71(2):226–232. https://doi.org/10.1016/j.jadohealth.2022.02.013
5. Delnevo CD, Giovenco DP, Villanti AC. Assessment of menthol and nonmenthol cigarette consumption in the US, 2000 to 2018. *JAMA Netw Open*. 2020;3(8):e2013601. https://doi.org/10.1001/jamanetworkopen.2020.13601
6. Delnevo CD, Miller Lo E, Giovenco DP, Cornacchione Ross J, Hrywna M, Strasser AA. Cigar sales in convenience stores in the US, 2009–2020. *JAMA*. 2021;326(23):2429–2432. https://doi.org/10.1001/jama.2021.19692
7. Ganz O, LaVake M, Hrywna M, King Jensen JL, Delnevo CD. National trends in sales and price for commercial tobacco and nicotine products: 2018–2022. *JAMA Netw Open*. 2024;7(3):e241384. https://doi.org/10.1001/jamanetworkopen.2024.1384
8. Federal Trade Commission. Federal Trade Commission Cigarette Report for 2022. 2023. Available at: https://www.ftc.gov/news-events/news/press-releases/2023/10/ftc-releases-reports-cigarette-smokeless-tobacco-sales-marketing-expenditures-2022. Accessed October 7, 2024.
9. Matthes BK, Kumar P, Dance S, Hird T, Carriedo Lutzenkirchen A, Gilmore AB. Advocacy counter-strategies to tobacco industry interference in policymaking: a scoping review of peer-reviewed literature. *Global Health*. 2023;19(1):42. https://doi.org/10.1186/s12992-023-00936-7
10. Weixel N. Top Biden officials meet with Black, public health leaders following menthol ban delay. *The Hill*. December 20, 2023. Available at: https://thehill.com/policy/healthcare/4370407-top-biden-officials-meet-with-black-public-health-leaders-following-menthol-ban-delay. Accessed April 17, 2024.
11. Baumgaertner E, Stockton B, Lindsay R. How Big Tobacco used George Floyd and Eric Garner to stoke fear among Black smokers. *Los Angeles Times*. April 25, 2022. Available at: https://www.latimes.com/world-nation/story/2022-04-25/inside-big-tobaccos-strategy-to-stoke-fear-among-black-smokers-facing-menthol-bans. Accessed April 1, 2024.
12. NIH Reporter. The unvarnished truth: pursuing health equity by correcting disinformation targeting African Americans about the FDA's proposed ban on menthol cigarettes and flavored cigars. 2025. Available at: https://reporter.nih.gov/search/sg9oE2OHvUOIPsHaGt6BRQ/project-details/11023115. Accessed March 3, 2025.
13. The Internet Archive. Wayback Machine. October 2001. Available at: http://web.archive.org. Accessed March 2025.
14. Miller Lo EJ, Young WJ, Ganz O, Talbot EM, O'Connor RJ, Delnevo CD. Trends in overall and menthol market shares of leading cigarette brands in the USA: 2014–2019. *Int J Environ Res Public Health*. 2022;19(4):2270. https://doi.org/10.3390/ijerph19042270
15. Majmundar A, Moran MB. For or against tobacco control: sponsored tobacco advocacy messages on Facebook and Instagram. *Nicotine Tob Res*. 2021;23(11):1861–1868. https://doi.org/10.1093/ntr/ntab111
16. Lewis MJ, Ling PM. "Gone are the days of mass-media marketing plans and short term customer relationships": tobacco industry direct mail and database marketing strategies. *Tob Control*. 2016;25(4):430–436. https://doi.org/10.1136/tobaccocontrol-2015-052314
17. Weiner BJ, Lewis CC, Stanick C, et al. Psychometric assessment of three newly developed implementation outcome measures. *Implement Sci*. 2017;12(1):108. https://doi.org/10.1186/s13012-017-0635-3
18. Lewis MJ, Ackerman C, Ling P. 'Being politically active does not have to be difficult.' A content analysis of tobacco industry-sponsored advocacy websites. *Tob Control*. 2020;29(e1):e98–e105. https://doi.org/10.1136/tobaccocontrol-2019-055413
19. Brock B, Carlson SC, Moilanen M, Schillo BA. Reaching consumers: how the tobacco industry uses email marketing. *Prev Med Rep*. 2016;4:103–106. https://doi.org/10.1016/j.pmedr.2016.05.020
20. Osman A, Queen T, Choi K, Goldstein AO. Receipt of direct tobacco mail/email coupons and coupon redemption: demographic and socioeconomic disparities among adult smokers in the United States. *Prev Med*. 2019;126:105778. https://doi.org/10.1016/j.ypmed.2019.105778
21. US Department of Health and Human Services. *The Health Consequences of Smoking: 50 Years of Progress. A Report of the Surgeon General*. Atlanta, GA: National Center for Chronic Disease Prevention and Health Promotion, Office on Smoking and Health; 2014.
22. Kamisar B. Conservative group plans $10 million effort to soften Harris' Black voter support. *NBC News*. August 27, 2024. Available at: https://www.nbcnews.com/politics/2024-election/conservative-group-campaign-kamala-harris-black-voters-rcna168393. Accessed October 7, 2024.
23. Office of Management and Budget. OIRA Conclusion of EO 12866 Regulatory Review: Tobacco Product Standard for Menthol in Cigarettes. 2025. Available at: https://www.reginfo.gov/public/do/eoDetails?rrid=341411. Accessed February 18, 2025.
24. de Lacy-Vawdon C, Livingstone C. Defining the commercial determinants of health: a systematic review. *BMC Public Health*. 2020;20(1):1022. https://doi.org/10.1186/s12889-020-09126-1

Designating Cartels as Terrorist Organizations: The Wrong Path to Addressing the Illicit Fentanyl Crisis

Jack Wolthuis, BA, and Daniel G. Aaron, MD, JD

ABOUT THE AUTHORS

Jack Wolthuis is a student at the S.J. Quinney College of Law, University of Utah, Salt Lake City. Daniel G. Aaron is an associate professor of law at the S.J. Quinney College of Law.

On January 20, 2025, President Donald Trump signed a new executive order related to the ongoing opioid crisis titled "Designating Cartels and Other Organizations as Foreign Terrorist Organizations and Specially Designated Global Terrorists."[1] The order declares a national emergency over opioid-trafficking cartels and states that it is US policy to "ensure the total elimination of these organizations' presence in the United States."[1]

Public health officials have long recognized the importance of synthetic opioids, particularly fentanyl, to the current US opioid crisis.[2] Largely made in Mexico from precursors generated in China, fentanyl has become incorporated into the drug supply chain and contributed to one of the most serious health crises in US history, as well as a precipitous fall in US life expectancy.[3]

Health experts have advanced medical interventions—including expanded health care coverage, syringe exchanges, naloxone, government-sponsored drug treatment programs, and medication for opioid use disorder—as the principal solution to the opioid crisis. Public advocacy successfully pressed for elimination of the "X-waiver"—a bureaucratic hurdle that encumbered buprenorphine prescribing—through the passage of the 2023 Mainstreaming Addiction Treatment Act (part of the Consolidated Appropriations Act, Pub L No. 117-328, Div FF, Title I, §1262 [December 29, 2022]). Health interventions provided through medical care may have contributed to a landmark 14% decrease in overdose deaths in 2023.[4]

Simultaneously, some researchers hypothesize that the Joe Biden presidential administration's pursuit of cartels may offer a partial explanation for the decrease in overdose deaths.[4] Starting in 2021, the Biden administration used a whole of government approach to increase drug interdiction, and some informal evidence suggests that fentanyl is becoming rarer and more expensive.[4] Unfortunately, rigorous evidence-based review of the frequency of fentanyl use, street prices, and the impact of interdiction efforts has faced uphill challenges owing to the lack of transparency from the Drug Enforcement Administration and a shaky federal illicit opioid data infrastructure.[5]

It is curious that, as illicit entities have accumulated responsibility for US overdose deaths, there has not been a robust dialogue among health experts about using the legal system to take public health measures with respect to cartels. Public health experts have generally defended the sprawling litigation against opioid manufacturers,[6] which has gleaned more than $50 billion in settlement funds and has driven systemic change by holding actors accountable for exacerbating US addiction risk.

By contrast, historians and legal scholars have identified the perverse incentives for politicians to coopt "the war on drugs" and its purported public health underpinnings to target disfavored groups, including racial, ethnic, and religious minorities.[7] Drug enforcement has been criticized for contributing to community disruption, mass incarceration, and a high overdose rate in people released from jails and prisons.

During his campaign rallies, President Trump frequently invoked fentanyl and cartels in his rhetoric. In one campaign statement, he asserted that "drug cartels are waging war on America," lamented that "millions and millions of families and people are being destroyed," and warned that "drug kingpins and vicious traffickers will never sleep soundly again" (https://bit.ly/4knsaBu). On several occasions, he suggested that the United States take military action on Mexican soil and promised to push for designating cartels as terrorist groups.

INVOKING THE THREAT OF TERRORISM

The new executive order, signed on inauguration day, is notable for invoking threatening language about national security, health, and safety. It describes the cartels as waging a "campaign of assassination, terror, rape, and brute force" and "flood[ing] the United States with deadly drugs, violent criminals, and vicious gangs."[1] Although then secretary of Health and Human Services Xavier Becerra renewed the opioid public health emergency in September 2023, the new executive order uses national security powers: it requires cabinet officials to make a recommendation about which cartels to designate as terrorist organizations and to prepare to invoke a 1798 law called the Alien Enemies Act (https://bit.ly/3GZRBuA). The Alien Enemies Act, last used in World War II as legal authority to imprison persons of Japanese descent in internment camps, allows the United States to "apprehend," "secure," and "remove" the subjects of a "foreign nation or government" (https://bit.ly/3GZRBuA). When the president makes a declaration under this law, all subjects of the foreign nation may be apprehended regardless of their involvement in illegal conduct and with limited process.

Following this executive order, on February 20, the administration designated eight cartels as foreign terrorist organizations. On March 15, the administration invoked the Alien Enemies Act—even though a cartel is not a "foreign nation or government." It proclaimed that a Venezuela-based organization called Tren de Aragua is "perpetrating, attempting, and threatening an invasion or predatory incursion against the territory of the United States" (https://bit.ly/4mGqEg7) and that Venezuelan citizens older than 14 years in the organization could be "apprehended, restrained, secured, and removed as Alien Enemies" (https://bit.ly/4mGqEg7). By the following day, the White House claimed that officers had "arrested nearly 300 Tren de Aragua terrorists" and deported these "heinous monsters" to El Salvador (https://bit.ly/3YRvlJB). During these events, the American Civil Liberties Union filed a lawsuit alleging that the administration is using the Alien Enemies Act in an unlawful manner, bypassing standard immigration processes, and deporting individuals who are not members of Tren de Aragua. Later that day, a federal judge issued a temporary restraining order prohibiting these deportations; at the time of this writing, legal proceedings are ongoing.

FEAR AND POWER IN DRUG POLICY

There is reason to be concerned that the administration may be hoping to use antiterrorism legal authorities and the health and safety threat of cartels to generate fear and consolidate power. Political scientists have noted that security crises can significantly shift the political landscape. Such crises often lead to a surge in public support for the government, and in times of fear, citizens may be more willing to accept—or even approve of—authoritarian actions.[8] The United States has not seen a crackdown on terrorism since 9/11, which saw the passage of the USA Patriot Act (Pub L No. 107–56 [2001]), a law largely enforced against Muslim Americans that exacerbated Islamophobia in the United States.[9] In the weeks after 9/11, President George W. Bush expanded presidential power, and his approval rating reached 90%. Similarly, as one legal scholar has observed about the current administration, "routine policy matters are now cloaked in the language of imminent threat," with new executive orders invoking crises over energy, food prices, cartels, and border security.[10] Recent reporting suggests that this administration is considering an additional executive order designating fentanyl as a weapon of mass destruction, echoing President Bush's use of this language to marshal popular support.

Politicians throughout history have generally exercised restraint in their exercise of presidential power,[8,10] yet health and safety have at times been misused to frighten the US public and procure support for "law and order" politicians.[7,11] The invocation of the health and safety threat of cartels clashes with executive orders signed by the president that appear to contravene public health—orders that purport to withdraw from the World Health Organization; cut enrollment assistance programs for federal health care plans; rescind a Biden order building toward three affordable drug efforts; and crack down on diversity, equity, and inclusion programs nationwide. According to experts, leaving the World Health Organization risks the US having "far less protection from emerging outbreaks" and "heightened vulnerabilities to a wide range of global health threats."[12(p1029)] True public health is rooted in solidarity, community, and mutual protection and is invoked broadly—not selectively for political gain. Self-serving invocations of health and safety risk misusing the machinery of the state, sowing mistrust in government, and generating health inequity that could last for years to come, especially for vulnerable communities targeted by state power.

Today, misuse of presidential powers to fight cartels would likely disproportionately fall on immigrants living in the United States. Before his 2025 inauguration, the president threatened to use "elite squads of [immigration control], border patrol, and federal law enforcement officers to hunt down, arrest, and deport every last illegal alien gang member until there is not a single one left in this country" (https://bit.ly/4dsOoQD). Yet US citizens, not immigrants, represent 89% of convicted fentanyl traffickers and are 12 times more likely to be convicted of trafficking than noncitizens.[13] Threatening mass deportations could undermine the already precarious health status of immigrants by discouraging them from seeking health care while failing to address real causes of the US opioid crisis.

Anticartel efforts risk replicating the problems with antigang laws, which, in addition to failing to prevent gang involvement, provide law enforcement officers with broad discretion that has enabled disproportionate enforcement in minority communities.[14] Legal scholars have described how labels such as "gang," "immigrant," and "criminal" have acted as a neutralizer of solidarity by fomenting us versus them thinking—in opposition to core tenets in public health.[15,16] Indeed, as these developments in drug and cartel policy have taken place, the administration has simultaneously attempted to undermine US agencies with significant public health impact, including the US Agency for International Development (which Elon Musk called a criminal organization), the US Centers for Disease Control and Prevention, and the US Environmental Protection Agency.

Public health experts must be aware of efforts to misuse the machinery of the state[16] and must support evidence-based policy efforts for persons with addiction. Harm reduction efforts such as medication for opioid use disorder and syringe exchange programs have evidentiary support. We should also consider investing in greater international cooperation, which has historically provided some success in mitigating drug trafficking, and addressing poverty and other social determinants of opioid mortality.[17]

Additionally, efforts to address cartels—already in place during the Biden administration—could be expanded by reallocating resources from low-level enforcement to targeting key actors in the illicit drug supply chain for the most dangerous drugs.[2] Officials should be aware, however, that anticartel efforts could become more difficult if cartels are forced to turn to more potent synthetic opioids. Fentanyl is already exceptionally easy to produce and smuggle; small quantities can yield hundreds of thousands of pills. Nitrazenes, a class of synthetic opioid that can be 40 times more potent than fentanyl, are likely to proliferate in the United States if law enforcement targets only fentanyl. The current administration's application of tariffs to Mexican goods, intended in part to pressure Mexico to curb fentanyl trafficking, is liable to fall into this trap. To push the illicit drug supply in a safer direction, law enforcement could pair anticartel efforts with clear communication to cartels about safer drugs that will be deprioritized for enforcement.

THE FUTURE OF DRUG POLICY

The international opioid crisis is complex and multifactorial. In the long term, we must shift from fear-based policymaking to international health equity. Although pursuing cartels has some merit, the current administration's approach appears to be aimed not at securing health and safety but at drawing political support through social stratification as it dismantles US domestic and international public health infrastructure. Claiming foreign citizens in the United States are members of criminal organizations eligible for deportation, stirring up fears of terrorism, and withdrawing from the World Health Organization will only hamper the long-term cooperation needed to address the opioid crisis. AJPH

CORRESPONDENCE

Correspondence should be sent to Daniel G. Aaron, 383 South University St, Salt Lake City, UT 84112 (e-mail: Daniel.Aaron@law.utah.edu). Reprints can be ordered at https://www.ajph.org by clicking the "Reprints" link.

PUBLICATION INFORMATION

Full Citation: Wolthuis J, Aaron DG. Designating cartels as terrorist organizations: the wrong path to addressing the illicit fentanyl crisis. *Am J Public Health*. 2025;115(8):1211–1214.

Acceptance Date: March 31, 2025.

DOI: https://doi.org/10.2105/AJPH.2025.308142

ORCID iDs:

Jack Wolthuis https://orcid.org/0009-0008-4375-4407

Daniel G. Aaron https://orcid.org/0000-0003-4490-7504

CONTRIBUTORS

The authors contributed equally to this work.

ACKNOWLEDGMENTS

We are grateful to Kif Augustine-Adams, Ivan Meitus chair and professor of law at the Brigham Young University School of Law; Kelly Gillespie, professor of law at the Saint Louis University School of Law; and Beau Kilmer, codirector of the RAND Drug Policy Research Center, for their comments on this article.

CONFLICTS OF INTEREST

The authors have no conflicts of interest to disclose.

REFERENCES

1. White House. Designating cartels and other organizations as foreign terrorist organizations and specially designated global terrorists. January 20, 2025. Available at: https://www.whitehouse.gov/presidential-actions/2025/01/designating-cartels-and-other-organizations-as-foreign-terrorist-organizations-and-specially-designated-global-terrorists. Accessed February 10, 2025.

2. Frank RG, Pollack HA. Addressing the fentanyl threat to public health. *N Engl J Med.* 2017;376(7):605–607. https://doi.org/10.1056/NEJMp1615145
3. Aaron DG. Public health in the opioid litigation. *Loy U Chi Law J.* 2021;53:11–87.
4. Hoffman J, Weiland N. What's behind the remarkable drop in US overdose deaths. *New York Times.* November 21, 2024. Available at: https://www.nytimes.com/2024/11/21/health/overdose-deaths-decline-drug-supply.html. Accessed December 18, 2024.
5. Pardo B, Kilmer B. Giving drug policy decision-makers the data they need. June 24, 2022. Available at: https://www.rand.org/pubs/testimonies/CTA2133-1.html. Accessed January 22, 2025.
6. Aaron DG. Opioid accountability. *Tenn Law Rev.* 2022;89:611–678. https://doi.org/10.2139/ssrn.3854060
7. Oliva J, El-Sabawi T. The "new" drug war. *Va Law Rev.* 2024;110:1103–1168. https://doi.org/10.2139/ssrn.4529699
8. Levitsky S, Ziblatt D. *How Democracies Die.* New York, NY: Crown; 2018.
9. Beydoun KA. Islamophobia: toward a legal definition and framework. *Colum Law Rev.* 2016;116:108–125.
10. Johnson BJ. Normalizing emergencies. *Yale J Regul.* February 6, 2025. Available at: https://www.yalejreg.com/nc/normalizing-emergencies-by-brandon-j-johnson. Accessed February 7, 2025.
11. Aaron DG, Francis LP. Health law and bigotry distractions. *J Law Med Ethics.* 2024;52(2):350–363. https://doi.org/10.1017/jme.2024.92
12. Gostin LO, Meier BM, Pace L. A world without WHO—a crossroads for US global health leadership. *JAMA.* 2025;333(12):1028–1029. https://doi.org/10.1001/jama.2024.28827
13. Bier DJ. US citizens were 89% of convicted fentanyl traffickers in 2022. August 23, 2023. Available at: https://www.cato.org/blog/us-citizens-were-89-convicted-fentanyl-traffickers-2022. Accessed December 11, 2024.
14. Hayat FN. Abolish gang statutes with the power of the Thirteenth Amendment: reparations for the people. *UCLA Law Rev.* 2023;70:1120–1205.
15. Canon D. *Pleading Out: How Plea Bargaining Creates a Permanent Criminal Class.* New York, NY: Basic Books; 2022.
16. Parmet WE. Immigration law as a social determinant of health. *Temple Law Rev.* 2020;92(4):931–952.
17. Dasgupta N, Beletsky L, Ciccarone D. Opioid crisis: no easy fix to its social and economic determinants. *Am J Public Health.* 2018;108(2):182–186. https://doi.org/10.2105/AJPH.2017.304187

The Power of Community in Promoting Water Safety in Rural Madagascar

Sydney Brown

ABOUT THE AUTHOR

The author is with the College of Public Health, University of South Florida, Tampa.

Entering the modest home of Madame Charlotte, an elderly Malagasy woman from Toamasina, Madagascar, I was greeted by the familiar scent of sea air mixed with the warmth of sun-soaked earth after weeks of rain. I was ready for my first participant interview, with questions in hand; however, the conversation quickly took a pleasantly unexpected turn. Instead of diving into the prepared list of queries, we began to chat about home décor—something in which neither of us anticipated finding common ground. Her eyes lit up as she highlighted various handmade items within her home, each piece telling a story of its own. I shared how I also valued the small details that made a house feel like a home. We laughed and exchanged stories about our origins: two women from different worlds, connected by a shared appreciation for life's intricacies.

Then she brought up a name from last year's project—a young woman from my team. "How is she doing?" she asked with genuine interest. Momentarily taken aback, I realized it had been nearly a year since that brief interaction, yet Madame Charlotte remembered her so clearly. This moment illuminated the profound significance of building connections and community.

Community building formed the cornerstone of our three-year project aimed at reducing biofilm growth in water storage containers in rural eastern coastal Madagascar. Biofilm, a slimy layer of bacteria and other microorganisms that forms on surfaces in contact with water, poses significant health risks by contaminating stored water and making it unsafe for consumption. This issue is particularly critical in regions with limited access to clean water, where such contamination can lead to waterborne diseases and exacerbate existing public health challenges. From the beginning, we worked closely with local partners, stakeholders, and community members. We hired local staff and trained students in qualitative inquiry and community-based research to help ensure that our efforts were both scientifically valid and sound and culturally relevant. We also collaborated with public health social marketers and environmental engineers to minimize the pitfalls of parachute science.

When I transitioned in my interview with Madame Charlotte to the questionnaire on water cleanliness, I anticipated the usual brief responses. Instead, she elaborated extensively on her water use, describing her daily routine and the challenges of ensuring clean water for her family. She pointed out nuances I had not considered—how scrubbing heavy containers left her with aching joints and how she often worried that younger family members might not continue the laborious task when she could no longer do it herself. These detailed insights were invaluable, transforming what I had expected to be a routine interview into a conversation rooted in trust and mutual respect.

This trust was not incidental; it was the result of years of participant observation in which we immersed ourselves in the community's daily lives. We washed dishes, collected water, and participated in everyday routines, building rapport and demonstrating our commitment to understanding their world. Conversations with local friends and coworkers provided vital insights into water use and safety practices and the broader cultural context in which these practices were embedded. Trust, we learned, is the cornerstone of effective public health interventions. Without it, even the most carefully designed strategies can fail to resonate with the people they aim to help.

As Madame Charlotte and I concluded the interview, she showed me her latest creation—handcrafted pillows she had made herself. Each one was more intricate than the last, showcasing her skill and creativity. She handed one to me, encouraging me to feel the fabric's softness and observe the careful stitching. Seeing the pride in her eyes as she shared this part of herself, I fully grasped the depth of our connection. We were no longer strangers from different countries but, rather, newly bonded women setting out together on a journey toward improved health and connection.

Our collaboration with a well-established local nonprofit organization in Madagascar was foundational to the project's success. This organization was deeply embedded within the community and served as a bridge for developing trust and sensitivity between our team

AJPH August 2025, Vol. 115, No. 8

and the residents. Rather than imposing solutions, we actively worked to dismantle the hierarchical power dynamics that often characterize such projects. This meant prioritizing local leadership in every stage of the intervention, from designing the cleaning protocol to training local staff and students. For example, we appointed a local school teacher, renowned for her ability to connect with diverse groups, as the lead communications specialist. She spearheaded community meetings, facilitated feedback sessions, and helped adapt messaging strategies to align with local cultural norms and languages, ensuring the initiative's reach and resonance.

By ensuring that decision-making authority rested within the community, we sought to counteract the paternalistic tendencies often rooted in postcolonial development practices. This approach reinforced a sense of ownership among community members, enabling them to see themselves not as passive recipients of aid but as architects of their own health solutions. In a country grappling with the enduring legacies of colonialism, this shift in power dynamics was more than symbolic; it was a necessary step toward fostering self-reliance and sustainability. The project's importance resides not only in its tangible outcomes—reduced biofilm growth and improved water safety—but also in its role as a model for equitable, community-driven public health interventions that honor the agency and expertise of local populations.

This experience highlighted the transformative power of radical hope—hope that is active, rooted in trust, and nurtured through creativity and community engagement. We had been welcomed into this community, not as outsiders collecting data but as individuals genuinely invested in the community's well-being. Witnessing hope evolve into actionable change is why I joined the public health workforce. Standing in Charlotte's well-decorated home, I knew we were on the right path.

The principles applied in this project offer critical lessons for public health students and professionals. To engage communities effectively, it is essential to prioritize trust building and local partnerships. This requires moving beyond top-down approaches and embracing strategies that involve listening, learning, and collaborating with those most affected by public health challenges. For me, this process underscored the importance of cocreation and cultural resonance in public health work. It deepened my understanding of the complexities of community engagement and solidified my commitment to centering equity and sustainability in future projects. I know I help create a healthier, more equitable future, one that honors the agency of those we aim to serve, by reimagining public health as a collaborative, community-driven endeavor. AJPH

CORRESPONDENCE

Correspondence should be sent to Sydney Brown, 3400 E Fletcher Ave, Tampa, FL 33613 (e-mail: sydneylaurenbrown@usf.edu). Reprints can be ordered at https://www.ajph.org by clicking the "Reprints" link.

PUBLICATION INFORMATION

Full Citation: Brown S. The power of community in promoting water safety in rural Madagascar. *Am J Public Health.* 2025;115(8):1215–1216.

Acceptance Date: December 8, 2024.

DOI: https://doi.org/10.2105/AJPH.2024.307974

ORCID iD:
Sydney Brown https://orcid.org/0009-0008-7941-8915

ACKNOWLEDGMENTS

This material is based on work supported by the National Science Foundation (NSF) through grant 2107114.

I express my heartfelt gratitude to my incredible team, who have truly become like family to me. Your unwavering support, camaraderie, and shared passion have made this journey both meaningful and inspiring.

A special thank you to my principal investigators, particularly Mahmooda Pasha, for your continued guidance, mentorship, and encouragement. Your dedication and belief in my potential have been invaluable, and I am deeply grateful for the opportunities and knowledge you have shared with me.

Note. Any opinions, findings, conclusions, or recommendations expressed in this editorial are those of the author and do not necessarily reflect the views of NSF.

CONFLICTS OF INTEREST

The author declares no conflicts of interest.

Tackling Wicked Problems: The Power of Community Among the Unhoused

Kelly Marnfeldt, Louise Xie, and Angela Zhang

ABOUT THE AUTHORS

Kelly Marnfeldt is with the Leonard Davis School of Gerontology, University of Southern California, Los Angeles. Louise Xie is with the Annenberg School for Communication and Journalism, University of Southern California, Los Angeles. Angela Zhang is with the Department of Population and Public Health Sciences, Keck School of Medicine, Los Angeles, and the Spatial Sciences Institute, Dornsife College of Letters, Arts, and Sciences, University of Southern California, Los Angeles.

> Every human being has the right to safe, clean, affordable, and accessible water adequate for human consumption, cooking, and sanitary purposes.[1]
>
> (California State Legislature, 2012)

> We have been fighting for drinking water for 20 years. People need to have an image of that fight. It's not enough to highlight water justice. The state is in violation of its own law, and we're still at "pilot programs."
>
> (Los Angeles Community Action Network member)

In September 2012, California became the first state to recognize access to water as a human right, affirming that all residents are entitled to safe, clean, and accessible water.[1] Thirteen years after the passage of this bill, the unhoused community in Skid Row, Los Angeles, continues to fight for water justice.

Skid Row covers 50 blocks in Los Angeles and is home to one of the highest concentrations of unhoused people in the city.[2] Many Skid Row residents have to walk two to three large blocks just to access clean drinking water. For the unhoused, there is virtually no access to water for toileting, bathing, cooking, washing clothes, or cleaning, and access to hot water does not exist. The contrast between the legal promise and the reality could not be more stark, making lack of access to safe, adequate water for hygiene and sanitation an urgent health crisis for the residents of Skid Row and an ever-escalating "wicked problem."[3]

Traditional public health approaches are insufficient to solve today's complex challenges, necessitating more participatory approaches.[4–6] Unlike top-down approaches focusing on the dissemination of scientific expertise, participatory approaches are inherently collaborative. They deepen our understanding of existing problems and underlying causes, identify provisional solutions agreeable to all parties, and facilitate the implementation of these solutions.[6] Nowhere is the failure of traditional approaches to health inequities more evident than in Skid Row.

Along with five other students, we recently had the opportunity to collaborate on a community-engaged project with the Los Angeles Community Action Network (LA CAN), a nonprofit dedicated to serving and empowering Skid Row residents through a long-standing partnership with a faculty member.

Our work in Skid Row was informed by and further advances the Burke et al. social ecological model.[7] The political, racial, and socioeconomic challenges in Skid Row are "co-constitutive," simultaneously shaping and being shaped by individual and collective experiences. Often operating "outside conscious awareness," these dynamics have a profound impact on community health.[7] Water justice, therefore, is rooted in residents' lived experiences and Skid Row's historic and political landscape.

THE PROCESS

To ensure that our research responded to and accurately depicted the problem of water injustice in Skid Row, we deployed a community-based participatory research (CBPR) approach in partnership with LA CAN. CBPR aims to catalyze social change and improve community health equity by involving community members and researchers in all phases of research as collaborators.[8]

Our collaboration with LA CAN began with a tour through Skid Row. Along the way, staff pointed out the limited spaces where community members take showers, wash their hands, and refill water. Because the unhoused population is often depicted as a monolith, this initial walkthrough was crucial for us to understand the diversity of lived experiences in Skid Row.

The tour established the foundation for our collaboration as co-researchers.

AJPH August 2025, Vol. 115, No. 8

LA CAN staff shared stories of residents' creativity and ingenuity in meeting their water needs, such as using makeshift tools to open fire hydrants, transporting large water containers with walkers or strollers, collecting rainwater with plastic sheets, and purifying water through solar still techniques.

The conversations with the Skid Row community during our walking tour highlighted insecurity related to water for hygiene and sanitation and inspired the codesign of four "community data wrangling" water workshops. With LA CAN, we created data visualizations of residents' lived experiences that became a blueprint for community-engaged research. This process underscored that collaboration and capacity building are measures of progress in creating actionable strategies for change.

Recognizing that water injustice would not be solved overnight, we viewed our work as a stepping stone toward water justice. Our workshops leveraged community insights and expertise to analyze water access in Skid Row, capturing lived experiences through murals, R Studio–generated maps, water diaries, and photovoice journals.

RETHINKING EXPERTISE

Early on, it became clear that an understanding of water injustice was embedded in the lived experience of our community partners. For example, we initially focused on the utilitarian uses of water (e.g., drinking, cleaning, washing). However, after our first meeting with community members, we learned that a core value was the therapeutic aspect of hot water, not only for cleaning and bathing but also for reflection and restoration. Without community input, we would have overlooked the significance of the lack of hot water. Research that draws on the insights of those with lived experience ensures that research questions are specific and relevant, that the methods used are appropriate for the population, and that the results can be translated into meaningful action.

These community workshops were an important milestone in relationship building and helped us develop a shared understanding of the research, the tools required, and the language needed to make it meaningful to those affected. They also challenged us to envision creative, public-facing outcomes not foreseen in traditional approaches. Practically, the workshops served as a curriculum that could be used to document and investigate other issues for broader change identified by staff and community members, including food and housing insecurity.

Our planning meetings with LA CAN were most fruitful when we were asked to envision a world where all of our water needs are met rather than limiting ourselves to a narrow research question. We built trust by establishing a shared vision of the future and elevating the community's priorities. Our experiences align with CBPR principles, according to which translational outcomes are best achieved by engaging partners in defining research aims rather than imposing researcher-defined questions.[9,10]

When working with community members, many of whom are engaged with or actively involved in the process of changing the deleterious conditions they confront daily, novel questions emerge and competing priorities are often present. Yet, the flexible and dynamic process required to build community is what made the work sustainable and relevant. Among the students involved, developing relationships and sharing knowledge with community partners fostered hope for change and provided a foundation for continued collaboration with our new partners as this project came to a close. As one workshop participant shared, "Collaborations [are about] sharing knowledge. . .an exchange of expertise, exchange the skills we all have; [it's] not about extracting, it's about teaching each other."

PROPOSING SOLUTIONS

Our collaboration with LA CAN has highlighted proximate steps to incentivize greater community building in public health. First, public health researchers should recognize that CBPR is rigorous and particularly powerful when engaging underserved populations. As previous literature and our experiences have shown, CBPR specifically addresses the local relevance of public health problems.[9]

Second, public health researchers need to view community building as a prerequisite to meaningful collaboration and building hope. Effective community building is an iterative process of building trust with diverse partners, with each interaction serving as an opportunity for deeper engagement. Furthermore, as evidenced by our collaboration, community building across sectors increases the mutual understanding and shared vision required to address wicked problems that evade resolution through traditional, siloed approaches.

Finally, if community building is to be valued in public health research, students need support for the time commitment and best practices required. Our experience with LA CAN was enabled by a multidisciplinary university course and a long-standing partnership between our professor and LA CAN. Without these structural components, students seldom have the opportunity to engage with local communities in a rigorous and equitable manner. We hope that community-focused courses grounded in participatory research become a standard offering accessible to all students rather than a rare privilege. At the conclusion of this class, several students continued to partner and volunteer with LA CAN on new projects, a testament to the lasting impact of this collaboration.

CONCLUSION

As with many other issues in Skid Row, water injustice is complex and co-constitutive, actively shaping and shaped by residents' individual and collective experiences. Thus, as researchers, we can sustainably address the ever-shifting reality of social problems only through active dialogue with community members.

Our project with LA CAN has greatly affected us professionally and personally. Guided by the local community, we witnessed the living embodiment of the gap in public health scholarship in which success is measured through data extraction for publication, thus neglecting the deeper engagement necessary for systemic change. Although data are essential, so is the lived experience behind the numbers. Counting the number of water bottles distributed or meals served in Skid Row addresses the emergency but ignores the system. Stories must be part of the data, specifically stories of the lived experience of those who call Skid Row home. They are the experts on what is needed and what it means to achieve water justice in their community. Community building is essential for creating sustainable, hopeful solutions in public health. AJPH

CORRESPONDENCE

Correspondence should be sent to Angela Zhang, Spatial Sciences Institute, University of Southern California, 3616 Trousdale Pkwy, AHF B55, Los Angeles, CA 90089 (e-mail: awzhang@usc.edu). Reprints can be ordered at https://www.ajph.org by clicking the "Reprints" link.

PUBLICATION INFORMATION

Full Citation: Marnfeldt K, Xie L, Zhang A. Tackling wicked problems: the power of community among the unhoused. *Am J Public Health*. 2025;115(8):1217–1219.

Acceptance Date: December 22, 2024.

DOI: https://doi.org/10.2105/AJPH.2025.308007

ORCID iDs:

Kelly Marnfeldt https://orcid.org/0000-0003-3047-8016

Louise Xie https://orcid.org/0009-0000-0811-2873

Angela Zhang https://orcid.org/0000-0001-5172-6192

CONTRIBUTORS

The authors contributed equally to the ideation, writing, and editing of this article.

ACKNOWLEDGMENTS

Funding for the work described in this article was provided by a University of Southern California Generative Artificial Intelligence research grant; a University of Southern California Visions and Voices, Arts in Action grant; and a University of Southern California Equity Research Institute community-engaged research grant.

We express our gratitude to the Los Angeles Community Action Network, particularly Pete White, Todd Cunningham, and our team of co-researchers, whose collaboration, dedication, and innovative spirit made this research possible. Their commitment to empowering housed and unhoused people in the Skid Row community and willingness to share their expertise were invaluable in shaping our experience. We also thank François Bar, whose guidance and support was instrumental in the development of this research.

CONFLICTS OF INTEREST

The authors declare that they have no conflicts of interest to disclose regarding this research.

REFERENCES

1. California State Legislature. California Assembly Bill No. 685, Chapter 524. Available at: http://www.leginfo.ca.gov/pub/11-12/bill/asm/ab_0651-0700/ab_685_bill_20120925_chaptered.pdf. Accessed January 14, 2025.
2. Ward JM, Garvey R, Hunter SB. Recent trends among the unsheltered in three Los Angeles neighborhoods. Available at: https://www.rand.org/content/dam/rand/pubs/research_reports/RRA1800/RRA1890-2/RAND_RRA1890-2.pdf. Accessed January 14, 2025.
3. Rittel HWJ, Webber MM. Dilemmas in a general theory of planning. *Policy Sci*. 1973;4(2):155–169. https://doi.org/10.1007/BF01405730
4. Fischer F. Citizen participation and the democratization of policy expertise: from theoretical inquiry to practical cases. *Policy Sci*. 1993;26(3):165–187. https://doi.org/10.1007/BF00999715
5. Lasker RD, Weiss ES. Broadening participation in community problem solving: a multidisciplinary model to support collaborative practice and research. *J Urban Health*. 2003;80(1):14–47. https://doi.org/10.1093/jurban/jtg014
6. Head BW, Alford J. Wicked problems: implications for public policy and management. *Adm Soc*. 2015;47(6):711–739. https://doi.org/10.1177/0095399713481601
7. Burke NJ, Joseph G, Pasick RJ, Barker JC. Theorizing social context: rethinking behavioral theory. *Health Educ Behav*. 2009;36(suppl 5):55S–70S. https://doi.org/10.1177/1090198109335338
8. Israel BA, Schulz AJ, Parker EA, Becker AB. Review of community-based research: assessing partnership approaches to improve public health. *Annu Rev Public Health*. 1998;19:173–202. https://doi.org/10.1146/annurev.publhealth.19.1.173
9. Israel BA, Eng E, Schulz AJ, Parker EA. *Methods in Community-Based Participatory Research for Health*. 2nd ed. Jossey-Bass; 2005.
10. Unertl KM, Schaefbauer CL, Campbell TR, et al. Integrating community-based participatory research and informatics approaches to improve the engagement and health of underserved populations. *J Am Med Inform Assoc*. 2016;23(1):60–73. https://doi.org/10.1093/jamia/ocv094

The Escalating War on Immigrants Is a Public Health Crisis

Luisa N. Borrell, DDS, PhD, and Farzana Kapadia, PhD, MPH

ABOUT THE AUTHORS

Luisa N. Borrell is with the Graduate School of Public Health & Health Policy, The City University of New York, New York, and the Department of Surgery, Medical and Social Sciences, Universidad de Alcalá, Alcalá de Henares, Madrid, Spain, and is an associate editor of AJPH. *Farzana Kapadia is with the School of Global Public Health, New York University, New York, and is an associate editor of* AJPH.

AJPH August 2025, Vol. 115, No. 8

Between 2017 and 2021, the presidential administration of Donald Trump implemented a range of exclusionary policies and tactics to restrict immigration and limit immigrant rights.[1,2] These policies and practices included declaring an emergency at US borders, drastically reducing and temporarily suspending refugee admission, trying to end birthright citizenship, restricting the practice of releasing immigrants held in detention while awaiting immigration proceedings, preventing asylum seekers from entering the United States, increasing scrutiny of work permits, targeting sanctuary cities, denying public benefits to immigrants, and expanding detentions and deportations.

At the very beginning of his second term, on January 20, 2025, Trump issued 10 executive orders that either reinstated immigration policies from his first term or introduced new exclusionary measures.[3] The latest round of aggressively harmful policies includes seeking to end birthright citizenship, ending humanitarian programs, and limiting or ending funding for nongovernmental organizations that provide support to immigrants. In this editorial, we highlight specific economic and political actions whose only purpose is to restrict or prevent immigrants from accessing federal programs and health care services and call on the public health community to monitor and report on how these actions affect the health and well-being of immigrant communities.

PROTECTING THE HEALTH OF IMMIGRANTS

Aggressive immigration enforcement strategies will continue to exacerbate poor physical and mental health outcomes among immigrants and their families by increasing and perpetuating fear, discrimination, limited access to health care services,[4] and family separation.[5] Strategies to protect the health and well-being of immigrants must include upstream interventions that address entrenched power imbalances by improving access to public benefits that enable immigrants to live safe, healthy, and productive lives.

First, policies expanding the types of services provided in federally qualified health centers to provide health care access to immigrants, particularly undocumented immigrants, are needed.[6] Similarly, immigration policies that continue to legitimize excluding immigrants from access to legal employment, education, and housing must be rescinded or scaled back, given their direct relationship to increasing health inequities in immigrant populations. Additionally, facilitating more pathways, rather than curtailing legitimate pathways, to attain legal status for immigrants residing in the United States is warranted to prevent family separation and disruption.

Second, current media discourse and misinformation about immigrants is perpetuating fear and stigmatization of this population, leading to poor mental health.[7] Changing such discourses and narratives will improve mental health and facilitate the integration of immigrants into their communities. For example, inflammatory rhetoric and public misconceptions about immigration should be countered through evidence-based policies and public education efforts.[8] Such efforts are increasingly necessary to reduce the dehumanizing narratives about recent immigrants in the public discourse[9] and contribute to creating a more supportive environment for immigrants and, ultimately, affect health outcomes.

Finally, immigrant communities tend to informally engage in collective strategies to help navigate the effects of immigration policies. These strategies should be identified and fostered through partnerships with nonprofit organizations that advocate for immigrant populations and provide them with the information they need to navigate the system.[10] Protecting immigrant health from the devastating policies being enacted under the second Trump administration will require multilayered and multifaceted approaches that include protecting access to health care, housing, food, education, and employment—key social determinants of health. In addition, campaigns to reverse and reduce fear and stigmatization and strengthen community-based initiatives and advocacy to empower immigrant communities are warranted.

CHARTING A RESEARCH AND POLICY AGENDA

To understand how these exclusionary policies affect the health and well-being of immigrants, their families, and their communities, we expect submissions to *AJPH* that examine how immigration policies—such as the proposed changes to the public charge rule, limiting access to health insurance coverage under the Affordable Care Act for Deferred Action for Childhood Arrivals recipients, preventing access to federally funded housing, and limiting access to Supplemental Nutrition Assistance Program benefits—will affect health outcomes. Furthermore, based on this information and knowledge, we call for evidence-based policy recommendations and potential interventions to reduce health inequities among immigrant populations, challenge misconceptions about immigration, promote evidence-based discourse, and explore community-based initiatives and partnerships to support immigrant populations. AJPH

CORRESPONDENCE

Correspondence should be sent to Luisa N. Borrell, DDS, PhD, Department of Epidemiology & Biostatistics, Graduate School of Public Health & Health Policy, The City University of New York, 55 West 125th St, Room 530, New York, NY 10027 (e-mail: Luisa.Borrell@sph.cuny.edu).

PUBLICATION INFORMATION

Full Citation: Borrell LN, Kapadia F. The escalating war on immigrants is a public health crisis. *Am J Public Health*. 2025;115(8):1220–1221.

Acceptance Date: April 13, 2025.

DOI: https://doi.org/10.2105/AJPH.2025.308158

ORCID iDs:
Luisa N. Borrell https://orcid.org/0000-0002-0560-4853

Farzana Kapadia https://orcid.org/0000-0003-3459-767X

CONTRIBUTORS

The authors contributed equally to this editorial.

CONFLICTS OF INTEREST

The authors have no conflicts of interest to declare.

REFERENCES

1. Friedman AS, Venkataramani AS. Chilling effects: US immigration enforcement and health care seeking among Hispanic adults. *Health Aff (Millwood)*. 2021;40(7):1056–1065. https://doi.org/10.1377/hlthaff.2020.02356
2. Miller DP, John RS, Yao M, Morris M. The 2016 presidential election, the public charge rule, and food and nutrition assistance among immigrant households. *Am J Public Health*. 2022;112(12):1738–1746. https://doi.org/10.2105/AJPH.2022.307011
3. Mayer-Brown. Trump 2.0: executive order tracker. 2025. Available at: https://www.mayerbrown.com/en/insights/resource-centers/washington-update/trump-2-executive-order-tracker. Accessed March 8, 2025.
4. Janevic T, Birnie L, Belfon K, et al. Immigrant inequities in uninsurance and postpartum Medicaid extension: a quasi-experimental study in New York City, 2016–2021. *Am J Public Health*. 2025;115(5):732–735. https://doi.org/10.2105/AJPH.2024.307968
5. Young MDT, Sudhinaraset M, Tafolla S, Nakphong MK, Yan Y, Kietzman KG. The "disproportionate costs" of immigrant policy on the health of Latinx and Asian immigrants. *Soc Sci Med*. 2024;353:117034. https://doi.org/10.1016/j.socscimed.2024.117034
6. Parker E, Schut RA, Boen C. The promise and limits of inclusive public policy: federal safety net clinics and immigrant access to health care in the US. *Soc Forces*. 2024;103(3):992–1017. https://doi.org/10.1093/sf/soae111
7. Espinoza-Kulick M, Espinoza-Kulick A, González E, Takahashi J. Immigration policy is health policy: news media effects on health disparities for Latinx immigrant and Indigenous groups. *Health Promot Pract*. 2023;24(5):818–827. https://doi.org/10.1177/15248399221150816
8. Boateng FD, Pryce DK, Chenane JL. I may be an immigrant, but I am not a criminal: examining the association between the presence of immigrants and crime rates in Europe. *Int Migr Integr*. 2021;22:1105–1124. https://doi.org/10.1007/s12134-020-00790-1
9. Gonçalves I. Promoting hate speech by dehumanizing metaphors of immigration. *Journalism Pract*. 2023;18(2):265–282. https://doi.org/10.1080/17512786.2023.2212661
10. LeBrón AMW, Schulz AJ, Gamboa C, Reyes Á, Viruell-Fuentes EA, Israel BA. Mexican-origin women's individual and collective strategies to access and share health-promoting resources in the context of exclusionary immigration and immigrant policies. *BMC Public Health*. 2024;24(1):1757. https://doi.org/10.1186/s12889-024-19204-3a

Time Scarcity, Health Behaviors, and Unconditional Cash in Los Angeles

Amy Castro, PhD, Mira Philips, MSc, Isabelle Kim, MSW, Stacia West, PhD, and Bo-Kyung Elizabeth Kim, PhD

Unconditional cash interventions, such as guaranteed income, are a proposed solution for mediating the adverse health outcomes associated with financial scarcity. To test this, the City of Los Angeles, California, conducted a mixed-methods, randomized controlled trial in which they gave 3202 people $1000 with no strings attached for 12 months in 2022. Although the quantitative findings demonstrated mixed health effects, the qualitative findings highlighted how recipients viewed their well-being as an insurance policy against scarcity and reallocated time to preventive health behaviors when receiving a guaranteed income. (*Am J Public Health*. 2025;115(8):1222–1225. https://doi.org/10.2105/AJPH.2025.308125)

AJPH August 2025, Vol. 115, No. 8

Differences in socioeconomic status contribute to health disparities, with people in poverty experiencing worse health than those with higher incomes.[1–3] Poverty is associated with increased morbidity, diminished quality of life, food insecurity,[1–4] and time scarcity.[5,6] Time is an important resource for health promotion,[5,6] and time scarcity prevents healthy behaviors and is linked to negative health outcomes.[5] Although time scarcity causes similar effects among most individuals, those with higher incomes are more likely to be able to relieve their time deficit by paying for such things as stress reduction, childcare, and household help.[5] The intersection of time scarcity and financial scarcity amplifies negative health outcomes among the most disadvantaged, particularly those lacking paid leave and strong work benefits.[7]

STUDY OBJECTIVE

Unconditional cash transfers, such as guaranteed income, are increasingly being tested in the United States as a remedy for alleviating hardship and its associated health stressors. Guaranteed income payments are a fixed amount of recurring cash payments that are predictable, contain no restrictions on how recipients use the funds, and are associated with a range of positive health outcomes.[1] Conditional cash payments are more commonly tested in low- and middle-income countries and are associated with some positive health outcomes and increased use of preventive health services. They require behavioral compliance and periodic means testing, and they often include restrictions on how cash can be spent. In the United States, conditional cash payments can be associated with administrative burdens and stigma, which can deter eligible recipients. By contrast, guaranteed income is perceived as less stigmatizing, more efficient, and more likely to engender self-determination.[8,9]

A randomized controlled trial (RCT) of guaranteed income in Stockton, California, provides causal evidence of positive health outcomes for recipients, including lower mental distress, more energy, and improved physical functioning.[10] The recipients reported reductions in time scarcity, but it is not clear from this study how this affected health behaviors. We built on that inquiry through a substrand of a mixed-methods RCT of guaranteed income.

RESEARCH QUESTION

In January 2022, the City of Los Angeles began providing 3202 treatment group participants with a monthly guaranteed income of $1000 for 12 months. This substrand of the larger RCT asked to what degree guaranteed income alleviates time scarcity and alters health behaviors.

PARTICIPANTS, SAMPLE, GEOGRAPHIC LOCATION, SETTING, AND YEAR OF STUDY

The RCT consisted of 3202 individuals in the treatment group and 4992 in the control group. Eligibility criteria included Los Angeles residency, being aged 18 years or older, being pregnant or having at least one dependent child (younger than 18 years or a student younger than 24 years), and having an income at or below the federal poverty level. The mean annual income was $14 273 for the treatment group and $14 476 for the control group, indicating that the majority were living in deep poverty. The qualitative sample (n = 34) mirrored the larger RCT. Interviewees were predominantly women in their 30s, with six reporting being married. The majority of participants identified as Hispanic (n = 17), seven identified as Black, and six identified as non-Hispanic White. We asked the single-item self-rated screener, "In general, would you say that your health is excellent, very good, good, fair, or poor?" and provided probes to elicit rationale. Interviewees described a range of diagnosed health conditions predating the experiment, including hypertension (7), diabetes (6), asthma (4), anxiety (7), depression (4), posttraumatic stress disorder (4), back or neck injury (5), and high-risk pregnancy (4). Participants could select multiple responses. Complete RCT demographics are provided in the appendix (available as a supplement to the online version of this article at http://www.ajph.org).

METHODS

Consistent with a parallel mixed-methods design,[11] in an analogous substrand, we explored health behaviors. For recruitment, we relied on convenience sampling through a notification distributed via the Qualtrics survey platform (Qualtrics, Provo, UT). We performed semistructured interviews lasting 1.5 to 2.5 hours at the midpoint of disbursements and four months after the final payment. We recorded and professionally transcribed all interviews, during which participants used aliases. We compensated participants for their time with a $50 gift card. Participants chose their own interview location. We recruited 35 recipients to participate in round 1 interviews; 1 participant canceled, yielding 34 participants. We recruited the same participants for round 2, with 25 responding and 3 canceling, leaving us with 22 respondents. Interview prompts focused on health behaviors, finances, decision-making, well-being trajectories, and parenting. We performed all coding in Dedoose (SocioCultural Research Consultants, Redondo Beach, CA) without the use of artificial intelligence. Coding involved a thematic analysis approach at the semantic level,[12,13] and we used grounded theory methods for latent and theoretical coding. Full details are provided in the preanalysis plan found in the appendix.

KEY FINDINGS

The primary RCT contained a range of well-being outcomes that are outside the scope of this inquiry and that indicated few statistically significant changes attributable to the guaranteed income. By contrast, the qualitative substrand provided a better picture of health behaviors and stressors that the quantitative data masked. Of those interviewed, 2 rated their health as excellent, 3 as very good, 9 as good, 12 as fair, and 4 as poor; 2 declined to answer. Participants attributed their ratings to the burden of unpaid care work, along with the lack of time and material resources to proactively manage their health. More importantly, their responses indicated a degree of health literacy, including the ability to access and understand information pertinent for health decision-making; however, without guaranteed income, they were unable to act on the information. Except for two, all interviewees reported that they had health insurance and a health care provider but that lack of child care in conjunction with unpredictable or inflexible work hours and severe financial hardship created resource and time barriers to accessing care.

The data from this study highlight how participants viewed their bodies as insurance policies against market risks and indicate that the participants were aware that they were at risk for multiple conditions connected to social determinants of health. Recipients reacted to this risk with a stepwise approach to health behaviors that overlapped with the alleviation of time scarcity and having more control over their time. For example, Nelli (White, 30s) credited the guaranteed income for enabling her to focus enough to "remember to take my medicine every day," and Michelle (Hispanic, 20s) attributed her mindset shift directly to the guaranteed income, saying:

> I'm able to look at things in a more positive way just because I have control of my time. . . . I have learned to kind of manage my eating habits, my exercise habits, a little better than I have before. I've gotten into this mentality that however I'm feeling, I should still be able to accomplish one to two tasks a day.

These changes unfolded along a distinct time line, with participants explicitly situating their health behaviors and goals in the time frame of the 12-month intervention. In the first six months, participants focused on using the guaranteed income to relieve material hardship and offset acute financial stress in their networks. Participants reported that, as material hardship lessened, they had more time between months 6 and 9 to allocate to preventive health behaviors. This included purchasing healthier foods, increasing consumption of fruits and vegetables, prioritizing sleep, resuming exercise, choosing walking over public transit, increasing compliance with treatment plans abandoned because of cost and time scarcity, and prioritizing their mental health through therapy.

Interviewees linked their health risks with stress and finances; for example, Yolanda (Black, 50s), said, "People die from stress. Some people have so much stress because they don't know how they're going to feed their family, pay their rent, and keep the lights on, and all that can kill people." Stress and financial difficulties motivated participants to use the guaranteed income to address burgeoning health problems and improve their quality of life. These shifts were particularly pronounced for participants with chronic back and neck pain, which they attributed to poor working conditions and the physical burden of unpaid care work for children and elders.

EVALUATION, TRANSFERABILITY, AND ADVERSE EFFECTS

We did not identify any adverse or unintended consequences in this study, but the dissonance between the quantitative and qualitative findings indicates the need for future research that tests the degree to which unconditional cash can mediate the relationship between health literacy and social determinants of health.

SCALABILITY

As unconditional cash programs proliferate, important opportunities exist to test the consequences of guaranteed income on downstream health outcomes, as well as to better understand how changes in health promotion behaviors are linked to the alleviation of time scarcity. Of note, programs implementing guaranteed income for individuals most vulnerable to chronic disease or at high health risk may find a mixed-methods design to be useful in terms of detecting small, but positive health behavior changes.

PUBLIC HEALTH SIGNIFICANCE

Our findings indicate that guaranteed income may function as a protective health factor and an avenue for health literacy by alleviating time and financial constraints. A growing body of evidence illustrates that health literacy can serve as a mediating social determinant of health,[14] but there is comparatively little evidence on the underlying mechanisms driving these outcomes.[15] The World Health Organization defines health literacy as individual-level knowledge and behaviors along with the ability to use it,[16] but this relationship is mediated by the structural environment. These data indicate that guaranteed income provided a pathway through structural constraints, enabling participants to quickly prioritize lifestyle changes and act on health goals. The speed at which these changes occurred indicates that the absence of resources, and subsequently time, may be a larger barrier to health behaviors than a lack of personal health knowledge. AJPH

ABOUT THE AUTHORS

Amy Castro and Stacia West are with the Center for Guaranteed Income Research, School of Social Policy & Practice, University of Pennsylvania, Philadelphia. Mira Philips and Isabelle Kim are PhD candidates in the School of Social Policy & Practice, University of Pennsylvania, Philadelphia. Stacia West is also with the College of Social Work, University of Tennessee, Knoxville. Bo-Kyung Elizabeth Kim is with the Department of Community Health Sciences, Fielding School of Public Health, University of California, Los Angeles.

CORRESPONDENCE

Correspondence should be sent to Amy Castro, 3701 Locust Walk, Philadelphia, PA 19104 (e-mail: amycastro@sp2.upenn.edu). Reprints can be ordered at http://www.ajph.org by clicking the "Reprints" link.

PUBLICATION INFORMATION

Full Citation: Castro A, Philips M, Kim I, West S, Kim BKE. Time scarcity, health behaviors, and unconditional cash in Los Angeles. *Am J Public Health*. 2025;115(8):1222–1225.

Acceptance Date: March 15, 2025.

DOI: https://doi.org/10.2105/AJPH.2025.308125

ORCID iDs:

Amy Castro https://orcid.org/0000-0002-2074-3501

Isabelle Kim https://orcid.org/0000-0002-5901-7347

Stacia West https://orcid.org/0000-0001-8806-2318

Bo-Kyung Elizabeth Kim https://orcid.org/0000-0001-8851-5073

CONTRIBUTORS

A. Castro and M. Philips analyzed the data. A. Castro, M. Philips, and I. Kim collected and interpreted the data. A. Castro, S. West, and B-. E. Kim designed and conceptualized the study. All authors wrote the article.

ACKNOWLEDGMENTS

This research was funded by the City of Los Angeles, California and Mayors for a Guaranteed Income.

The authors wish to thank Abigail Marquez, Aaron Strauss, and the City of Los Angeles, Community Investment for Families Department, for their partnership designing and implementing the intervention. We acknowledge MoCaFi for their role disbursing the guaranteed income on the Angelos card.

CONFLICTS OF INTEREST

The authors have no conflicts of interest to declare.

HUMAN PARTICIPANT PROTECTION

The University of Pennsylvania's institutional review board determined this research to be exempt.

REFERENCES

1. Sun S, Huang J, Hudson DL, Sherraden M. Cash transfers and health. *Annu Rev Public Health.* 2021;42:363–380. https://doi.org/10.1146/annurev-publhealth-090419-102442
2. Braveman PA, Cubbin C, Egerter S, Williams DR, Pamuk E. Socioeconomic disparities in health in the United States: what the patterns tell us. *Am J Public Health.* 2010;100(suppl 1): S186–S196. https://doi.org/10.2105/AJPH.2009.166082
3. Adler NE, Stewart J. Health disparities across the lifespan: meaning, methods, and mechanisms. *Ann N Y Acad Sci.* 2010;1186:5–23. https://doi.org/10.1111/j.1749-6632.2009.05337.x
4. Gundersen C, Ziliak JP. Food insecurity and health outcomes. *Health Aff (Millwood).* 2015; 34(11):1830–1839. https://doi.org/10.1377/hlthaff.2015.0645
5. Jabs J, Devine CM. Time scarcity and food choices: an overview. *Appetite.* 2006;47(2):196–204. https://doi.org/10.1016/j.appet.2006.02.014
6. Strazdins L, Griffin AL, Broom DH, et al. Time scarcity: another health inequality? *Environ Plan A.* 2011;43(3):545–559. https://doi.org/10.1068/a4360
7. Venn D, Strazdins L. Your money or your time? How both types of scarcity matter to physical activity and healthy eating. *Soc Sci Med.* 2017;172:98–106. https://doi.org/10.1016/j.socscimed.2016.10.023
8. Lagarde M, Haines A, Palmer N. Conditional cash transfers for improving uptake of health interventions in low- and middle-income countries: a systematic review. *JAMA.* 2007;298(16):1900–1910. https://doi.org/10.1001/jama.298.16.1900
9. Thomas CC, Walton GM, Reinhart EC, Markus HR. Mitigating welfare-related prejudice and partisanship among US conservatives with moral reframing of a universal basic income policy. *J Exp Soc Psychol.* 2023;105:104424. https://doi.org/10.1016/j.jesp.2022.104424
10. West S, Castro A. Impact of guaranteed income on health, finances, and agency: findings from the Stockton randomized controlled trial. *J Urban Health.* 2023;100(2):227–244. https://doi.org/10.1007/s11524-023-00723-0
11. Tashakkori A, Johnson RB, Teddlie C. *Foundations of Mixed Methods Research: Integrating Quantitative and Qualitative Approaches in the Social and Behavioral Sciences.* 2nd ed. Thousand Oaks, CA: SAGE; 2020.
12. Charmaz K. *Constructing Grounded Theory.* 2nd ed. Thousand Oaks, CA: SAGE; 2014.
13. Braun V, Clarke V. Thematic analysis. In: Cooper H, Camic PM, Long DL, et al., eds. *APA Handbook of Research Methods in Psychology, Vol 2: Research Designs: Quantitative, Qualitative, Neuropsychological, and Biological.* Washington, DC: American Psychological Association; 2012:57–71. https://doi.org/10.1037/13620-004
14. Nutbeam D, Lloyd JE. Understanding and responding to health literacy as a social determinant of health. *Annu Rev Public Health.* 2021;42:159–173. https://doi.org/10.1146/annurev-publhealth-090419-102529
15. Berete F, Gisle L, Demarest S, et al. Does health literacy mediate the relationship between socioeconomic status and health related outcomes in the Belgian adult population? *BMC Public Health.* 2024;24:1182. https://doi.org/10.1186/s12889-024-18676-7
16. World Health Organization. Health literacy. August 5, 2024. Available at: https://www.who.int/news-room/fact-sheets/detail/health-literacy. Accessed October 28, 2024.

Breaking Barriers: Advancing Employment Opportunities for Black Women

Cynthia Tucker, DrPH, Tamika L. Foust, MBA, MHRM, Nicole Baldwin, BS, and Tamecia Moore, MPH

Employment has emerged as a critical focus in HIV interventions for Black women. A multilevel, community-based employment initiative in Chicago, Illinois, focused on justice-involved Black women with HIV. This program addressed complex barriers through bundled interventions, including navigation services and case management, with a major focus on employment. The evaluation demonstrated improvements in employment outcomes and health care access. The initiative's success underscores its potential as a model for addressing the complex intersecting challenges faced by Black women with HIV.
(*Am J Public Health*. 2025;115(8):1226–1228. https://doi.org/10.2105/AJPH.2025.308153)

AJPH August 2025, Vol. 115, No. 8

The Black Women First initiative—part of the Special Projects of National Significance Program funded by the Department of Health and Human Services Office of the Assistant Secretary for Health Minority HIV/AIDS Fund—aims to address the complex needs of Black women with HIV.[1] The initiative, which encompasses 12 demonstration sites and is supported by an evaluation and technical assistance provider, recognized the complex challenges faced by this population, including employment discrimination, limited health care access, and adherence barriers.[2]

INTERVENTION AND IMPLEMENTATION

We examined the AIDS Foundation of Chicago's Black Women First initiative demonstration project which developed and evaluated a comprehensive employment program for Black women with HIV who are justice involved. The program sought to improve employment opportunities, health care access, medical adherence, and overall well-being. The program's objectives included the following:

- Addressing employment services and opportunities,
- Improving health care access,
- Enhancing medical treatment adherence, and
- Promoting long-term stability and health.

Black women with HIV face significant challenges related to unemployment, underemployment, and barriers to HIV treatment and care.[2] This initiative adopted a comprehensive, multilevel approach to address these interconnected issues among justice-involved women.

The intervention was implemented with a fivefold approach:

1. Community engagement. Black women (n = 53) were engaged in listening sessions and creating community advisory boards to inform the design and implementation of the interventions.[3,4]
2. The HIV Workforce Taskforce. Partnerships were developed with employers, academic institutions, and community organizations to support participants and facilitate hiring.[5] This component strengthened partnerships with various stakeholders and organized job readiness and resource fairs, which were attended by more than 100 Black women and addressed employment discrimination and challenges related to criminal backgrounds.[6]
3. The Women's Connection Summit of Hope. The summit provided access to employment opportunities, case management, health services (e.g., sexually transmitted infection and hepatitis C virus testing), housing support, and legal services.[7] Participants received

professional attire, grooming training, and capacity-building resources.

4. Capacity building and training. "Thoughtful Thursdays," a bimonthly employment-training series covered topics such as ethical artificial intelligence usage, effective communication, and navigating workplace discrimination.
5. Direct services and community partnerships. Individualized support was offered through mentorship, job coaching, and resume building in collaboration with workforce development organizations.

This multipronged approach integrated community involvement, strategic partnerships, skill development, and direct support services.[3]

PLACE, TIME, AND PERSONS

The intervention was implemented in Chicago, Illinois, from 2021 to 2025. The target population was unemployed and underemployed Black justice-involved women with HIV.

PURPOSE

This program sought to underscore the critical importance of comprehensive, community-driven interventions in addressing the multifaceted social determinants affecting Black women with HIV. Specifically, the AIDS Foundation of Chicago recognized that employment plays a crucial role in addressing poverty and improving access to health care, transportation, housing, and social support for Black women. By employing a multilayered approach, it effectively confronted the intersecting challenges faced by this population, yielding positive outcomes and disrupting cycles of marginalization. The program's community-centered design involved Black women in shaping interventions tailored to their specific needs, fostering trust and relevance.[8] The fivefold framework, including community engagement, a workforce taskforce, summits, capacity building, and direct services, addressed various aspects of participants' lives while promoting dignity and empowerment.[3]

EVALUATION AND ADVERSE EFFECTS

Our evaluation of the AIDS Foundation of Chicago's program under the Black Women First initiative revealed significant positive outcomes and some unintended consequences.

Community engagement efforts successfully engaged 53 Black women in listening sessions, ensuring the development of tailored programming that addressed their specific needs. Job resource fairs proved valuable, as more than 100 Black women attended three events that offered crucial skill-building opportunities, personalized coaching, and inspirational panel discussions. The Summit of Hope expos were particularly effective, as they reached more than 400 Black women and proved essential resources; notably, 67 women obtained new identification cards, enabling their access to care and supportive services. In terms of employment outcomes, the program facilitated 35 job interviews, resulting in 15 new employment opportunities, with all participants receiving tailored coaching and updated resumes. Strategic partnerships, such as the collaboration with Jumphire in Chicago, led to an eight-week apprenticeship program, creating pathways to full-time employment and venue space for one of the Summit of Hope events.

However, the evaluation also identified unintended outcomes. The initial virtual format of the job resource fair, necessitated by the COVID-19 pandemic, inadvertently excluded participants who lacked smartphones. This issue was addressed in subsequent events by providing smartphones and cell phone service plans and offering in-person options. The security policy measures at the Summit of Hope expos involved searches of attendees on probation, which may have caused unintended trauma for some participants. To lessen trauma to participants, information and registration entry procedures for future Summit of Hope events will be sent to all participants in advance.

SUSTAINABILITY

The intervention's sustainability is based on strategic partnership development, innovative funding approaches, and direct community engagement. Multilevel partnerships created a robust support network. The program also braided resources from multiple funding streams. Direct community engagement ensured that the intervention remained responsive to the evolving needs of Black women with HIV who are justice involved.

PUBLIC HEALTH SIGNIFICANCE

This intervention demonstrates how intersectional, community-driven approaches can effectively address complex public health challenges and can serve as a model for future interventions targeting marginalized populations, emphasizing the importance of addressing social determinants of health comprehensively. In conclusion, the AIDS Foundation of Chicago's program marks a significant advancement in addressing the needs of Black women with HIV by focusing on employment and a holistic approach to improving health outcomes and overall quality of life for marginalized populations. *AJPH*

ABOUT THE AUTHORS

All authors are with the AIDS Foundation of Chicago, Chicago, IL.

CORRESPONDENCE

Correspondence should be sent to Cynthia Tucker, DrPH, AIDS Foundation of Chicago, 200 W. Monroe St, Suite 1150, Chicago, IL 60606 (e-mail: ctucker@aidschicago.org). Reprints can be ordered at http://www.ajph.org by clicking the "Reprints" link.

PUBLICATION INFORMATION

Full Citation: Tucker C, Foust TL, Baldwin N, Moore T. Breaking barriers: advancing employment opportunities for Black women. *Am J Public Health*. 2025;115(8):1226–1228.

Acceptance Date: April 9, 2025.

DOI: https://doi.org/10.2105/AJPH.2025.308153

ORCID iDs:

Cynthia Tucker https://orcid.org/0000-0003-0645-5308

Tamecia Moore https://orcid.org/0000-0002-9691-2690

CONTRIBUTORS

The authors contributed equally to this work.

ACKNOWLEDGMENTS

This study is funded by the Health Resources and Services Administration (HRSA) of the US Department of Health and Human Services (HHS; grant U90HA39727).

We would like to thank the AIDS Foundation of Chicago, the community partnerships team, and the evaluation team members who worked on the HRSA Black Women First study and the demonstration sites. In addition, we would like to thank Serena Rajabiun, PhD, and Corliss Heath, PhD, who encouraged all sites to employ innovation while meeting specific project aims.

Note. The contents of this article are those of the authors and do not necessarily represent the official views of or an endorsement by HRSA, HHS, or the US government.

CONFLICTS OF INTEREST

The authors have no conflicts of interest to disclose.

HUMAN PARTICIPANT PROTECTION

Ethics approvals were obtained from the University of Massachusetts, Lowell and the Boston University Charles River Campus institutional review boards (protocol numbers 20-147 and 5832X).

REFERENCES

1. Health Resources and Services Administration. Improving care and treatment coordination: focusing on Black women with HIV—evaluation and technical assistance provider. 2020. Available at: https://www.hrsa.gov/grants/find-funding/HRSA-20-115. Accessed May 22, 2025.
2. Chinn JJ, Martin IK, Redmond N. Health equity among Black women in the United States. *J Womens Health (Larchmt)*. 2021;30(2):212–219. https://doi.org/10.1089/jwh.2020.8868
3. Farhang L, Morales X. Building community power to achieve health and racial equity: principles to guide transformative partnerships with local communities. *NAM Perspect*. 2022;2022:10.31478/202206d. https://doi.org/10.31478/202206d
4. Rocco M, Meshesha M, Scott J, et al. Using participatory art approaches to promote health and empower client voice: examples from the Black Women First initiative. March 2023. Available at: https://targethiv.org/sites/default/files/media/documents/2023-03/Cleared-BWF_Participatory Arts_IssueBrief_031723-508.pdf. Accessed May 22, 2025.
5. AIDS Foundation Chicago. HIV workforce and employment. Available at: https://www.aidschicago.org/our-work/hiv-workforce-and-employment. Accessed February 1, 2025.
6. Hoven H, Backhaus I, Gerő K, Kawachi I. Characteristics of employment history and self-perceived barriers to healthcare access. *Eur J Public Health*. 2023;33(6):1080–1087. https://doi.org/10.1093/eurpub/ckad178
7. Conway P. Women's Connection Summit of Hope lives up to its name. June 21, 2024. Available at: https://www.aidschicago.org/womens-connection-summit-of-hope-lives-up-to-its-name. Accessed February 1, 2025.
8. Chelak K, Chakole S. The role of social determinants of health in promoting health equality: a narrative review. *Cureus*. 2023;15(1):e33425. https://doi.org/10.7759/cureus.33425

Global LGBTQ+ Public Health in the Face of Legal Persecution

Stewart Landers, JD, MCP, and B. Ethan Coston, PhD, MA

ABOUT THE AUTHORS

At the time this editorial was written, Stewart Landers was with the Health Services Division, JSI Research & Training Institute, Boston, MA. B. Ethan Coston is with the Gender, Sexuality and Women's Studies Department, Virginia Commonwealth University, Richmond. Both authors are AJPH associate editors.

See also Global LGBTQ+ Public Health in the Face of Legal Persecution, pp. 1231–1270.

The condition of lesbian, gay, bisexual, transgender, and queer (LGBTQ+) people's health and well-being across the globe varies greatly, and there is much that is not known. Although many volumes of work have been published on LGBTQ+ health in the United States, Canada, and the so-called Global North, research articles, program analyses, and political perspectives centering people of the global majority have been largely and problematically excluded or ignored.

For more than two decades, the US government has focused increasing attention on the health and human rights of LGBTQ+ people globally, including through the 2011 presidential memorandum on international initiatives to advance the human rights of lesbian, gay, bisexual, and transgender persons (updated in 2021[1]) and diplomatic engagement in United Nations and World Health Organization initiatives and sustainable development goals (e.g., the 2008 Declaration on Human Rights, Sexual Orientation and Gender Identity). However, with all of the progress made, there have been setbacks, including recriminalization and new anti-LGBTQ+ laws passed in many places, and the world we are living in today remains precarious and often deadly for LGBTQ+ people.

As of March 2025,[2] 64 countries had criminalized private, consensual, same-sex sexual activity; 12 countries had jurisdictions that can impose the death penalty for private, consensual same-sex activity[3]; and 14 countries criminalized the gender identity or expression of transgender people. Just as in the United States, LGBTQ+ people globally face numerous health care inequities owing to stigma and bias, violence, discriminatory policies, and other sociopolitical forces and bad-faith actors. This special section, featuring eight articles that examine global LGBTQ+ health amid struggles for decriminalization and legal recognition, explores many aspects of these pressing public health issues.

Two of our contributions look to Asia, where support for LGBTQ+ rights continues to grow, although, as in the United States, challenges remain. On January 23, 2025, Thailand became the second Asian country to legalize same-sex marriage (following Taiwan, which established that right on May 19, 2019). Yiu Tung Suen (p. 1196) scans the status of same-sex marriage across Asia and notes that the current debate focuses primarily on whether same-sex marriage conflicts with traditional societal values rather than on its well-documented public health benefits. Care coordination for LGBTQ+ people also remains a pressing concern for our contributors. Lodge et al. (p. 1245) use key informant interviews in Mumbai and New Delhi conducted among transgender women with HIV, community leaders, health providers, and researchers to explore how stigma, poverty, and lack of gender-affirming care hinder access to essential HIV medical care.

In many countries in Africa, the trend toward repression of LGBTQ+ people through legal means has paralleled what is happening in the United States; this is perhaps unsurprising given that the same organizations are funding these often Christian Nationalist political agendas. In 2023, legislation passed in Uganda that criminalized homosexuality and targeted other queer identities, including the use of capital punishment for "serial offenders" or for transmission of "terminal" illnesses such as HIV. Uganda is not alone in legislating harsh penalties for same-sex acts and identities. Similar laws that carry sentences of capital punishment or life imprisonment can be found in Mauritania, Somalia, Nigeria, Sudan, Tanzania, and Zambia.

Tucker et al. (p. 1264) describe how US-based right-wing organizations reacted to the growing global movement for sexual and reproductive health and rights and how the rights of sexual and gender minorities developed and expanded at meetings such as the 1994 International Conference on Population and Development and the 1996 Beijing Conference.

In particular, they note that the activities of these organizations do not have their origins within the African nations themselves—Kenya in this case—but rather contort colonial logics in an attempt to convince community members that LGBTQ+ rights are actually "non-African."

Wallach et al. (p. 1254) explore the same dynamic in postcolonial Belize, Jamaica, Kenya, Singapore, Dominica, and Saint Vincent and the Grenadines and the role that strategic litigation can perform in improving the social climate and therefore the health of sexual and gender minorities. A coalition of public health experts, legal professionals, and local advocacy groups is needed if such litigation is to be effective.

Finally, Ogunbajo et al. (p. 1231) separately explore human rights abuses and their impact on LGBTQ+ people's lack of access to essential health and mental health services in Nigeria, Kenya, and Ghana. The conditions faced by LGBTQ+ people in these countries are likely to be further aggravated by the discontinuation of foreign aid through the United States Agency for International Development.

Transnationalism is the final theme that runs through many of the articles in this collection. In addition to the work of Wallach et al., Ide-Lamberts and Onyeise (p. 1236) explicitly looks at the duality of US residents confronting complex transnational pressures. Faced with different evolving legal, cultural, and religious contexts in the United States and their country of origin, they encounter minority stressors in both contexts. Navigating the social and legal dimensions of human rights and access to health care services is a challenge for LGBTQ+ individuals trying to find their way in a new country while maintaining connections to and juggling the challenges of supporting their old life.

Although *AJPH* has always published articles that examine public health challenges and successes in other countries, a global focus is needed more now than ever. It is not just the spread of infectious diseases that knows no national boundaries or colonial borders; dissemination of ideas themselves, of moral panics, and of visions about what constitutes good health occurs widely through our communities, networks, and the digital sphere.

In today's marketplace of ideas, public health practitioners might assume agreement on the value of clean air, clean water, and healthy, affordable food. Yet, even these basics of public health are mired in an increasing environment of disinformation. Each of a growing number of pressing public health issues need to be better understood, ferociously documented, and unapologetically advocated for in the public sphere. Continuing after this issue, let it be known: *AJPH* welcomes well-argued and evidence-based research, analysis, practice, and opinion articles from every corner of the globe. *AJPH*

CORRESPONDENCE

Correspondence should be sent to Stewart Landers, 44 Farnsworth St, Boston, MA 02210 (e-mail: stewartjaylanders@gmail.com). Reprints can be ordered at https://www.ajph.org by clicking the "Reprints" link.

PUBLICATION INFORMATION

Full Citation: Landers S, Coston BE. Global LGBTQ+ public health in the face of legal persecution. *Am J Public Health*. 2025;115(8):1229–1230.

Acceptance Date: March 16, 2025.

DOI: https://doi.org/10.2105/AJPH.2025.308122

ORCID iDs:

Stewart Landers https://orcid.org/0009-0005-5101-4108

B. Ethan Coston https://orcid.org/0000-0002-6511-4362

CONTRIBUTORS

S. Landers co-conceptualized the theme for this special section, drafted the road map editorial, and revised the editorial throughout the publication process. B. E. Coston co-conceptualized the theme for this special section and reviewed and edited several drafts of the editorial.

CONFLICTS OF INTEREST

There are no conflicts of interests from any funding or affiliation-related activities.

REFERENCES

1. The White House. Memorandum on advancing the human rights of lesbian, gay, bisexual, transgender, queer, and intersex persons around the world. Available at: https://bidenwhitehouse.archives.gov/briefing-room/presidential-actions/2021/02/04/memorandum-advancing-the-human-rights-of-lesbian-gay-bisexual-transgender-queer-and-intersex-persons-around-the-world/#:~:text=That%20memorandum%2C%20for%20the%20first,bisexual%2C%20and%20transgender%20persons%20everywhere. Accessed March 14, 2025
2. Human Dignity Trust. Map of jurisdictions that criminalize LGBT people. Available at: https://www.humandignitytrust.org/lgbt-the-law/map-of-criminalisation. Accessed March 14, 2025.
3. Dahir AL. Where being gay is punishable by death, aid cuts are "heartbreaking." Available at: https://www.nytimes.com/2025/03/04/world/africa/usaid-africa-uganda-lgbtq.html. Accessed March 14, 2025.

Barriers to Gender-Affirming Care, Health Care Services, and Experiences of Health Care Provider Bias Among Transgender People in Nigeria

Adedotun Ogunbajo, PhD, MPH, MHS, Temitope Oke, PhD, MSW, Calvin Fitch, PhD, Arjee Restar, PhD, MPH, Alphonso Barney, MS, Olakunle Oginni, PhD, and DeMarc Hickson, PhD, MPH

See also Global LGBTQ+ Public Health in the Face of Legal Persecution, pp. 1229–1270.

In the current study, we explored barriers to accessing gender-affirming care among transgender and gender-diverse (TGD) people in Nigeria. Between February and September 2021, we conducted focus group discussions with 25 adult TGD individuals residing in Nigeria. We found (1) a lack of trans-competent health care providers, (2) high medical costs, (3) limited access to accurate health information, (4) experiences of transphobia, and (5) a lack of trans-specific programming. Health care services that cater to the unique needs of TGD people in Nigeria are needed. (*Am J Public Health*. 2025;115(8):1231–1235. https://doi.org/10.2105/AJPH.2025.308057)

In sub-Saharan Africa, the health of transgender and gender-diverse (TGD) populations—individuals whose current gender identity or gender expression do not align with their birth-assigned sex—remains largely understudied.[1–3] In Nigeria, sexual- and gender-minority (SGM) communities experience stigma, violence, and discrimination, which might hinder access to health care services. Previous work has demonstrated that access to gender-affirming care (GAC) improves the mental health and well-being of TGD populations.[4–7] However, the health care experiences of the TGD population in Nigeria remain understudied.

STUDY OBJECTIVE

To characterize barriers to accessing GAC among TGD in Nigeria, we carried out a qualitative study that explored (1) barriers to GAC services, (2) health care experiences of TGD populations, and (3) health care providers' (HCPs') bias.

RESEARCH QUESTION

What are the barriers to accessing GAC, including negative experiences in health care settings and HCP bias, among TGD in Nigeria?

PARTICIPANTS, SAMPLE, GEOGRAPHIC LOCATION, SETTING, AND YEAR OF STUDY

Between February and September 2021, we conducted three focus group discussions with 25 TGD individuals. The participants, recruited through convenience sampling, resided in Abuja (n = 17) or Lagos (n = 8), Nigeria.

METHODS

The study inclusion criteria were (1) being aged 18 years or older, (2) identifying as TGD (having a current gender identity that differs from birth-assigned sex), and (3) residence in either Lagos or Abuja. Recruitment was conducted in collaboration with two nonprofit organizations that provide health and advocacy services to SGM communities in Lagos and Abuja. Health outreach workers, key opinion leaders, and community activists shared study promotional materials with the target population during programming events (HIV testing outreach, peer educator sessions) and by sharing with members of their social network (via text message, phone calls, and social media posting). They provided study contact information to potential participants. Recruitment strategies utilized for SGM

AJPH August 2025, Vol. 115, No. 8

communities in the United States, such as clubs and bars, cannot be deployed in this setting because of the illegality of such establishments in Nigeria.

To maintain confidentiality, we obtained verbal informed consent from all participants before study enrollment. All focus group discussions were conducted in the private offices of the partner organizations. After conducting a detailed literature review and consulting with academic researchers, we developed a focus group guide capturing several thematic areas. The discussions were digitally recorded and lasted about 1.5 hours. Participants received 5000 Naira (US $10).

All interview transcripts were transcribed verbatim by a Nigeria-based transcription company. We utilized a qualitative content analysis approach to analyze the transcripts (NVIVO 12).[8] First, a study team member (A. O.) read 20% of the transcripts and created an outline of preliminary emergent themes. We defined themes as codes with similar patterns of response. Next, a draft codebook was developed and circulated to the study team for review, who provided iterative feedback until a refined codebook emerged. Next, one team member (A. O.) coded all transcripts. We utilized the consolidated criteria for reporting qualitative research (COREQ) checklist to ensure the systematic application of qualitative data analysis and summary of our findings.[9]

KEY FINDINGS

The majority (52%) of participants were aged 25 years or older, 80% were transgender women, and 20% were transgender men. While 76% had at least a high-school diploma, 96% had a monthly income of 50 000 Naira (US $100) or lower. Most (68%) were single, 40% were unemployed, and 24% had unstable housing.

A synopsis of the emergent themes is discussed here, and representative quotes are provided in Box 1.

Barriers to Gender-Affirming Health Care Services

Three key themes emerged in barriers to accessing GAC: (1) difficulty finding competent and affirming HCPs to assist with the gender-affirmation process, (2) transgender individuals often being forced to seek out information and self-administer hormones, and (3) hormone therapy being expensive.

Participants described knowing that GAC, specifically hormone therapy, should be prescribed, administered, and monitored by a trained medical professional, but widespread transphobia in Nigeria made it difficult to find HCPs who were willing and able to provide these services. While some participants expressed some knowledge about the clinical requirements to administer GAC, others noted how transphobia permeates Nigerian society and inhibits access to GAC, specifically hormones.

Participants discussed the dearth of accessible information on hormone therapy. As a consequence, because of limited health information and a stigmatizing health care environment, participants turned to social media as a source of information. While some participants mentioned engaging with people on the Internet about hormone therapy but not getting enough information about hormone dosage and how to self-administer, others built an online community of transgender women to deepen their knowledge about hormone therapy. A few participants described having gained access to hormone therapy. These individuals often self-administered because of HCPs' inability to provide GAC services. One participant commented on the dangers of self-administration and the potential for overdosing because of limited information and lack of medical guidance.

Participants noted the high cost of hormone therapy as a major barrier and that many people are forced to pay for these medications themselves or resort to crowdfunding platforms (e.g., GoFundMe) to raise money.

Experiences Within the Health Care Setting

Four key themes emerged regarding navigating the health care system for other non-GAC health services: (1) lack of health care service options for transgender individuals, (2) health facilities often misgendering transgender individuals, (3) health centers lacking the appropriate medications needed by transgender populations, and (4) having positive health care experiences at community-based organizations compared to traditional health care settings.

Participants described the lack of options for general health care services tailored to the unique needs of TGD people, especially compared to sexual-minority men who have access to more tailored services. There were also some expressed apprehensions about seeking health services at facilities that serve the general public. One participant discussed the fear of their transgender identity being discovered during a medical examination.

Several participants relayed experiences of nonaffirmation, such as being intentionally misgendered and being incorrectly classified as a gay man by HCPs. It was especially hurtful when these comments came from staff

BOX 1— Illustrative Quotes From Focus Group Discussion With 25 Transgender People in Abuja and Lagos, Nigeria, Conducted in February–September 2021

Theme and Subtheme	Illustrative Quote
Barriers to gender-affirming health care services	
It is difficult to find competent and accepting health care providers (HCPs) to assist with the gender-affirmation process.	"I have challenges, because with taking hormonal pills, with the research I did online, you can't just place yourself on hormonal pills yourself, you have to . . . there is a protocol like, a consultant that you need to talk to, because they will have to check your liver, your kidney. . . ." (26-year-old transgender woman) "Some transgender women might be HIV-positive, you know, if you are HIV-positive and you still want to take hormonal pills you will have to seek for a consultant, to check maybe this hormonal pill . . . you have to balance both; it can be a lot." (30-year-old transgender woman)
Transgender individuals are often forced to seek their own information and self-administer their own hormones.	"You can chat up [people] online through social media about something like hormones, but they don't give you like a specific dosage or how to actually self-medicate?" (32-year-old transgender man) "When I got information about the drug, it was online. I was always conversing with other trans girls outside the state, so they were telling me 'use this, use that' . . . I just kept searching." (25-year-old transgender woman) "With the hormonal therapy, I am presently on hormones . . . and I am self-medicating because nobody will want to prescribe anything for you." (24-year-old transgender man)
Hormone therapy is expensive.	"As a trans person, it's not easy getting hormone therapy in Nigeria, a bottle of the pill cost about 46,000 Naira [about $95]. I have trans friends that have started their hormonal therapy and sometimes tell me that they've spent a lot of money trying to get their pills, they have GoFundMe to fund all of that." (22-year-old transgender woman)
Experiences within the health care setting as a transgender community member	
There is a lack of health care service options for transgender individuals.	"As a trans-identified person, zero [health care centers], but for MSM [men who have sex with men], there are abundance of health care services and all of that but, as a trans-identified person, zero." (30-year-old transgender man) "The doctors found out about you like they have to strip you of your clothes, and they found out, what are you going to do about that?" (26-year-old transgender woman)
Health facilities often misgender transgender individuals.	"I've gone to care in that facility, they don't want to accept my gender, that I'm a trans woman. . . . It's the same community organization, which supposed to be for us, and a staff working there will sit me down and start telling me, my life that I'm living is bullshit, I don't get it." (30-year-old transgender woman) "If I wanted to get health care services, I just claimed to be a gay man, which is cringeworthy to begin with." (22-year-old transgender man)
Health centers lack the appropriate medications needed by transgender populations.	"After going to hospital and them not having the medication that I needed, I have to go and take natural herbs." (27-year-old transgender woman)
Positive health care experiences occur at community-based organizations (CBOs).	"Well. In general hospital it's zero for me, yes . . . it's zero for me, but when it comes to CBOs, they are not homophobic, they're not transphobic, so they are fine, at least." (26-year-old transgender woman)
Health care provider bias	
There is unequal access to hormone therapy based on gender identity.	"My understanding is that most of these drugs are multipurpose drugs; they don't have one use. They [HCPs] don't give the drugs to people who want to transition; they give it to men who are struggling with testosterone issues." (29-year-old transgender man)
Individuals experience prejudicial treatment from health care providers.	"When you go to the hospital, you see someone that is trained to not look at you but to only look at what brought you here. Once they see you, they already judge you from your head, your shoes. They have misplaced priority and don't have the emotional intelligence to deal with this issue." (32-year-old transgender woman)

members at facilities expected to be inclusive and accepting of the SGM community. One participant recalled being forced to misgender themselves to receive health care services.

Another participant mentioned seeking out alternative medicines because of health care centers not having the appropriate medications. Lastly, some participants reported having a more positive health care experience at community-based organizations that specifically serve SGM communities.

Health Care Provider Bias

Two key themes emerged in participants' experiences of bias among HCPs: (1) unequal access to hormone therapy based on gender identity, and (2) experiences of prejudicial treatment from HCPs.

Participants indicated that accessing hormones for health issues was easier for cisgender people with endocrine problems compared with transgender people seeking these hormones for

GAC. Participants also discussed experiencing prejudice from HCPs attributable to their reason for presenting at the medical setting or their outward appearance.

EVALUATION, TRANSFERABILITY, AND ADVERSE EFFECTS

This first-of-its-kind study, to our knowledge, shone light on the barriers to health care access experienced by TGD people in Nigeria, which might be applicable to similar countries across sub-Saharan Africa. This study also highlights the possibility of developing TGD-specific health services by organizations that have primarily served the SGM community but largely excluded TGD groups. In addition, future studies should investigate the longitudinal effects of limited access to GAC on the health and wellness of TGD populations in Nigeria and across the African continent.

SCALABILITY

The development, testing, and scaling of interventions aimed at addressing health disparities among TGD in Nigeria is desperately needed. Specifically, we need to design and conduct randomized controlled trials investigating the efficacy of different health care delivery models (e.g., traditional health care setting, peer-to-peer, telehealth) and sensitivity training to address health disparities among TGD people in Nigeria.

PUBLIC HEALTH SIGNIFICANCE

To our knowledge, there are no programs within any major hospital systems in Nigeria specifically catering to the unique health care needs of TGD people. A recently published study exploring access to HIV services among TGD individuals in Nigeria found a lack of transgender-inclusive and gender-affirming HIV services, which perpetuated experiences of stigma and discrimination.[10] There is a dire need for accessible, competent, and comprehensive gender-affirming health care services—including social, psychological, legal, and medical services. It is also important to consider the potential for self-administered GAC because of limited access to hospital-based care and the potential negative consequences that have been found, including both inadequate hormone concentrations[11] and excessive hormone dosing.[12]

Given the inevitable public backlash and potential for increased violence against TGD Nigerians in response to a TGD-centered hospital or clinic, community-based organizations that serve sexual minority men should expand their service offerings to include TGD-specific health care. Program offerings should include case management, gender-affirming primary care including HIV prevention and care services, and social and mental health service programs.[13] Specifically, SGM health organizations should explore offering free or low-cost GAC to TGD populations in Nigeria, as cost is a major barrier. In addition, advocacy for policy change must co-occur with health promotion programs for this community. Most importantly, these programs should employ TGD individuals as staff members and hold regular staff training in cultural sensitivity and effective communication with TGD clients. AJPH

ABOUT THE AUTHORS

Adedotun Ogunbajo, Temitope Oke, Alphonso Barney, and DeMarc Hickson are with Us Helping Us, People Into Living Inc, in Washington, DC. Calvin Fitch is with the Department of Psychiatry, Massachusetts General Hospital, Harvard Medical School, Boston. Arjee Restar is with the Department of Epidemiology, University of Washington, Seattle. Olakunle Oginni is with the Wolfson Centre for Young People's Mental Health, Division of Psychological Medicine, and Clinical Neuroscience, Cardiff University, Cardiff, United Kingdom.

CORRESPONDENCE

Correspondence should be sent to Adedotun Ogunbajo, PhD, MPH, MHS, Us Helping Us, People into Living Inc, 3636 Georgia Ave NW, Washington, DC 20010 (e-mail: dotunogunbajo@gmail.com). Reprints can be ordered at https://www.ajph.org by clicking the "Reprints" link.

PUBLICATION INFORMATION

Full Citation: Ogunbajo A, Oke T, Fitch C, et al. Barriers to gender-affirming care, health care services, and experiences of health care provider bias among transgender people in Nigeria. *Am J Public Health*. 2025;115(8):1231–1235.

Acceptance Date: February 3, 2025.

DOI: https://doi.org/10.2105/AJPH.2025.308057

ORCID iDs:

Adedotun Ogunbajo https://orcid.org/0000-0002-3074-6431

Olakunle Oginni https://orcid.org/0000-0002-2340-9429

CONTRIBUTORS

A. Ogunbajo and T. Oke participated in conceptualization, investigation, formal analysis, and methodology. T. Oke and D. Hickson participated in funding acquisition. T. Oke participated in project administration. A. Ogunbajo wrote the original draft. All authors participated in writing, reviewing, and editing and read and approved the final article.

ACKNOWLEDGMENTS

This study was partly funded by the Us Helping Us, People into Living Inc. A. Ogunbajo acknowledges salary support from US National Institutes of Health grant K01MH129165.

Most importantly, we thank all the participants of the study for their bravery in telling their stories, even in the face of intense discrimination and marginalization. We would also like to thank the staff at Improved Sexual Health and Rights Advocacy Initiative and Trans Global Nigeria.

CONFLICTS OF INTEREST

The authors have no conflicts of interest to disclose.

HUMAN PARTICIPANT PROTECTION

The study protocol was approved by the Pearl Institutional Review Board.

REFERENCES

1. Jobson GA, Theron LB, Kaggwa JK, Kim H-J. Transgender in Africa: invisible, inaccessible, or ignored? *SAHARA J*. 2012;9(3):160–163. https://doi.org/10.1080/17290376.2012.743829
2. Chakrapani V. Need for transgender-specific data from Africa and elsewhere. *Lancet HIV*. 2021;8(5):e249–e250. https://doi.org/10.1016/S2352-3018(20)30344-1
3. Crowell TA, Fast PE, Bekker LG, Sanders EJ. Involvement of African men and transgender women who have sex with men in HIV research: progress, but much more must be done. *J Int AIDS Soc*. 2020;23(suppl 6):e25596. https://doi.org/10.1002/jia2.25596
4. Jarrett BA, Peitzmeier SM, Restar A, et al. Gender-affirming care, mental health, and economic stability in the time of COVID-19: a multi-national, cross-sectional study of transgender and nonbinary people. *PLoS One*. 2021;16(7):e0254215. https://doi.org/10.1371/journal.pone.0254215
5. Hughes LD, Kidd KM, Gamarel KE, Operario D, Dowshen N. "These laws will be devastating": provider perspectives on legislation banning gender-affirming care for transgender adolescents. *J Adolesc Health*. 2021;69(6):976–982. https://doi.org/10.1016/j.jadohealth.2021.08.020
6. Mann S, Campbell T, Hien ND. Access to gender-affirming care and transgender mental health: evidence from Medicaid coverage. *Am J Health Econ*. 2024;10(2). https://doi.org/10.1086/728080
7. Nobili A, Glazebrook C, Arcelus J. Quality of life of treatment-seeking transgender adults: a systematic review and meta-analysis. *Rev Endocr Metab Disord*. 2018;19(3):199–220. https://doi.org/10.1007/s11154-018-9459-y
8. Elo S, Kyngäs H. The qualitative content analysis process. *J Adv Nurs*. 2008;62(1):107–115. https://doi.org/10.1111/j.1365-2648.2007.04569.x
9. Tong A, Sainsbury P, Craig J. Consolidated criteria for reporting qualitative research (COREQ): a 32-item checklist for interviews and focus groups. *Int J Qual Health Care*. 2007;19(6):349–357. https://doi.org/10.1093/intqhc/mzm042
10. Tun W, Pulerwitz J, Shoyemi E, et al. A qualitative study of how stigma influences HIV services for transgender men and women in Nigeria. *J Int AIDS Soc*. 2022;25(suppl 1):e25933. https://doi.org/10.1002/jia2.25933
11. Salakphet T, Mattawanon N, Manojai N, Muangmool T, Tangpricha V. Hormone concentrations in transgender women who self-prescribe gender-affirming hormone therapy: a retrospective study. *J Sex Med*. 2022;19(5):864–871. https://doi.org/10.1016/j.jsxm.2022.02.023
12. Baba T, Endo T, Ikeda U, et al. Self-administration of gender-affirming hormones and supratherapeutic dosing are relatively common in Japanese transgender women. *J Obstet Gynaecol Res*. 2022;48(8):2208–2213. https://doi.org/10.1111/jog.15231
13. Morenz AM, Goldhammer H, Lambert CA, Hopwood R, Keuroghlian AS. A blueprint for planning and implementing a transgender health program. *Ann Fam Med*. 2020;18(1):73–79. https://doi.org/10.1370/afm.2473

The Effects of LGBTQ+ Persecution on Transnational African Immigrants

Kelechi Ibe-Lamberts, PhD, and Destiny Onyeise, MA

ABOUT THE AUTHORS

Kelechi Ibe-Lamberts is a faculty member at the Division of Community Health Sciences, School of Public Health, University of Illinois–Chicago. Destiny Onyeise is a doctoral student in the School of Medicine and Public Health, University of Wisconsin–Madison.

See also Global LGBTQ+ Public Health in the Face of Legal Persecution, pp. 1229–1270.

The persecution of LGBTQ+ (lesbian, gay, bisexual, transgender, queer or questioning, and all subsects) individuals is a global issue and an infringement on universal human rights. This is most prevalent in Africa, with several African countries enacting laws that criminalize or stigmatize individuals based on their sexuality, sexual orientation, or gender identity.[1] Countries such as Nigeria, with its Same-Sex Marriage Prohibition Bill in 2014, and Uganda, with its Anti-Homosexuality Act in 2023, have recently drawn attention for their anti-LGBTQ+ laws. These legal and cultural attitudes provoke harsh actions toward members of these communities. Anti-LGBTQ+ laws in countries such as Uganda and Nigeria impose severe penalties, including imprisonment and, in some cases, death for those in same-sex relationships. What provides the impetus for these laws and such notions? These laws are deeply rooted in colonial era penal codes imposed by British colonizers, including antisodomy laws, which were first applied in India and New Zealand.[2]

Despite the "end" of colonial rule, 33 of 55 African nations still criminalize homosexuality.[3] Many of these legal frameworks exhibit deeply ingrained cultural and religious beliefs that often portray LGBTQ+ norms and identities as immoral and unnatural. As a result, African LGBTQ+ individuals in these regions face not only legal discrimination but also social ostracization, violence, and the constant threat of persecution. These hostile environments often lead to an exodus of African LGBTQ+ individuals to other countries to seek refuge. African immigrants have been one of the fastest growing immigrant populations in the United States for the past few decades.[4] Immigration numbers are up; however, this does not negate the sustained, cross-border connections that remain between home and host country and the impact these connections have on the immigrants' mental and physical health and welfare.

Transnationalism, the process by which immigrants maintain strong connections and engage in activities that transcend borders, allows the development and sustenance of multifaceted ties to both native country and host country.[5,6] Although well known in anthropological and even economic arenas, the notion of transnationalism remains in its nascent stages in the context of migration and health, especially in the Black diaspora. Many transnational immigrants make significant efforts to resist assimilation and negotiate acculturation to the host land by maintaining relationships and ties in their homelands that allow them to retain their cultural identity. For transnational African LGBTQ+ immigrants, the impact of anti-LGBTQ+ laws extends across borders. Even while living in countries with more progressive protections, LGBTQ+ immigrants face psychological trauma and isolation, knowing their home countries still criminalize their identities. Tied to families and communities back home through regular communication, financial commitment, or frequent visits, they may face rejection or live in secrecy, deepening their sense of alienation. This dual existence—seeking acceptance abroad while staying connected to cultures that deny their humanity—takes a lasting toll on their mental and emotional health, shaping the course of their transnational lives as a member of the LGBTQ+ community.

The intersecting identities of Black, immigrant, and LGBTQ+ individuals often amplify the weight of discrimination borne by these individuals.[7,8] When combined with cultural expectations regarding gender roles (i.e., standards and norms that dictate what is acceptable behavior for both genders), the pressure can push many beyond their allostatic load, intensifying the mental and emotional toll they bear, which can catalyze additional physical health issues. Despite the hostility that they face, many of these individuals remain connected to their homeland because of cultural responsibilities and

AJPH August 2025, Vol. 115, No. 8

caregiving ties. They may support family members abroad via remittances and other forms of economic assistance, even as they navigate cultural norms in the United States as members of the LGBTQ+ community.

AFRICAN LGBTQ+ IMMIGRANTS

Although African LGBTQ+ immigrants frequently send remittances back home, they experience more economic insecurity than their counterparts because of perceived discrimination and limited work opportunities. Often, immigrants and refugees struggle to find jobs they want and are left unemployed or working in jobs that are physically demanding or require strenuous labor; sex work is another avenue to income.[9] Like most people, African LGBTQ+ immigrants desire a sense of self-efficacy. Yet, they face more obstacles than do those who do not share their identities, which prevents them from feeling empowered and satisfied in life. The discrimination and limited job opportunities increase stress among African LGBTQ+ immigrants because they affect their sense of self and hinder their ability to send adequate remittances to their family in their home country, who depend on them for financial support. Despite this continuing connection, complexities arise when their home country and family members in their homeland hold anti-LGBTQ+ attitudes.

It can feel lonely navigating a new country, but when you do not receive emotional support and acceptance from family members back home and have not found a supportive community in your new environment, the journey of life can feel daunting and unbearable. Sometimes, African LGBTQ+ immigrants internalize the homophobic sentiments from their home and host countries, which further perpetuates internal struggle and perceived alienation.[10,11] African LGBTQ+ immigrants encounter unique stressors stemming from their intersecting identities as African immigrants and sexual and gender minorities. As a result of the feelings of isolation and rejection and other unique stressors, this community faces a multitude of risk factors for experiencing mental health issues.

According to current literature, LGBTQ+ immigrants and refugees report high levels of mental health challenges, including issues with anxiety, depression, posttraumatic stress, and increased substance use, which can be attributed to home and host country discrimination and economic and environmental instability (e.g., housing insecurity, low social support, financial burdens).[10,11] Factors that contribute to the high prevalence of mental health issues could be mitigated if home and host countries stopped intentionally ignoring, excluding, and persecuting this community.

SOCIAL AND MENTAL RESPONSES

Although being transnational allows individuals to access resources from both their home and host countries, it also presents challenges from both sides. Even in a new country, safety is not guaranteed; the persecution of LGBTQ+ individuals in the United States remains evident, with numerous reports of hate crimes.[12] Furthermore, many states have enacted anti-LGBTQ+ policies that hinder progress toward inclusion and equity, highlighting the complex and perilous journey faced by these individuals.[13] In some states, such policies prohibit LGBTQ+-affirming curriculums in schools (which includes, e.g., book censorship) and exclude transgender students from sports teams. Notably, at the federal level, there are no laws that protect sexual and gender minorities from discrimination in public settings.

African LGBTQ+ immigrants face unique challenges that often make it harder for them to find safety and cope with persecution compared with other marginalized groups. Cultural norms and religious beliefs complicate their experience, as many come from backgrounds where homosexuality is stigmatized or condemned. This hostile environment forces them to create their own networks to gain essential support and refuge, so they often use social media platforms such as Clubhouse Facebook and WhatsApp group forums to connect with like-minded individuals across the diaspora.

Despite the potential for connection, many African LGBTQ+ immigrants find themselves in a "no-man's-land," caught between two worlds that often fail to offer safety, acceptance, and belonging. Research indicates that African immigrants generally have low utilization of mental health services,[14] and this is likely even lower among transnational African LGBTQ+ individuals because of distrust in these systems and cultural stigmas.

PATHWAYS TO HEALING AND ADVOCACY

In the host country, specific clinical and policy recommendations may promote the adequate provision of services to better address the needs of African LGBTQ+ immigrants. Clinical recommendations include using a trauma-informed and intersectional framework.[14] For health care professionals, one of the most important things to consider is the intersectional background of their patients. It is imperative that clinicians not provide conventional mental health avenues such as psychiatric therapy (e.g., cognitive behavioral therapy) and psychiatric medications (e.g., antidepressants) as the only solutions. Some transnational African LGBTQ+ immigrants are unaccustomed to actively seeking Western treatments to improve their mental health, so conventional medications and therapies may not be an avenue they will be familiar or comfortable with.[15] Consequently, if prescribed an unfamiliar remedy, the patient may misunderstand its use, question its effectiveness, or find it disruptive, leading to poor adherence and reduced health benefits.

So rather than insisting on these methods, clinicians should tailor recommendations to the transnational experience of African LGBTQ+ immigrants and provide appropriate paths for their holistic healing. Clinicians can practice patient-centered care to ensure high patient satisfaction and return to follow-ups. Because some African cultures use other healing and coping mechanisms, such as dancing,[16] building community, and engaging in spirituality practices,[15] to improve patient trust and promote holistic care, clinicians should prioritize the individual patient's needs and be willing to prescribe alternatives to conventional therapies. One way clinicians can demonstrate this is by familiarizing themselves with identity-affirming organizations and community support networks to refer patients to when needed.

Social support can be associated with spirituality—another key aspect of the unique transnational experience among African LGBTQ+ immigrants. Many either bring or reject their cultural and spiritual practices when they immigrate. Notably, religious leaders, groups, and institutions in many African countries do not support policies that promote the rights of LGBTQ+ individuals. In 2019, Ghanaian religious leaders successfully opposed a "comprehensive sexuality education" curriculum and had it removed from schools out of fear it would encourage youths to adopt more LGBTQ+ ideologies and dissent from existing socially acceptable moral codes.[17] Immigrating from a country that has widespread religious opposition to LGBTQ+ rights, African LGBTQ+ immigrants have unique and potentially complicated ties with their spirituality.

For those who seek solace in faith, finding a truly inclusive and identity-affirming religious group can "help foster social connections and promote resilience."[14] Persistent engagement with a supportive group and a continued routine of practicing one's faith may offer many psychosocial and mental health benefits. As a result, it becomes necessary for clinicians, social workers, and community members to be aware of this and promote LGBTQ+-affirming religious and spiritual organizations that may help African LGBTQ+ individuals build community.

Furthermore, the social determinants of health that critically affect African LGBTQ+ immigrants should be prioritized through multidisciplinary collaboration among public (government), private (for profit), and voluntary (e.g., nonprofit) health, housing, job, education, and legal sectors.[14] For example, host countries can improve immigration laws to extend access to quality health care services to all immigrants and assist with providing educational workshops and relevant information about this. The United States has taken one step toward this goal by introducing bill H.R. 5008: the HEAL for Immigrant Families Act of 2023.

In African countries, existing LGBTQ+-affirming organizations should continue their efforts and use any influence they have or that stakeholders who support them have to encourage transnational advocacy of LGBTQ+ rights within and outside their local area. There are several LGBTQ+ nongovernmental organizations and activists in African nations that produce and disseminate knowledge (e.g., research gaps on African sexuality) challenging harmful stereotypes and homophobic rhetoric; encourage open dialogue and discourse regarding the existence and protection of LGBTQ+ individuals in their country; and offer health-related services (e.g., for HIV/AIDS).[17,18] It is necessary for stakeholders and allies to continue to support and finance these nongovernmental organizations because they are single-handedly transforming their local political and social landscape, which has ramifications for regional, national, and global communities.

CONCLUSIONS

With the growing population of African immigrants and consequently LGBTQ+ African immigrants,[10] we urge the global community to acknowledge the mistreatment of African LGBTQ+ immigrants and urge key local and national actors to invest in their present and future. Educating oneself, particularly through partnership research and initiatives with African LGBTQ+ immigrants, on the intersectionality of sexual identity, race, gender, and immigration status and the unique stressors of this community is strongly encouraged. This intersectionality explains the transnational experience of African LGBTQ+ immigrants. Navigating homophobia and prejudice both in their host countries and from their home countries diminishes the overall physical, mental, spiritual, and psychosocial well-being of African LGBTQ+ immigrants. AJPH

CORRESPONDENCE

Correspondence should be sent to Kelechi Ibe-Lamberts, University of Illinois Chicago, School of Public Health, Community Health Sciences, 1603 W. Taylor St, Chicago, IL 60612 (e-mail: klamber4@uic.edu). Reprints can be ordered at https://www.ajph.org by clicking the "Reprints" link.

PUBLICATION INFORMATION

Full Citation: Ibe-Lamberts K, Onyeise D. The effects of LGBTQ+ persecution on transnational African immigrants. *Am J Public Health*. 2025;115(8): 1236–1239.

Acceptance Date: February 12, 2025.

DOI: https://doi.org/10.2105/AJPH.2025.308076

ORCID iDs:
Kelechi Ibe-Lamberts https://orcid.org/0000-0003-4324-6652

Destiny Onyeise https://orcid.org/0009-0008-9644-2247

CONTRIBUTORS

The authors contributed equally to writing the editorial.

CONFLICTS OF INTEREST

The authors have no conflicts of interest to disclose.

REFERENCES

1. Ssenyonjo M. Sexual orientation and the criminalisation of private consensual sexual acts between adults of the same gender. *Int Hum Rights Law Rev*. 2023;12(2):143–212. https://doi.org/10.1163/22131035-12020001
2. Novak A. *Transnational Human Rights Litigation: Challenging the Death Penalty and Criminalization of Homosexuality in the Commonwealth*. Cham, Switzerland: Springer International Publishing; 2020. https://doi.org/10.1007/978-3-030-28546-3
3. Bertolt B. The invention of homophobia in Africa. *J Arts Soc Sci Humanit*. 2019;5(3):651–659. https://doi.org/10.15520/jassh53418
4. Palarino JV. The immigrant health advantage: an examination of African-origin Black immigrants in the United States. *Popul Res Policy Rev*. 2021; 40(5):895–929. https://doi.org/10.1007/s11113-021-09647-6
5. Ibe-Lamberts K, Tshiwaka DI. The interplay between transnationalism and health behavior of African immigrants in America. In: Rodriquez S, ed. *Migrants: Public Attitudes, Challenges and Policy Implications*. Hauppauge, NY: Nova Science Publishers; 2017:29–58.
6. Vertovec S. Transnationalism and identity. *J Ethn Migr Stud*. 2001;27(4):573–582. https://doi.org/10.1080/13691830120090386
7. Robinson M, Ross LE. Gender and sexual minorities: intersecting inequalities and health. *Ethn Inequal Health Soc Care*. 2013;6(4):91–96. https://doi.org/10.1108/EIHSC-01-2014-0003
8. Bharat B, Chenneville T, Gabbidon K, Foust C. Considerations for psychological research with and for people of color and oppressed intersecting identities in the United States. *Transl Issues Psychol Sci*. 2021;7(4):363–377. https://doi.org/10.1037/tps0000285
9. Abreu RL, Gonzalez KA, Lindley L, Capielo Rosario C, Lockett GM, Teran M. "Why can't I have the office jobs?": immigrant Latinx transgender peoples' experiences with seeking employment. *J Career Dev*. 2023;50(1):20–36. https://doi.org/10.1177/08948453211062951
10. Ogunbajo A, Anyamele C, Restar AJ, Dolezal C, Sandfort TGM. Substance use and depression among recently migrated African gay and bisexual men living in the United States. *J Immigr Minor Health*. 2019;21(6):1224–1232. https://doi.org/10.1007/s10903-018-0849-8
11. Golembe J, Leyendecker B, Maalej N, Gundlach A, Busch J. Experiences of minority stress and mental health burdens of newly arrived LGBTQ* refugees in Germany. *Sex Res Soc Policy*. 2021; 18(4):1049–1059. https://doi.org/10.1007/s13178-020-00508-z
12. Coston L. Hate crimes against LGBT people in the United States. In: *Oxford Research Encyclopedia of Politics*. Oxford, UK: Oxford University Press; 2020. https://doi.org/10.1093/acrefore/9780190228637.013.1320
13. Fandel KJ. The consequences of homophobia: analysis of discriminatory medical and legislative policies and their influence on health disparities. 2024. Available at: https://red.library.usd.edu/honors-thesis/339. Accessed October 19, 2024.
14. D'souza F, Blatman Z, Wier S, Patel M. The mental health needs of lesbian, gay, bisexual, and transgender (LGBT) refugees: a scoping review. *J Gay Lesbian Ment Health*. 2022;26(4):341–366. https://doi.org/10.1080/19359705.2022.2109333
15. Moonsamy A, Gurayah T. Cultural perspectives and experiences of mental healthcare in Kwa-Zulu Natal, South Africa. *S Afr J Occup Ther*. 2024;54(1): 34–44. https://doi.org/10.17159/2310-3833/2024/vol54no1a5
16. Monteiro NM, Wall DJ. African dance as healing modality throughout the diaspora: the use of ritual and movement to work through trauma. *J Pan Afr Stud*. 2011;4(6):234–252.
17. Mogotsi I, Otchere YO, Botchway I, Muthoni Y, Gariseb R, Ramalepe LM. Psychosocial correlates of LGBTIQ+ experiences in selected African countries: reimagining LGBTIQ+ research. *J Soc Issues*. 2024;80(3):1079–1111. https://doi.org/10.1111/josi.12640
18. Moland N, Pizmony-Levy O. Rigid culture and social change: how African NGOs educate about LGBTI rights. *Comp Educ Rev*. 2024;68(2):212–237. https://doi.org/10.1086/729665

The Public Health Implications of Ghana's Anti-LGBTQ+ Bill: A Lesson From Nigeria

Eberechukwu Peace Akadinma, RN, MA, and Sean Hillier, PhD

ABOUT THE AUTHORS

Eberechukwu Peace Akadinma is a PhD student in the Health Policy Program, McMaster University, Hamilton, Ontario, Canada. Sean Hillier is with the Faculty of Health and the Centre for Indigenous Knowledges and Languages, York University, Toronto, Ontario, Canada.

See also Global LGBTQ+ Public Health in the Face of Legal Persecution, pp. 1229–1270.

AJPH August 2025, Vol. 115, No. 8

On February 28, 2024, Ghana's parliament passed a bill criminalizing the country's lesbian, gay, bisexual, transgender, and queer (LGBTQ+) community. Unlike Nigeria (often colloquially referred to as Ghana's sister country), whose anti-LGBTQ+ law primarily outlaws same-sex marriages, Ghana's new bill imposes punishments on all sexual and gender minorities. The bill seeks to punish the country's LGBTQ+ community and its allies with imprisonment, financial penalties, and other harsh punitive measures.[1] Since its passing, various international leaders have called on the president to veto the legislation,[2] with the country's finance minister emphasizing the potential adverse economic repercussions.[3] Recently the country's supreme court dismissed legal challenges against the bill, stating that the case could not be reviewed unless it became legislation.[4] The bill now awaits presidential approval to formalize its enactment into law.

Although it is worth exploring the interplay of culture, religion, and morality and how these factors act as both vehicles and drivers of anti-LGBTQ+ sentiment in the country, the lens that informs this work and the arguments it puts forward focuses exclusively on public health. In this work, we contend that Ghana's new bill must be seen for its potential public health consequences, particularly in terms of the country's efforts to mitigate HIV/AIDS and other sexually transmitted and bloodborne infections, and must therefore be vetoed. We draw parallels between Ghana and Nigeria given the similarities in the countries' histories—shaped by colonial legacies and homophobic laws—as well as evidence on the public health repercussions observed in Nigeria after the enactment of its anti-LGBTQ+ law. In addition, we urge Ghana to learn from Nigeria's mistakes for the future of its public health.

BACKGROUND

The criminalization of homosexuality in Ghana dates back to the Offenses Against the Person Act of 1861, introduced by the British colonial government, under which sodomy was punishable by 10 years of imprisonment to life in prison.[5] Three years after the country's independence, in 1960, Ghana introduced the Criminal Offenses Act, with section 104(1)(b) of the act criminalizing same-sex activity by categorizing it as "unnatural carnal knowledge."[5] Although that act was rarely enforced, Coleman et al.[6] noted that 2006 marked the first public debate on the threat homosexuality posed to Ghanaian society. This debate was sparked by a radio announcement from the Gay and Lesbian Association of Ghana that the country would host an international conference of gays and lesbians in its capital, Accra.[6]

In 2011, the debate regarding homosexuality in Ghana was again rekindled, partly as a result of threats from the United Kingdom and United States administrations to withdraw foreign aid support from African countries that failed to uphold LGBTQ+ rights.[6–8] Subsequent debates on criminalizing homosexuality in the country received little attention until 2021, shortly after the Ghanian legislature passed a resolution allowing for individual parliamentarians to introduce the Private Member's Bill.[9]

In any parliamentary system, bills are typically introduced by the executive branch of the government. However, a Private Member's Bill resolution allows individual members of parliament to introduce bills.[10] With the Private Member's Bill resolution in effect in 2021, Samuel George introduced the country's current anti-LGBTQ+ bill under the guise of "human sexual rights and Ghanaian family values." As Appiagyei-Atua[11] acutely noted, the bill's name is a stark irony as its contents, replete with biblical references, explicitly and unequivocally condemn the existence of LGBTQ+ individuals.[11] The bill asserts that not only is homosexuality foreign to Ghana, but it is also "taboo, inhuman, and alien"[1] to Ghanaian society. In addition, the bill highlights a perceived gap in the 1960 Criminal Offenses Act, which did not outlaw advocacy, claiming that such a gap allowed for LGBTQ+ advocates to "sponsor and promote the proliferation of those sexual activities."[1]

The bill further alleges instances in which "young persons are promised travel opportunities, allowances, and other gifts to cause them to engage in or advocate for LGBTTQQIAAP+."[1] The reasons for the bill's adoption of the acronym LGBTTQQIAAP+ (lesbian, gay, bisexual, transgender, transsexual, queer, questioning, intersex, asexual/aromantic, ally, and pansexual), despite its relatively limited usage, remains unclear. However, the intent behind its use is evident: to trivialize and ridicule sexual and gender diversity while simultaneously ensuring the comprehensive criminalization and prohibition of all sexual orientations and gender identities. Correspondingly, the bill calls for several punitive measures including imprisonment, disbanding of LGBTQ+ and advocacy groups, and even medical intervention for individuals who are intersex or questioning their gender identity.[1]

Since the bill's first introduction in 2021, several arbitrary police arrests have occurred, notably the arrest of 21 LGBTQ+ activists for organizing a meeting on human rights.[12] After its parliamentary hearing in 2022 and subsequent deliberations, the Ghanaian parliament passed the bill on February 28, 2024, and it now awaits presidential approval to be formally enacted into law. The likelihood that the bill will become law is high, as now-president John Mahama has expressed support for it, citing religious convictions.[13] If the bill is enacted, LGBTQ+ individuals and their allies in the country will face both state-sanctioned and extralegal punishments. Critics have characterized the bill as draconian, attributing its emergence to a confluence of factors including colonial legacies, religiosity, and political tensions.[14] Furthermore, as noted, the bill shares deep parallels with the history and climate of homophobia in Nigeria. Within this broader context emerges valuable lessons for Ghana regarding the impact of the forthcoming legislation on its public health system.

NIGERIA: A NATION BOUND IN UNFREEDOM

Akin to Ghana, the first anti-LGBTQ+ law in Nigeria dates back to the Criminal Code Act introduced by the British colonial government in 1914, which criminalized homosexuality with imprisonment of seven to 14 years.[15] However, the Same-Sex Marriage Prohibition Act (SSMPA) remains the focal point of conversations surrounding homosexuality in the country.[8]

Nigeria's anti-LGBTQ+ law resulted from a combination of local and global events.[8] For instance, the discourse on recriminalizing homosexuality in Nigeria began in the early 2000s, coinciding with trends in the criminalization or recriminalization of homosexuality across the continent, often described as a "wave of homophobia."[16] Likewise, at the national level, the enactment of anti-LGBTQ+ legislation in the country occurred alongside heightened religious campaigns against the LGBTQ+ community and coincided with the then president's bid for reelection.[8]

The SSMPA was first introduced in 2006 by Bayo Ojo, Nigeria's then minister of justice, but was rejected in 2007.[17] At the time, the bill proposed a five-year prison sentence for same-sex marriages.[17] In 2008 a revised bill was introduced, proposing a three-year jail sentence for people in same-sex relationships and a five-year sentence for aiding or witnessing a gay marriage.[17] Akanle et al.[17] noted that the 2008 bill not only criminalized homosexuals in the country but also failed to acknowledge same-sex marriages certified internationally. Then-president Goodluck Ebele Jonathan signed the SSMPA into law on December 17, 2013, and the legislation came into effect in 2014. The SSMPA carries penalties of 14 and 10 years of imprisonment, respectively, for the country's LGBTQ+ members and allies.[17]

Since the enactment of the SSMPA in Nigeria, several studies have demonstrated its debilitating impacts on the well-being and overall livability of LGBTQ+ individuals in the country.[18,19] For instance, immediately after the legalization of the SSMPA, Schwartz et al.[20] reported a 44.4% decrease in participation in baseline study procedures for HIV prevention and treatment services. The authors also observed an increase in individuals avoiding health care and reporting fear of seeking health care.[20] Similarly, Human Rights Watch[21] reported a decline in participation in HIV treatment programs, with HIV-positive individuals hesitant to pick up their antiretroviral medications.

Also, several other studies have shown a reluctance among men who have sex with men to test or seek treatment for HIV and other sexually transmitted and bloodborne infections as a result of fear of stigma and discrimination.[22,23] Although there is an overall downward trend in the incidence of HIV infections in the country, the prevalence of HIV among men who have sex with men and transgender individuals remains on the rise.[24] The public health consequences of Nigeria's legislation are a cautionary tale for Ghana regarding the likely impacts of its own discriminatory laws.

GHANA'S NEW BILL AND ITS PUBLIC HEALTH IMPLICATIONS

Since Ghana's passing of the new bill, various international leaders have called on the president to veto the legislation,[2] and, as noted, the country's finance minister has emphasized the potential adverse economic repercussions, including the possibility of losing $3.8 billion in World Bank financing over the next five to six years.[3] Although the concerns about potential economic repercussions are valid given the West's history of threatening African countries with aid withdrawal,[25] there are three critical weaknesses related to these concerns.

First, a closer look at Uganda and Nigeria reveals that threats to withdraw foreign aid are often hollow, with foreign aid increasing in some instances amid worsening violence against LGBTQ+ people.[26] Second, several studies have demonstrated that threatening to withdraw foreign aid is largely ineffective in ensuring compliance from recipient countries.[27,28] Third, foreign aid, as with the threat of its withdrawal, is a neocolonial and neoliberal machination to advance imperialism rather than genuine support.[8] Consequently, as research has demonstrated, the threat of aid withdrawal is often perceived by the receiving country as Western interference.[8] This perception further endangers LGBTQ+ individuals, who are construed as products of Westernization or, in the phrasing of Ghana's new bill, "threats of infiltration of foreign cultures."[1]

However, little has been said about the undeniable consequences the bill will have for Ghana's public health system, particularly its public health efforts to mitigate HIV/AIDS and other sexually transmitted and bloodborne infections. Ghana has made tremendous progress in eradicating HIV, including ratifying Project 95-95-95, the Joint United Nations Programme on HIV/AIDS initiative aimed at ensuring that, by 2025, 95% of HIV-positive individuals are aware of their status, 95% are on antiretroviral therapy, and 95% are successful in achieving viral suppression.[29] In addition, the country has implemented national HIV testing coverage to reduce the costs of HIV tests as well as an HIV self-testing program to enable citizens to check their status from the comfort of their homes.[29]

Despite these successes, the testing coverage rate among men who have sex with men is 26.6%,[29] a figure that is bound to worsen if the bill is formalized into law. Furthermore, the forthcoming legislation categorizes HIV as the "gay disease."[1] Although HIV/AIDS does not exclusively affect LGBTQ+ populations, such a categorization reveals the intersectional stigma that some LGBTQ+ people face as a result of their status as queer or living with HIV.[30] Moreover, women with HIV/AIDS in Ghana outnumber men with HIV/AIDS, and HIV transmission among women occurs largely through sexual contact with their male partners.[31] Considering the widespread gender inequality and moralization of HIV/AIDS in the country,[31] enacting the bill will increase challenges in accessing testing, treatment, and care for all people living with HIV or at high risk of HIV transmission, regardless of their sexual or gender orientation.

WAYS FORWARD: CALL TO ACTION

Considering the risks that Ghana's new bill poses to the country's public health, we present some actionable steps to mitigate its adverse effects on both individual and public health. Note that these steps are not exhaustive but are instead crucial starting points to be applied in Ghana, Nigeria, and elsewhere.

Now, more than ever, there is a need to strengthen both national and international LGBTQ+ alliances.[8] In the face of the ongoing erosion of sexual rights and freedoms, these organizations, with their skills and expertise, are uniquely positioned to organize, advocate, and push back against state-sponsored anti-LGBTQ+ sentiment.[32] Those in power must unite in solidarity with the LGBTQ+ community in Ghana and urge the country's leaders to reaffirm their commitment to protecting citizens' rights by vetoing the bill.

Correspondingly, there is an urgent need to advocate for legal protections for allied and health care providers who care for the LGBTQ+ community. Several health workers and peer educators in Nigeria have voiced concerns over the real threat of police arrests with respect to their ability to care for the LGBTQ+ community.[21] Although Ghana's new bill does not explicitly implicate medical workers, the indirect threat to health care providers is unmistakable, necessitating a need for guaranteed protection from legal consequences. Furthermore, as this new bill undermines public health efforts, health care professionals in the country face a significant challenge: any public health effort to mitigate HIV/AIDS in

AJPH August 2025, Vol. 115, No. 8

Ghana that does not contend with the bill is fundamentally defective.

Research demonstrates that nongovernmental organizations are the primary health care providers for sexual and gender minorities in countries with discriminatory laws, primarily because of the widespread fear of discrimination and stigma associated with their sexuality and, in some cases, their lack of access to dignity-based care.[33–35] This finding, then, underscores the urgent need to strengthen community-based health initiatives tailored to support and address the unique health needs of LGBTQ+ individuals.

Furthermore, in accordance with findings from studies in Nigeria highlighting the reluctance of sexual minority men to seek testing for sexually transmitted and bloodborne infections[22,23] alongside the broader psychosocial harms caused by the country's anti-LGBTQ+ law,[18,36] community-based health initiatives must prioritize comprehensive mental health and well-being support, HIV/AIDS prevention and treatment, and sexual and reproductive health services. In addition, these programs should include peer support networks and strategic outreach services to improve health care accessibility, especially for individuals who experience isolation and those who are reluctant to test and disclose their health status.[22]

Most important, we recognize Ghana's anti-LGBTQ+ bill as a product of misguided personal, religious, and political convictions. The focus on its potential economic repercussions is parochial; instead, a stronger emphasis must be placed on the personhood and rights of LGBTQ+ people in Ghana. Criminalizing a marginalized group is a blatant abuse of power and a violation of fundamental human rights. We call on the Ghanaian as well as the Nigerian government to abandon and repeal laws that dehumanize and endanger sexual and gender minorities and commit to protecting all citizens equally. The Nigerian and Ghanaian governments must ensure that laws are rooted in equality and human dignity principles. Recognizing and affirming the humanity of LGBTQ+ individuals is not only a moral and ethical duty but a necessary step toward building a society that values the personhood of all, regardless of their sexual orientation or gender identity. AJPH

CORRESPONDENCE

Correspondence should be sent to Eberechukwu Peace Akadinma, 1280 Main St W, Hamilton, Ontario, Canada L8S 4L8 (e-mail: akadinme@mcmaster.ca). Reprints can be ordered at https://www.ajph.org by clicking the "Reprints" link.

PUBLICATION INFORMATION

Full Citation: Akadinma EP, Hillier S. The public health implications of Ghana's anti-LGBTQ+ bill: a lesson from Nigeria. *Am J Public Health*. 2025; 115(8):1240–1244.

Acceptance Date: February 12, 2025.

DOI: https://doi.org/10.2105/AJPH.2025.308075

ORCID iDs:
Eberechukwu Peace Akadinma https://orcid.org/0000-0002-0111-2720

Sean Hillier https://orcid.org/0000-0003-3874-9212

CONTRIBUTORS

E. P. Akadinma contributed to writing, conceptualizing, drafting, editing, and revising. S. Hillier contributed to writing, drafting, editing, and revising.

ACKNOWLEDGMENTS

We thank Beverley Giblon for her generosity throughout the writing process. We also thank all of the peer reviewers for their intellectual acuity and generous reading of the article.

CONFLICTS OF INTEREST

The authors have no conflicts of interest to disclose.

REFERENCES

1. United Nations in Ghana. Draft bill on Proper Sexual Rights and Ghanaian Family Values Bill 2021: an analysis by UN independent human rights experts. Available at: https://ghana.un.org/en/139914-draft-bill-proper-sexual-rights-and-ghanaian-family-values-bill-2021-analysis-un-independent. Accessed March 13, 2024.
2. US Department of State. Ghanaian parliament's passage of legislation undermines human rights. Available at: https://www.state.gov/ghanaian-parliaments-passage-of-legislation-undermines-human-rights. Accessed November 12, 2024.
3. Africanews Ghana: finance ministry warns country stands to lose $3.8B over controversial anti-LGBTQ bill. Available at: https://www.africanews.com/2024/03/04/ghana-finance-ministry-warns-country-stands-to-lose-38-billion-over-controversial-anti-lgb. Accessed March 14, 2024.
4. BBC. Ghana anti-LGBT bill: supreme court dismisses legal challenges. Available at: https://www.bbc.com/news/articles/crrw2r8epw8o. Accessed December 25, 2024.
5. Atuguba RA. Homosexuality in Ghana: morality, law, human rights. *J Politics Law*. 2019;12(4):113. https://doi.org/10.5539/jpl.v12n4p113
6. Coleman TE, Ako EY, Kyerematen JG. A human rights critique of Ghana's Anti-LGBTIQ+ Bill of 2021. *Afr Hum Rights Law J*. 2023;23(1):96–125. https://doi.org/10.17159/1996-2096/2023/v23n1a5
7. Baisley E. Framing the Ghanaian LGBT rights debate: competing decolonisation and human rights frames. *Can J Afr Stud*. 2015;49(2):383–402. https://doi.org/10.1080/00083968.2015.1032989
8. Peace AE. A discursive attempt toward the political economy of homophobia in Nigeria. *J Hum Rights*. 2024;23(5):512–529. https://doi.org/10.1080/14754835.2024.2416123
9. Graphic Online. Private Member's Bill: key to parliamentary effectiveness. Available at: https://www.graphic.com.gh/features/opinion/private-member-s-bill-key-to-parliamentary-effectiveness.html. Accessed March 13, 2024.
10. Cavari A, Rosenthal M, Shpaizman I. Reevaluating the policy success of Private Members Bills. Available at: https://journals.sagepub.com/doi/full/10.1177/20531680231181750. Accessed March 13, 2024.
11. Appiagyei-Atua K. Ghana's new anti-homosexuality bill violates everyone's rights, not just LGBTIQ+ people. Available at: http://theconversation.com/ghanas-new-anti-homosexuality-bill-violates-everyones-rights-not-just-lgbtiq-people-expert-224888. Accessed March 12, 2024.
12. CBC Radio. 21 people were arrested in Ghana during an LGBTQ rights event. Advocates want them freed. Available at: https://www.cbc.ca/radio/asithappens/as-it-happens-the-wednesday-edition-1.6041507/21-people-were-arrested-in-ghana-during-an-lgbtq-rights-event-advocates-want-them-freed-1.6041510. Accessed March 13, 2024.
13. Reuters. Ghana's opposition leader expresses anti-LGBTQ stance ahead of December elections. Available at: https://www.reuters.com/world/africa/ghanas-opposition-leader-expresses-anti-lgbtq-stance-ahead-dec-elections-2024-01-31. Accessed December 25, 2024.
14. Human Rights Watch. Ghana: president should veto anti-LGBT bill. Available at: https://www.hrw.org/news/2024/03/05/ghana-president-should-veto-anti-lgbt-bill. Accessed March 12, 2024.
15. Sogunro AO. Advocacy, social control, and the criminalisation of same-sex relationships: the

evolution and enforcement of "anti-gay laws" in Nigeria. Available at: https://repository.up.ac.za/bitstream/handle/2263/78375/Sogunro_Advocacy_2020.pdf?sequence=1&isAllowed=y. Accessed March 12, 2024.

16. Thoreson RR. Troubling the waters of a 'wave of homophobia': political economies of anti-queer animus in sub-Saharan Africa. *Sexualities.* 2014;17(1–2):23–42. https://doi.org/10.1177/1363460713511098
17. Akanle O, Adejare GS, Fasuyi J. To what extent are we all humans? Of culture, politics, law and LGBT rights in Nigeria. In: Steyn M, Mpofu W, eds. *Decolonising the Human: Reflections From Africa on Difference and Oppression.* Wits University Press; 2021:46–64.
18. Ogunbajo A, Restar A, Edeza A, et al. Poor sleep health is associated with increased mental health problems, substance use, and HIV sexual risk behavior in a large, multistate sample of gay, bisexual and other men who have sex with men (GBMSM) in Nigeria, Africa. *Sleep Health.* 2020;6(5):662–670. https://doi.org/10.1016/j.sleh.2020.02.010
19. Giwa SAO, Logie CH, Karki KK, Makanjuola OF, Obiagwu CE. Police violence targeting LGBTIQ+ people in Nigeria: advancing solutions for a 21st century challenge. *Greenwich Soc Work Rev.* 2020;1(1):36–49. https://doi.org/10.21100/gswr.v1i1.1108
20. Schwartz SR, Nowak RG, Orazulike I, et al. The immediate effect of the Same-Sex Marriage Prohibition Act on stigma, discrimination, and engagement on HIV prevention and treatment services in men who have sex with men in Nigeria: analysis of prospective data from the TRUST cohort. *Lancet HIV.* 2015;2(7):e299–e306. https://doi.org/10.1016/S2352-3018(15)00078-8
21. Isaack W, Buchanan J. "Tell me where I can be safe": the impact of Nigeria's Same Sex Marriage (Prohibition) Act. Available at: https://www.hrw.org/report/2016/10/20/tell-me-where-i-can-be-safe/impact-nigerias-same-sex-marriage-prohibition-act. Accessed March 12, 2024.
22. Dirisu O, Sekoni A, Vu L, et al. 'I will welcome this one 101%, I will so embrace it': a qualitative exploration of the feasibility and acceptability of HIV self-testing among men who have sex with men (MSM) in Lagos, Nigeria. *Health Educ Res.* 2020;35(6):524–537. https://doi.org/10.1093/her/cyaa028
23. Rodriguez-Hart C, Bradley C, German D, et al. The synergistic impact of sexual stigma and psychosocial well-being on HIV testing: a mixed-methods study among Nigerian men who have sex with men. *AIDS Behav.* 2018;22(12):3905–3915. https://doi.org/10.1007/s10461-018-2191-5
24. World Health Organization. HIV country profiles. Available at: https://cfs.hivci.org. Accessed January 9, 2025.
25. Asongu SA, Nwachukwu JC. Is the threat of foreign aid withdrawal an effective deterrent to political oppression? Evidence from 53 African countries. *J Econ Issues.* 2017;51(1):201–221. https://doi.org/10.1080/00213624.2017.1287510
26. Comstock AL. Gay rights and US foreign aid: a look at Nigeria and Uganda. Available at: https://scholarworks.arcadia.edu/cgi/viewcontent.cgi?article=1014&context=agsjournal. Accessed January 9, 2025.
27. Dasandi N, Erez L. The flag and the stick: aid suspensions, human rights, and the problem of the complicit public. *World Dev.* 2023;168:106264. https://doi.org/10.1016/j.worlddev.2023.106264
28. McElhose R. Are threats to impose financial sanctions an effective approach for the United States to protect LGBTQ rights in Africa? *Emory Int Law Rev Recent Dev.* 2023;37:1.
29. Boakye DS, Adjorlolo S. Achieving the UNAIDS 95-95-95 treatment target by 2025 in Ghana: a myth or a reality? *Glob Health Action.* 2023;16(1):2271708. https://doi.org/10.1080/16549716.2023.2271708
30. Abubakari GM, Dada D, Nur J, et al. Intersectional stigma and its impact on HIV prevention and care among MSM and WSW in sub-Saharan African countries: a protocol for a scoping review. *BMJ Open.* 2021;11(8):e047280. https://doi.org/10.1136/bmjopen-2020-047280
31. Owusu AY. A gendered analysis of living with HIV/AIDS in the Eastern Region of Ghana. *BMC Public Health.* 2020;20(1):751. https://doi.org/10.1186/s12889-020-08702-9
32. Weiss ML, Bosia MJ, Blasius M, et al. *Global Homophobia: States, Movements, and the Politics of Oppression.* 1st ed. Champaign, IL: University of Illinois Press; 2013.
33. Ndione AG, Procureur F, Senne JN, et al. Sexuality-based stigma and access to care: intersecting perspectives between healthcare providers and men who have sex with men in HIV care centres in Senegal. *Health Policy Plan.* 2022;37(5):587–596. https://doi.org/10.1093/heapol/czac010
34. Holland CE, Papworth E, Billong SC, et al. Access to HIV services at non-governmental and community-based organizations among men who have sex with men (MSM) in Cameroon: an integrated biological and behavioral surveillance analysis. *PLoS One.* 2015;10(4):e0122881. https://doi.org/10.1371/journal.pone.0122881
35. Immigration and Refugee Board of Canada. The situation of sexual and gender minorities in Nigeria (2014–2018). Available at: https://irb.gc.ca:443/en/country-information/research/Pages/situation-gender-minorities-nigeria.aspx. Accessed February 10, 2023.
36. Ogunbajo A, Iwuagwu S, Williams R, et al. Experiences of minority stress among gay, bisexual, and other men who have sex with men (GBMSM) in Nigeria, Africa: the intersection of mental health, substance use, and HIV sexual risk behavior. *Glob Public Health.* 2021;16(11):1696–1710. https://doi.org/10.1080/17441692.2020.1834598

Transgender Women in India: A Syndemic and Intersectional Framework Addressing HIV Care Gaps

William Lodge II, PhD, MSc, Shruta Rawat, MSc, Alpana Dange, MS, MA, MPhil, Madina Agénor, ScD, MPH, Vivek R. Anand, MBA, Don Operario, PhD, Matthew J. Mimiaga, ScD, MPH, and Katie B. Biello, PhD, MPH

See also Global LGBTQ+ Public Health in the Face of Legal Persecution, pp. 1229–1270.

The prevalence of HIV among transgender women (TGW) in India is disproportionately high, estimated at 4% to 8% in comparison with the national average of 0.2%. Despite free antiretroviral therapy (ART) provided by the government, TGW encounter multilevel barriers—including stigma, poverty, and lack of gender-affirming care—that hinder HIV care access and retention. Existing behavioral frameworks fail to address the compounded effects of systemic oppression on the health of TGW with HIV in India.

We present a conceptual framework integrating syndemic theory and intersectionality to examine structural and syndemic factors shaping HIV care barriers. Informed by key informants—including TGW with HIV, community leaders, health providers, and Indian researchers—the framework highlights how systemic marginalization, particularly through discriminatory policies, shapes social position and exacerbates inequities in HIV care outcomes. It also underscores the role of community mobilization and collective action in overcoming these barriers.

The framework provides a foundation for interventions tailored to the needs of TGW. By centering community-driven strategies and addressing structural inequities, it offers a pathway to improve HIV care engagement and health outcomes among TGW in India. (*Am J Public Health.* 2025;115(8):1245–1253. https://doi.org/10.2105/AJPH.2025.308046)

AJPH August 2025, Vol. 115, No. 8

Transgender women (TGW) in India are individuals who identify as female and were assigned male at birth. This diverse community includes hijras, kinnars, and aravanis,[1] who hold unique cultural and spiritual roles in Hinduism and Islam across South Asia and are often recognized as a "third gender." Despite these important cultural identities, the term TGW is commonly used in national legal and policy contexts.[1–4]

India has the third-largest population of people with HIV, and TGW are disproportionately affected.[5] HIV prevalence among TGW in India is significantly higher than the national average of 0.2%, ranging from 4% to as high as 8%.[6,7] This disparity underscores the impact of intersecting structural barriers and social inequities on health outcomes. Although HIV can be managed with ongoing antiretroviral therapy (ART), achieving maximal benefit requires consistent engagement with the health care system and adherence to ART.[8] Adherence to prescribed ART reduces morbidity and mortality among people with HIV and lessens the likelihood of sexual transmission through maintenance of viral suppression.[9]

India's ART program is the second largest in the world and includes direct access to diagnostic facilities and free first-, second-, and third-line ART.[10] However, despite no-cost ART and expanded HIV testing, TGW experience significant structural and systemic barriers to engaging with these services.[11–13] ART coverage among TGW remains at 58%, far below the Joint United Nations Programme on HIV/AIDS target of 95%.[14]

One study of TGW and men who have sex with men reported that only 63% were fully adherent to ART (i.e., took 100% of prescribed doses).[13]

However, the study data were not stratified by gender, and there are no available data on viral suppression among TGW with HIV. Similarly, access to HIV prevention tools such as oral preexposure prophylaxis and postexposure prophylaxis is limited because they are not yet widely available or affordable, further exacerbating gaps in the HIV care continuum.[15] Integrating prevention as a key component of HIV care requires addressing these structural and operational barriers to ensure equitable access to and affordability of HIV prevention tools among TGW.[15] Given the high HIV prevalence among TGW in India, more research is needed to explore both the barriers to and supportive factors needed to improve HIV care outcomes in this population.

TGW in India face multilevel structural and psychosocial factors such as substance use, stigma, and poverty that cluster and interact. The clustering of these adverse health conditions is consistent with the concept of syndemics ("synergistic epidemics"), which worsen access to and engagement and retention in HIV care.[16] These systemic factors, in tandem with power dynamics and privilege through an intersectional lens, are crucial to examine given that such an assessment will contribute to a deeper understanding of HIV care outcomes among TGW.

Moreover, HIV responses have historically failed to address the unique needs of TGW.[17] For example, India's National AIDS Control Organization initially categorized TGW under the broader umbrella of men who have sex with men, failing to recognize the unique social and health care needs of TGW. It was not until 2006 that the organization introduced targeted HIV interventions specifically for TGW.[18] The earlier misclassification exemplifies how structural determinants—rooted in transphobia and exclusion—have hindered the development of effective health care responses. Even with targeted interventions now in place, societal and institutional barriers continue to impede access to and engagement in HIV care.[6]

Intersectionality offers a critical lens to examine syndemic factors in relation to HIV care outcomes by exploring how systems of oppression affect social positions, producing inequalities that contribute to syndemic factors and socioeconomic marginalization that drive disparities along the HIV care continuum.[19] Systems of oppression such as colonialism and transphobia have long-term ramifications for the social landscape of TGW in India. For example, colonialism and transphobia can be traced to the British colonial era when the Criminal Tribes Act of 1871 led to the criminalization and denial of civil rights.[20] Although the Supreme Court of India recognized transgender people as a "third gender" in 2014 and granted them entitlements such as education, housing, employment, and voting rights,[21] this historical precedent continues to influence cultural and societal values, resulting in social exclusion and discrimination that contribute to the increased disparities in HIV outcomes among TGW with HIV.[11,22–25]

Despite the availability of free ART through India's expansive program, significant barriers continue to impede access and adherence among TGW. The absence of data disaggregated by gender and the lack of published research on viral suppression among TGW underscore the need for more targeted investigations. Existing HIV care frameworks fall short of addressing the historical, legal, and cultural complexities affecting TGW.[26] To bridge this gap—in collaboration with TGW, community activists, and Indian researchers working directly with the TGW community—we propose a new, pragmatic framework that integrates the multifaceted barriers faced by TGW in India, accounts for intersecting systems of oppression, and aims to enhance HIV care engagement and retention.

THEORETICAL FOUNDATION

Our framework integrates 2 theoretical frameworks—syndemic theory and intersectionality—to provide a comprehensive understanding of the multilevel barriers that affect HIV care outcomes among TGW with HIV in India.

Syndemic Theory

Syndemic theory provides an approach to examine the role of these multilevel risk factors affecting HIV care outcomes among TGW. According to syndemic theory, various social constructs such as poverty and discrimination are intertwined with multiple concurrent adverse health conditions such as mental health disorders and substance use that magnify their effects on health vulnerability and disease severity.[27–29]

The theory has been used in India to explore HIV risk among gender and sexual minority groups and to inform interventions.[18,22,29–32] For instance, Chakrapani et al. found that TGW with a clustering of syndemic factors such as depression, alcohol use, and experiences of violence had higher odds of inconsistent condom use in the preceding month than those with no syndemic factors.[32] Although that study focused on HIV-related risk behaviors rather than HIV care outcomes, we can theorize how similar syndemic factors can also create barriers to accessing consistent treatment and adhering to ART, suggesting that syndemic theory could be applied to explore these challenges in future research in India.

Studies from other regions offer a clearer picture of how syndemic factors directly affect HIV care. For example, studies in the United States and Latin America have shown that psychosocial syndemic factors are associated with suboptimal ART adherence and detectable viral loads among men with HIV who have sex with men.[33–40] However, no studies to our knowledge have focused specifically on TGW living with HIV. Still, syndemic theory can be crucial in helping researchers and practitioners understand how to make meaningful improvements in HIV care.

Intersectionality

Syndemic theory has been criticized for its limited emphasis on social positions or historical contexts that drive health inequities.[41] Intersectionality addresses this gap by providing a more comprehensive examination of how multiple, intersecting social positions such as caste, gender, religion, and perceived skin color are situated within broader systems of power and privilege.[19]

Coined by Kimberlé Crenshaw, an African American legal scholar, this concept originated in Black feminist scholarship.[42] Intersectionality was pivotal in mobilizing women of color during the late 1960s and 1970s, especially within the Black feminist movement in the United States.[43] Its principles extend globally. The work of 19th-century Dalit social reformer Savitribai Phule and her advocacy against caste and gender discrimination in India exemplify the theory's broader relevance.[43]

Intersectionality has been used more broadly in social epidemiology and behavioral sciences to describe how these intersecting social positions are directly reflected in and informed by systems of power at the structural level (specifically in public health), leading to health inequities.[44] It has been used to help explain how TGW in India experience different HIV care outcomes on the basis of their social positions and these power structures.[11,45] More than a framework, it is a praxis aimed at dismantling oppressive systems through social justice.[46] Addressing barriers to HIV care through this lens also requires considering ways to break power structures as a means of improving HIV care outcomes among TGW.

Combining Theory and Intersectionality

A deeper examination of syndemic and intersectionality perspectives is crucial to unraveling the complex barriers to HIV care among TGW with HIV in India. Syndemic theory explains the clustering and interaction of psychosocial and contextual factors that give rise to health inequity. Still, it has been criticized for prioritizing biomedical factors while overlooking structural determinants such as power dynamics, historical trauma, and structural violence.[40] This limits its ability to address the deeper systems of oppression, such as colonialism and transphobia, that shape the health outcomes of TGW in India.

Conversely, intersectionality examines how multiple social positions intersect to create unique forms of marginalization but does not fully capture how these intersections interact with health outcomes. By combining syndemic theory with intersectionality, we and other scholars aim to address contextual and psychosocial clustering and the broader structural determinants rooted in systems of oppression that drive poor health outcomes.[19,47]

FRAMEWORK DEVELOPMENT

The development of our framework followed a community-engaged approach, integrating insights from key informants including health care experts providing health services to TGW, researchers, and TGW with HIV. To ensure that the framework was grounded in the realities of TGW in India, we conducted multiple feedback sessions in Mumbai and New Delhi with one of India's oldest lesbian, gay, bisexual, transgender, and queer community-based organizations. This participatory process provided essential input to shape several critical aspects of the framework, making it more relevant and reflective of lived experiences.

For example, a researcher with expertise in intersectionality and gender minorities suggested that we

> separate historically contingent systems of oppression (e.g., colonialism, capitalism, heteropatriarchy) and social inequities (e.g., religious discrimination, colorism, transphobia) with bidirectional arrows between these 2 boxes.

We restructured the framework by differentiating historically contingent systems from social inequities, highlighting their dynamic interaction with and influence on HIV care outcomes among TGW.

Feedback also emphasized the role of structural barriers in accessing ART.

According to a community member and activist,

> At the structural level, poverty as well as sociolegal and policy-level barriers are [having an impact]. . . . Lack of antidiscrimination laws will lead to TGW living in suboptimal housing and [having] inadequate access to clean water, triggering illnesses that affect health and adherence.

This observation was incorporated by demonstrating how sociolegal barriers and poverty contribute to syndemic conditions and ART adherence challenges, adding pathways to the framework from structural determinants to multilevel syndemic factors.

A community member and researcher who works with TGW highlighted the importance of acknowledging capitalism's role in the marginalization of TGW. According to that individual, "With capitalism, we would need to include points that draw an association between capitalism in Indian contexts and transphobia." This prompted us to elaborate further on how capitalist structures contribute to the social and economic marginalization of TGW, driving health inequities within the framework.

We also added internalized transphobia as an individual-level syndemic factor on the basis of the suggestion of a researcher and community activist who asked "At the individual level, would we also need to explore internalized transphobia as a contributing factor to syndemic conditions?" This addition allowed the framework to account for how internalized oppression affects health outcomes among TGW.

Finally, a TGW with HIV provided a nuanced perspective on caste:

> First of all, if I am a kinnar, if I am a transgender, then I don't belong to any caste. I am human, and everybody looks at me with this attitude only, and they all give me sympathy. They all respect me and worship me like a God.

The caste system, an ancient Hindu system, divided people into categories based on their occupations, such as the Brahmins (priests, teachers), Kshatriyas (warriors, rulers), Vaishyas (traders, merchants), Shudras (laborers), and Dalits, who were outside of the stratification (i.e., street sweepers, latrine cleaners).[48,49] This insight challenged our initial understanding of caste dynamics, suggesting that hijras and kinnars experience castes differently because of their cultural and spiritual significance. However, we retained caste within the framework to acknowledge the diversity of experiences among TGW. Further discussions revealed that although caste may not be as relevant for hijras or kinnars, it could significantly affect TGW, who do not belong to these traditional communities.

These inputs were gathered through in-person feedback sessions and comments on the development of the conceptual framework, ensuring that the framework was co-developed with and validated by community members and key stakeholders.

COMPONENTS OF THE CONCEPTUAL FRAMEWORK

Our conceptual framework illustrates the relationships among structural determinants (i.e., socioeconomic and political contexts) that are affected by systems of oppression, forming intersecting social positions rooted in inequities. These inequities have an impact on syndemic factors that contribute to suboptimal HIV care outcomes (e.g., HIV testing, access to ART, ART adherence, and viral suppression) among TGW with HIV in India (Figure 1).

HIV care outcomes represent key milestones in the continuum of care. For TGW with HIV in India, consistent HIV testing ensures early diagnosis, access to ART facilitates timely treatment, adherence to ART maintains optimal health, and viral suppression reduces morbidity, mortality, and onward transmission. However, as shown in Figure 1, each outcome is shaped by intersecting barriers, underscoring the need for targeted interventions to address these disparities and a conceptual framework to guide them in the context of India.

Structural Determinants

When considering systems of oppression and their relationship to structural determinants, we adapted the Conceptual Framework for Action on the Social Determinants of Health to fit within the Indian context,[50] following Yearby's reconfiguration of a similar framework in the United States. Yearby emphasized the importance of addressing the root causes of health disparities, including structural racism.[51] This adaption is crucial for understanding how intersecting systems of oppression—such as colonialism and transphobia—operate within India, producing and perpetuating health inequities among TGW.

Our adaptation includes 4 key domains: governance, social policies, public policy, and cultural and societal values. These determinants are interdependent and work in tandem to produce and reproduce social inequities that directly affect people's social positions.[43,46] By integrating the root causes of health disparities, colonialism, and transphobia, we underscore the role of these structural determinants in sustaining the marginalization of TGW. Colonial discriminatory policies such as

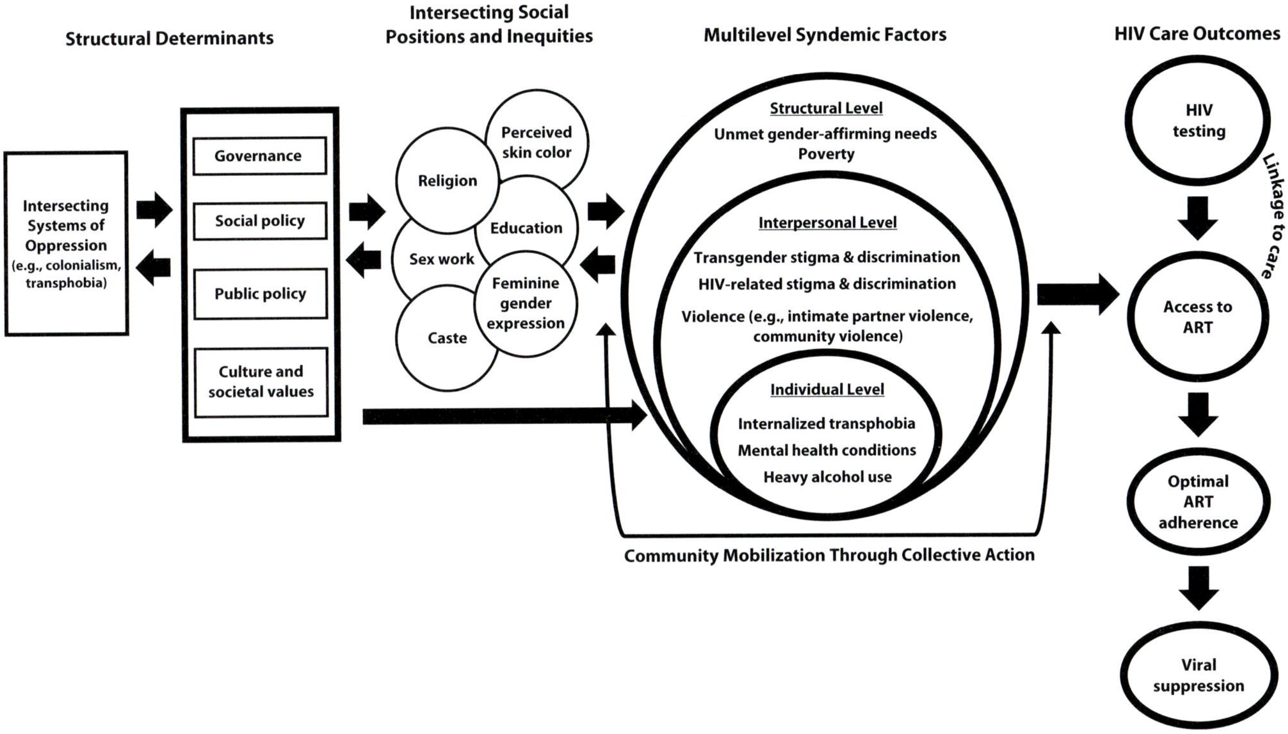

FIGURE 1— Syndemic and Intersectional Conceptual Framework Addressing HIV Care Gaps Among Transgender Women in India

Note. ART = antiretroviral therapy.

the Criminal Tribes Act of 1871 criminalized TGW, subjecting them to systematic discrimination. Their social positions and inequities were marked by social exclusion rooted in colonial-era policies that restricted their access to employment, education, and positions within the government.[1,52,53]

Intersecting Social Positions and Inequities

Intersecting social positions and inequities refer to the individual-level identities and social positions that intersect to shape the lived experiences of TGW. Broader structural determinants influence these positions, with a focus on how individual identities and inequities interact to affect health outcomes. In India, these intersecting social positions among TGW with HIV include caste, religion, occupation, skin tone, feminine gender expression, and education.[1] We selected these social positions for our framework because they mark precise fractions within the TGW community, often treated as a homogeneous population.[1] TGW with HIV are a diverse population made up of different religions (e.g., Hindu, Muslim), castes (e.g., Brahmins, Dalits), feminine gender expressions (i.e., ability to pass), skin tones (e.g., fair, dark), and employment status categories (e.g., sex work, traditional work called *badhai* [i.e., clapping one's hands and asking for alms]).[1]

For instance, although some TGW engage in sex work or begging as a means of survival, not all do. The bidirectional relationship between structural determinants and intersecting social positions is evident through the continued stigma and discrimination that limit opportunities for some TGW. As an example, sex work is technically legal, but the Immoral Traffic Prevention Act of 1959 renders certain activities punishable. These activities include brothel keeping, living off the earnings of sex work, and solicitation in areas in proximity to public places.[54] Under this legislation, TGW who depend on sex work for their livelihood remain vulnerable to arrest by law enforcement when they are found soliciting in public spaces or during police raids on hotels. Such laws further reinforce the historical discrimination against TGW.

Multilevel Syndemic Factors

In our conceptual framework, we intentionally incorporate syndemics within a socioecological approach, recognizing that multiple levels—individual, interpersonal, structural—intersect and cluster to magnify their impact on health outcomes.[55] Studies have shown that TGW in India face numerous barriers that contribute to poor health outcomes, including heavy alcohol use, mental health conditions, and internalized transphobia.[32,56,57] Interpersonal barriers such as stigma and discrimination related to TGW identity and HIV status as well as violence, including intimate partner violence and community and police violence, further compound health risks among TGW.[11,22,23,25]

Structural-level factors, such as unmet gender-affirming needs and poverty, are influenced by discrimination and stigma driven by structural determinants, which in turn have a direct impact on syndemic factors. For instance, despite the 2019 Transgender Protection Act's provisions against discrimination in education, employment, and property transactions, its lack of penalties and exclusion of civil and economic rights render it ineffective.[11,13,23–25,57] Similarly, health care stigma and discrimination experienced by TGW in India, as noted by Arora et al. and Chakrapani et al., exacerbate issues related to intersectional stigma based on social positions such as caste, sex work status, HIV, lack of gender affirmation, lack of education, and transgender identity, leading to inadequate access to and engagement in HIV care and treatment.[11,45] Understanding how these multilevel syndemic factors cluster and interact in the context of intersectionality at each level is crucial in providing interventions that can improve ART adherence and viral suppression in the HIV care cascade.

Community Mobilization Through Collective Action

Our model highlights ways to resist the impact of intersecting social positions on syndemic factors. It further helps in examining how these multilevel syndemic factors affect HIV care outcomes among TGW with HIV. Through its strengths-based approach, the framework effectively identifies protective factors against suboptimal HIV care outcomes and helps foster evidence-informed interventions.[58] This approach leverages existing social relationships (e.g., social support, volunteerism, activism) to combat stigma and improve health and well-being.[59]

In India, studies have indicated that social support systems can offer emotional, monetary, and psychosocial support to overcome multiple and intersecting forms of stigma.[60] Using a strengths-based approach, we offer a tool for others to examine multiple forms of resistance at the individual, interpersonal, and structural levels. In our conceptual framework, we call for moving away from social support and resilience as a unit of measure to using more actionable steps that inform interventions addressing barriers to HIV care that we see manifested in community mobilization.[61–63]

In many studies examining resilience and social support, findings often fall short of providing practitioners with actionable, scalable, cost-effective, and time-bound steps, as most studies define resilience at the individual level.[64] Our framework addresses this limitation by focusing on community mobilization through collective action. This includes engaging in lesbian, gay, bisexual, and transgender programs; pride events; support groups; and similar initiatives. Collective action is a form of community participation and resistance in which TGW work to improve the status and well-being of their community, which is crucial for effective community mobilization.[65,66]

For example, recent policies in India, such as the Support for Marginalized Individuals for Livelihood and Enterprise scheme, provide crucial support to TGW by offering scholarships, skill development programs, medical facilities, counseling services, and economic opportunities outside of sex work and begging.[67] However, if HIV care interventions incorporated peer navigation to ensure that TGW are accessing these governmental services—especially when education and literacy rates are low—it could significantly improve their engagement with the services and, consequently, enhance HIV care outcomes.[3] Peer navigators could help bridge the gap, ensuring that TGW can fully utilize the services designed to support them. By incorporating community mobilization into our framework, we acknowledge existing policies and encourage researchers and practitioners to focus on raising awareness and helping TGW benefit from these schemes. Community mobilization through collective action is essential for resisting barriers and improving health outcomes among TGW.

CONCLUSION

Our framework integrates syndemic theory and intersectionality to provide an understanding of barriers to ART adherence and viral suppression, highlighting how structural determinants and social positions affect multilevel syndemic factors. Intersectionality inherently addresses multilevel factors by conceptualizing how various systems of power and oppression intersect to shape lived experiences; our framework extends this conceptualization by explicitly focusing on how structural determinants and social positions affect multilevel syndemic factors specific to HIV care.

Furthermore, our conceptual framework is not merely an application of intersectionality but a novel approach that combines this perspective with syndemic theory to highlight the specific ways these barriers manifest, providing a deeper understanding of how to design targeted interventions and policies. Moreover, the use of community mobilization within the framework emphasizes the role of resistance and community action in overcoming such barriers. Developing interventions that leverage existing schemes such as Support for Marginalized Individuals for Livelihood and Enterprise and facilitate the access of TGW to these services encourages community mobilization through education and navigation, which may mitigate the impact of social positions on syndemic factors and the influence of syndemic factors on HIV care outcomes.

This framework has limitations. It requires empirical validation through both quantitative and qualitative studies. Although initial discussions with community partners and the existing literature have informed the framework, rigorous testing is necessary. The broad nature of our framework allows researchers and practitioners to focus on discrete pathways, such as the role of syndemic factors in ART adherence and the impact of structural determinants on HIV testing, while still acknowledging the overarching systems of power, including colonialism and transphobia, that shape these dynamics.

In addition, our framework was developed with input from key informants in New Delhi and Mumbai, 2 major cities with robust HIV diagnosis and treatment programs. However, it is important to note that the framework may need to be adapted in rural areas. Despite these limitations, the framework underscores the importance of understanding and addressing complex gender identities shaped by historical and social contexts.

Embedded in our conceptual framework are recommendations for advancing global health research and practice, specifically with respect to TGW with HIV and their engagement with HIV care. First, it is essential to consider the historical discrimination and stigma stemming from colonial exclusionary and discriminatory policies that continue to affect TGW with HIV. Second, HIV research often treats TGW in India as a monolith. By highlighting intersecting social positions and inequities, we advocate for research, interventions, and policies that account for these differences. Finally, although self-efficacy and resilience are important, our framework aims to draw attention to the need for community mobilization through peer navigation and community groups. By further exploring and validating this framework, we can make significant progress in addressing the disparities in HIV care faced by TGW, ultimately improving their quality of life. AJPH

ABOUT THE AUTHORS

William W. Lodge II is with the Jeb E. Brooks School of Public Policy, Cornell University, Ithaca, NY. At the time of this study, Shruta Rawat, Alpana Dange, and Vivek R. Anand were with The Humsafar Trust, Mumbai, Maharashtra, India. Madina Agénor is with the Department of Behavioral and Social Health Sciences, Brown University School of Public Health, Providence, RI. Don Operario is with the Department of Behavioral, Social, and Health Education Sciences, Emory University Rollins School of Public Health, Atlanta, GA. Matthew J. Mimiaga is with the Department of Epidemiology, Fielding School of Public Health, University of California, Los Angeles. Katie B. Biello is with the Department of Epidemiology, Brown University School of Public Health, Providence, RI.

CORRESPONDENCE

Correspondence should be sent to William Lodge II, PhD, MSc, Cornell University, Jeb E. Brooks School of Public Policy, 116 Reservoir Ave, MVR 2215, Ithaca, NY 14853 (e-mail: william.lodge@cornell.edu). Reprints can be ordered at https://www.ajph.org by clicking the "Reprints" link.

PUBLICATION INFORMATION

Full Citation: Lodge II W, Rawat S, Dange A, et al. Transgender women in India: a syndemic and intersectional framework addressing HIV care gaps. *Am J Public Health*. 2025;115(8):1245–1253.

Acceptance Date: January 25, 2025.

DOI: https://doi.org/10.2105/AJPH.2025.308046

ORCID iDs:

William Lodge II https://orcid.org/0000-0001-7058-2710

Katie B. Biello https://orcid.org/0000-0002-5017-5699

CONTRIBUTORS

W. Lodge II conceptualized the study and developed the framework. W. Lodge II and S. Rawat conducted key informant meetings that informed the framework's development. S. Rawat, A. Dange, and V. R. Anand contributed to the contextualization of the framework within the Indian health care landscape. M. Agénor and D. Operario provided critical revisions to strengthen the theoretical and methodological foundations. M. J. Mimiaga and K. B. Biello provided oversight and guidance on the conceptualization of the framework and the preparation of the article. All of the authors reviewed the final version of the article.

ACKNOWLEDGMENTS

We thank Jatin Chaudary and the study team at The Humsafar Trust for their valuable input on an earlier iteration of the conceptual model. We also extend our gratitude to the key informants—including researchers, activists, health care providers, and transgender women with HIV—who provided invaluable insights that informed the development of this framework.

CONFLICTS OF INTEREST

The authors have no conflicts of interest to disclose.

HUMAN PARTICIPANT PROTECTION

This study did not involve the collection of individual-level data but rather the development of a conceptual framework informed by key informant meetings. These discussions were conducted as part of a broader research collaboration and focused solely on participants' professional and expert opinions; no personal data were collected. As such, Brown University institutional review board review and approval were not required, as the key informant interviews did not meet the criteria for human participant research under the university's guidelines.

REFERENCES

1. Chakrapani V. Hijras/transgender women in India: HIV, human rights and social exclusion. Available at: https://www.undp.org/india/publications/hijras/transgender-india-hiv-human-rights-and-social-exclusion. Accessed September 6, 2024.

2. Jain D, Aher A, Shaikh S, Sarkar A, Tronic B. Negotiating violence: everyday queer experiences of the law. *Violence Gend.* 2020;7(4):141–149. https://doi.org/10.1089/vio.2020.0002
3. Dixit V, Garg B, Mehta N, Kaur H, Malhotra R. The third gender in a third world country: major concerns and the "AIIMS Initiative." *J Hum Rights Soc Work.* 2023;8(2):1–6. https://doi.org/10.1007/s41134-023-00238-3
4. Dutta A. An epistemology of collusion: hijras, kothis and the historical (dis)continuity of gender/sexual identities in eastern India. *Gend Hist.* 2012;24(3):825–849. https://doi.org/10.1111/j.1468-0424.2012.01712.x
5. National AIDS Control Organization. HIV estimates: 2023 factsheets. Available at: https://naco.gov.in/sites/default/files/HIV%20Estimates%202023%20Factsheets.pdf. Accessed August 26, 2024.
6. National AIDS Control Organization. White paper on comprehensive health related services for transgender persons. Available at: https://naco.gov.in/sites/default/files/Whitepaper_on_Transgender_Persons_Health.pdf. Accessed August 26, 2024.
7. National AIDS Control Organization. HIV sentinel surveillance 2016–17: technical brief. Available at: http://naco.gov.in/sites/default/files/HIV%20SENTINEL%20SURVEILLANCE_06_12_2017_0.pdf. Accessed August 26, 2024.
8. National AIDS Control Organization, Government of India. Annual report 2016–17. Available at: https://naco.gov.in/sites/default/files/NACO%20ANNUAL%20REPORT%202016-17.pdf. Accessed August 26, 2024.
9. Cohen MS, Chen YQ, McCauley M, et al. Prevention of HIV-1 infection with early antiretroviral therapy. *N Engl J Med.* 2011;365(6):493–505. https://doi.org/10.1056/NEJMoa1105243
10. National AIDS Control Organization. Prevention progress update 2020–21. Available at: https://naco.gov.in/sites/default/files/Prevention_Progress_Update.pdf. Accessed August 26, 2024.
11. Chakrapani V, Gulfam FR, Arumugam V, et al. Intersectional stigma and gender non-affirmation hinder HIV care engagement among transgender women living with HIV in India. *AIDS Care.* 2022;35(4):572–580. https://doi.org/10.1080/09540121.2022.2099511
12. Beattie TSH, Bhattacharjee P, Suresh M, Isac S, Ramesh BM, Moses S. Personal, interpersonal and structural challenges to accessing HIV testing, treatment and care services among female sex workers, men who have sex with men and transgenders in Karnataka state, South India. *J Epidemiol Community Health.* 2012:66(suppl 2):ii42–ii48. https://doi.org/10.1136/jech-2011-200475
13. Piña C, Dange A, Rawat S, et al. Antiretroviral treatment uptake and adherence among men who have sex with men and transgender women with HIV in Mumbai, India: a cross-sectional study. *J Assoc Nurses AIDS Care.* 2018;29(2):310–316. https://doi.org/10.1016/j.jana.2017.10.001
14. Joint United Nations Programme on HIV/AIDS. Key population atlas. Available at: https://kpatlas.unaids.org/dashboard. Accessed September 6, 2024.
15. Goswami S, Borate S, Marupuru S, Marupuru S. A scoping review of the current landscape of pre- and postexposure prophylaxis in India. *AIDS Patient Care STDS.* 2024;38(7):287–304. https://doi.org/10.1089/apc.2024.0078
16. Singer M, Clair S. Syndemics and public health: reconceptualizing disease in bio-social context. *Med Anthropol Q.* 2003;17(4):423–441. https://doi.org/10.1525/maq.2003.17.4.423
17. Poteat T, German D, Flynn C. The conflation of gender and sex: gaps and opportunities in HIV data among transgender women and MSM. *Glob Public Health.* 2016;11(7–8):835–848. https://doi.org/10.1080/17441692.2015.1134615
18. Chakrapani V, Lakshmi PVM, Newman PA, et al. Syndemic violence victimization, alcohol and drug use, and HIV transmission risk behavior among HIV-negative transgender women in India: a cross-sectional, population-based study. *PLOS Glob Public Health.* 2022;2(10):e0000437. https://doi.org/10.1371/journal.pgph.0000437
19. Quinn KG. The relationship between syndemics and intersectionality: a response to the commentary by Sangaramoorthy and Benton. *Soc Sci Med.* 2022;295:113784. https://doi.org/10.1016/j.socscimed.2021.113784
20. Singh H, Kumar P. Hijra: an understanding. *J Psychosom Res.* 2020;15(1):77–87. https://doi.org/10.32381/JPR.2020.15.01.6
21. Rao KS. *Do We Care?* Oxford University Press; 2017.
22. Chakrapani V, Newman PA, Shunmugam M, Logie CH, Samuel M. Syndemics of depression, alcohol use, and victimisation, and their association with HIV-related sexual risk among men who have sex with men and transgender women in India. *Glob Public Health.* 2017;12(2):250–265. https://doi.org/10.1080/17441692.2015.1091024
23. Willie TC, Chakrapani V, Hughto JMW, Kershaw TS. Victimization and human immunodeficiency virus-related risk among transgender women in India: a latent profile analysis. *Violence Gend.* 2017;4(4):121–129. https://doi.org/10.1089/vio.2017.0030
24. Ganju D, Saggurti N. Stigma, violence and HIV vulnerability among transgender persons in sex work in Maharashtra, India. *Cult Health Sex.* 2017;19(8):903–917. https://doi.org/10.1080/13691058.2016.1271141
25. Shaw SY, Lorway R, Bhattacharjee P, et al. Descriptive epidemiology of factors associated with HIV infections among men and transgender women who have sex with men in South India. *LGBT Health.* 2016;3(4):292–299. https://doi.org/10.1089/lgbt.2015.0023
26. Keene CM, Euvrard J, Amico KR, et al. Conceptualising engagement with HIV care for people on treatment: the Indicators of HIV Care and AntiRetroviral Engagement (InCARE) Framework. *BMC Health Serv Res.* 2023;23(1):435. https://doi.org/10.1186/s12913-023-09433-4
27. Oldenburg CE, Biello KB, Colby D, et al. Stigma related to sex work among men who engage in transactional sex with men in Ho Chi Minh City, Vietnam. *Int J Public Health.* 2014;59(5):833–840. https://doi.org/10.1007/s00038-014-0562-x
28. Tsai AC, Burns BFO. Syndemics of psychosocial problems and HIV risk: a systematic review of empirical tests of the disease interaction concept. *Soc Sci Med.* 2015;139:26–35. https://doi.org/10.1016/j.socscimed.2015.06.024
29. Chakrapani V, Kaur M, Tsai AC, Newman PA, Kumar R. The impact of a syndemic theory-based intervention on HIV transmission risk behaviour among men who have sex with men in India: pretest-posttest non-equivalent comparison group trial. *Soc Sci Med.* 2022;295:112817. https://doi.org/10.1016/j.socscimed.2020.112817
30. Tomori C, McFall AM, Solomon SS, et al. Is there synergy in syndemics? Psychosocial conditions and sexual risk among men who have sex with men in India. *Soc Sci Med.* 2018;206:110–116. https://doi.org/10.1016/j.socscimed.2018.03.032
31. Chakrapani V, Kaur M, Newman PA, Mittal S, Kumar R. Syndemics and HIV-related sexual risk among men who have sex with men in India: influences of stigma and resilience. *Cult Health Sex.* 2018;21(4):416–431. https://doi.org/10.1080/13691058.2018.1486458
32. Chakrapani V, Willie TC, Shunmugam M, Kershaw TS. Syndemic classes, stigma, and sexual risk among transgender women in India. *AIDS Behav.* 2019;23(6):1518–1529. https://doi.org/10.1007/s10461-018-2373-1
33. Biello KB, Oldenburg CE, Safren SA, et al. Multiple syndemic psychosocial factors are associated with reduced engagement in HIV care among a multinational, online sample of HIV-infected MSM in Latin America. *AIDS Care.* 2016;28(suppl 1):84–91. https://doi.org/10.1080/09540121.2016.1146205
34. Blashill AJ, Bedoya CA, Mayer KH, et al. Psychosocial syndemics are additively associated with worse ART adherence in HIV-infected individuals. *AIDS Behav.* 2015;19(6):981–986. https://doi.org/10.1007/s10461-014-0925-6
35. Fernández Y, Tapper A, Lodge W, Operario D. The utilization of syndemic theory in transgender literature: a structured literature review. Available at: https://home.liebertpub.com/trgh. Accessed September 6, 2024.
36. Friedman MR, Stall R, Silvestre AJ, et al. Effects of syndemics on HIV viral load and medication adherence in the Multicentre AIDS Cohort Study. *AIDS.* 2015;29(9):1087–1096. https://doi.org/10.1097/QAD.0000000000000657
37. Glynn TR, Safren SA, Carrico AW, et al. High levels of syndemics and their association with adherence, viral non-suppression, and biobehavioral transmission risk in Miami, a US city with an HIV/AIDS epidemic. *AIDS Behav.* 2019;23(11):2956–2965. https://doi.org/10.1007/s10461-019-02619-0
38. Harkness A, Bainter SA, O'Cleirigh C, Mendez NA, Mayer KH, Safren SA. Longitudinal effects of syndemics on ART non-adherence among sexual minority men. *AIDS Behav.* 2018;22(8):2564–2574. https://doi.org/10.1007/s10461-018-2180-8
39. Kuhns LM, Hotton AL, Garofalo R, et al. An index of multiple psychosocial, syndemic conditions is associated with antiretroviral medication adherence among HIV-positive youth. *AIDS Patient Care STDS.* 2016;30(4):185–192. https://doi.org/10.1089/apc.2015.0328
40. Pantalone DW, Valentine SE, Woodward EN, O'Cleirigh C. Syndemic indicators predict poor medication adherence and increased healthcare utilization for urban HIV-positive men who have sex with men. *J Gay Lesbian Ment Health.* 2018;22(1):71–87. https://doi.org/10.1080/19359705.2017.1389794
41. Sangaramoorthy T, Benton A. Intersectionality and syndemics: a commentary. *Soc Sci Med.* 2022;295:113783. https://doi.org/10.1016/j.socscimed.2021.113783
42. Crenshaw K. Mapping the margins: intersectionality, identity politics, and violence against women of color. *Stanford Law Rev.* 1991;43(6):1241. https://doi.org/10.2307/1229039
43. Collins PH. *Intersectionality as Critical Social Theory.* Duke University Press; 2019.

44. Bowleg L. The problem with the phrase women and minorities: intersectionality—an important theoretical framework for public health. *Am J Public Health.* 2012;102(7):1267–1273. https://doi.org/10.2105/AJPH.2012.300750
45. Arora L, Bhujang PM, Sivakami M. Understanding discrimination against LGBTQIA+ patients in Indian hospitals using a human rights perspective: an exploratory qualitative study. *Sex Reprod Health Matters.* 2022;29(2):2104678. https://doi.org/10.1080/26410397.2022.2104678
46. Collins PH. Intersectionality's definitional dilemmas. *Annu Rev Sociol.* 2015;41:1–20. https://doi.org/10.1146/annurev-soc-073014-112142
47. Smith LR, Patel VV, Tsai AC, et al. Integrating intersectional and syndemic frameworks for ending the US HIV epidemic. *Am J Public Health.* 2022;112(suppl 4):S340–S343. https://doi.org/10.2105/AJPH.2021.306634
48. Banerjee A, Bertrand M, Datta S, Mullainathan S. Labor market discrimination in Delhi: evidence from a field experiment. *J Comp Econ.* 2009;37(1):14–27. https://doi.org/10.1016/j.jce.2008.09.002
49. Meghani SA. HIV stigma, gay identity, and caste "untouchability": metaphors of abjection in my brother. . .Nikhil, the boyfriend, and "Gandu Bagicha." *J Med Humanit.* 2020;41(2):137–151. https://doi.org/10.1007/s10912-017-9437-5
50. Solar O, Irwin A. A conceptual framework for action on the social determinants of health. Available at: https://iris.who.int/bitstream/handle/10665/44489/9789241500852_eng.pdf?sequence=1. Accessed October 11, 2023.
51. Yearby R. Structural racism and health disparities. *J Law Med Ethics.* 2020;48(3):518–526. https://doi.org/10.1177/1073110520958876
52. Lal V. Not this, not that: the hijras of India and the cultural politics of sexuality. In: *Out Front: Lesbians, Gays, and the Struggle for Workplace Rights.* Vol. 61. Duke University Press; 1999: 119–140.
53. Li DH, Rawat S, Rhoton J, et al. Harassment and violence among men who have sex with men (MSM) and hijras after reinstatement of India's "sodomy law." *Sex Res Social Policy.* 2017;14(3):324–330. https://doi.org/10.1007/s13178-016-0270-9
54. Ministry of Women and Child Development. The Immoral Traffic (Prevention) Act, 1956. Available at: https://wcd.nic.in/sites/default/files/THE%20IMMORAL%20TRAFFIC%20%28PREVENTION%29%20ACT%2C%201956.pdf. Accessed October 11, 2023.
55. Sallis JF, Owen N, Fisher EB. Ecological models of health behavior. In: *Health Behavior and Health Education: Theory, Research, and Practice.* Jossey-Bass; 2008:465–485.
56. Bhattacharya S, Ghosh D. Studying physical and mental health status among hijra, kothi and transgender community in Kolkata, India. *Soc Sci Med.* 2020;265:113412. https://doi.org/10.1016/j.socscimed.2020.113412
57. Chakrapani V, Shunmugam M, Newman PA, Kershaw T, Dubrow R. HIV status disclosure and condom use among HIV-positive men who have sex with men and hijras (male-to-female transgender people) in India: implications for prevention. *J HIV AIDS Soc Serv.* 2015;14(1):26–44. https://doi.org/10.1080/15381501.2013.859113
58. Herrick AL, Stall R, Goldhammer H, Egan JE, Mayer KH. Resilience as a research framework and as a cornerstone of prevention research for gay and bisexual men: theory and evidence. *AIDS Behav.* 2014;18(1):1–9. https://doi.org/10.1007/s10461-012-0384-x
59. Poteat TC, Logie CH. A case for strengths-based approaches to addressing intersectional stigma in HIV research. *Am J Public Health.* 2022;112(suppl 4):S347–S349. https://doi.org/10.2105/AJPH.2021.306659
60. Chakrapani V, Newman PA, Mhaprolkar H, Kavi AR. *Sexual and Social Networks of Men Who Have Sex with Men (MSM) and Hijras in India: A Qualitative Study Final Report.* Mumbai, India: The Humsafar Trust; 2007.
61. Almeida-Brasil CC. Ceccato MDGB, Battistella Nemes MI, Crosland Guimarães MD, de Assis Acurcio F. Improving community mobilization in HIV treatment management: practical suggestions from patients in Brazil. *Rev Panam Salud Publica.* 2017;41:e119. https://doi.org/10.26633/RPSP.2017.119
62. Vijayakumar G. Collective demands and secret codes: the multiple uses of "community" in "community mobilization." *World Dev.* 2018;104:173–182. https://doi.org/10.1016/j.worlddev.2017.11.009
63. Blanchard AK, Lakkappa Mohan H, Shahmanesh M, et al. Community mobilization, empowerment and HIV prevention among female sex workers in South India. *BMC Public Health.* 2013;13:234. https://doi.org/10.1186/1471-2458-13-234
64. Dulin AJ, Dale SK, Earnshaw VA, et al. Resilience and HIV: a review of the definition and study of resilience. *AIDS Care.* 2018;30(suppl 5):S6–S17. https://doi.org/10.1080/09540121.2018.1515470
65. Breslow AS, Brewster ME, Velez BL, Wong S, Geiger E, Soderstrom B. Resilience and collective action: exploring buffers against minority stress for transgender individuals. *Psychol Sex Orientat Gend Divers.* 2015;2(3):253–265. https://doi.org/10.1037/sgd0000117
66. Suslovic B, Lett E. resilience is an adverse event: a critical discussion of resilience theory in health services research and public health. *Community Health Equity Res Policy.* 2024;44(3):339–343. https://doi.org/10.1177/2752535X231159721.
67. Government of India, Ministry of Social Justice and Empowerment. Support for Marginalized Individuals for Livelihood and Enterprise (SMILE): guidelines. Available at: https://socialjustice.gov.in/writereaddata/UploadFile/57291728283781.pdf. Accessed October 11, 2023.

Strategic Litigation, Public Health, and the Decriminalization of Same-Sex Sexual Intimacy: Lessons From Legal Challenges Across Former British Colonies

Sara Wallach, MPH, Jirair Ratevosian, DrPH, Tom Smith, MA, LLB, Katie Duval, BA (Oxon), MA, GDL, LPC, Stefan Baral, MD, and Chris Beyrer, MD

See also Global LGBTQ+ Public Health in the Face of Legal Persecution, pp. 1229–1270.

AJPH August 2025, Vol. 115, No. 8

Consistent data have demonstrated the harms of punitive laws criminalizing same-sex sexual intimacy in the context of both public health and human rights. However, as of January 2025, 61 United Nations member states criminalize consensual same-sex sexual acts among adults, with varying degrees of enforcement and severity.

We used 6 legal challenges across former British colonies in Africa, the Caribbean, and Asia to assess the role of strategic litigation in decriminalizing same-sex practices and where public health arguments, particularly regarding HIV, were central to these legal challenges. Successful decriminalization efforts in Belize and Dominica were contrasted by legal setbacks in Jamaica, Saint Vincent and the Grenadines, and Kenya.

Our findings emphasize the importance of integrating health-related evidence, country-specific data, and local civil society input into legal strategies, highlighting the critical role of collaboration between public health experts, legal professionals, and local advocacy groups. Future litigation efforts must carefully consider local contexts, engaging with communities to ensure both legal success and long-term societal change for LGBTQ+ (lesbian, gay, bisexual, transgender, queer or questioning, and all subsects) individuals. (*Am J Public Health*. 2025;115(8):1254–1263. https://doi.org/10.2105/AJPH.2025.308072)

In January 2025, 61 United Nations member states continue to criminalize, or de facto criminalize, consensual same-sex sexual intimacy among adults. Half of these countries are in Africa, with the remaining half spread throughout Asia, the Americas, and Oceania. These laws, like the countries to which they belong, are heterogeneous, differing in content, penalty severity, and degree of enforcement. Twenty-one countries punish violations with fines, whereas 7 explicitly invoke the death penalty. Some laws include prison sentences, with 9 countries specifying life in prison as punishment. Eight countries have laws that mention "flogging." Temporal variability in the enforcement of these laws is sometimes associated with political cycles or regional dynamics.[1]

Prosecution of these laws is not uncommon, and these efforts may change at the whims of individual politicians or media coverage. Police abuse and mistreatment has been widely reported, including the use of forced anal examinations to collect "evidence" for arrest. Anal examinations cannot be used to confirm anal sex and have been defined as a form of torture.[2] Furthermore, there are reports that police arbitrarily detain lesbian, gay, bisexual, transgender, queer or questioning, and all subsects (LGBTQ+)-perceived individuals for extortion. Instances of enforcement are likely to be underreported, and enforcement disproportionately affects poor and marginalized communities.[3]

Many current sodomy statutes are legacies of European colonial rule across Africa, Asia, and the Americas. British colonial rule codified the criminalization of sodomy through a section in the penal codes known as Section 377. This section criminalized same-sex behaviors between men, specifically "sodomy," "buggery," and other 18th–19th-century terms now understood to mean penile–anal and sometimes penile–oral intercourse. The language of these archaic statutes typically included terms such as intercourse "against the order of nature" or "unnatural" sex and variously included penile–anal or oral sex between men and women, including between married, consenting partners. Those trying to repeal these statutes must grapple with their vague and stigmatizing language.

All same-sex sexual intimacy criminalization laws between consenting adults, regardless of punishment or enforcement intensity, are violations of privacy rights, bodily autonomy, and other human rights. These laws legitimize negative beliefs about and attitudes toward homosexuality and the LGBTQ+ community and are a serious threat to the health, well-being, and full realization of rights to equality and nondiscrimination. Indeed, they explicitly violate the Universal Declaration of Human Rights, the Yogyakarta Principles, and the International Covenant on Civil and Political Rights.[4–6]

As a result, efforts are under way to eradicate these laws. In April 2024, the High Court of Dominica ruled that the Sexual Offenses Act was unconstitutional and limited individuals' rights to "liberty, freedom of expression, and protection of personal privacy."[7] In October 2023, Mauritius's Supreme Court ruled that its law criminalizing same-sex sexual intimacy violated individuals' natural way of being.[8] Similar laws have recently been successfully challenged (and subsequently overturned) in Barbados (2022), Antigua and Barbuda (2022), Angola (2021), and Gabon (2020).[1]

However, not all efforts to decriminalize same-sex sexual intimacy are successful, and some have resulted in increases in penalties for violations and greater enforcement. Decriminalization challenges have recently been denied, lost, or dismissed in Saint Vincent and the Grenadines (SVG; 2024), Malawi (2024), Jamaica (2023), Tunisia (2021), and Kenya (2019), and augmented criminalization laws have been introduced in Iraq (2024), Uganda (2023), and Turkmenistan (2022). Augmentations include harsher punishments, the prosecution of acquaintances such as landlords and health care workers, the expansion of what constitutes an "offense," and beyond.[1]

These legal challenges, lost and won, emphasize the importance of continued strategic litigation. Strategic litigation is litigation deliberately pursued to advance the protection and fulfillment of human rights.[9] Strategic litigation goals include challenging the validity of laws, promoting social and cultural transformations, securing reparations for those who have experienced violations, and raising awareness about violations. Strategic litigation can be enacted at local through international levels and via various rule-making bodies. It is often the only way discriminatory laws can be removed, as their persistence is generally supported by religious or conservative populaces, so governments may be concerned that proposals to remove punitive legislation will be politically unpopular. Having the laws removed through the courts circumvents this issue and therefore can be a necessary route even in countries where the government may, if only in private, support their elimination from the statute books.

We review our experience of strategic litigation for the decriminalization of same-sex sexual intimacy from a public health, HIV-centered perspective. We discuss our arguments, highlighting the common strategies and tactics we used and the differences in contexts that affected cases' outcomes. We also highlight the overall impact of our strategic litigation and opportunities and recommendations for the future.

THE CASES

The 6 cases[10–15] discussed here are those for which the Center for Public Health and Human Rights at Johns Hopkins University (CPHHR) was asked to submit expert testimony between the years of 2012 and 2022. CPHHR investigates human rights violations from an epidemiological perspective and develops rights-based approaches to dynamic public health issues.[16] Hogan Lovells International, LLP, a global law firm advocating "equality and opportunity," worked with us on the most recent case in SVG.[17]

We collected data on cases via filed petitions, official judgments, human rights databases, and news articles. We extracted filing dates, claimants' and defendants' details, interested parties' details, laws and their language, argument and judgment dates, judgments themselves, whether health had any weight in the decision, appeal dates and decisions, and points on which we felt the cases hinged. We also analyzed our testimonies for each case and any additional evidence we were asked to provide, extracted the health arguments, examined trends, and compared arguments across cases.

SYNTHESIS OF KEY TAKEAWAYS

Spanning Central America, the Caribbean, Africa, and Asia, the challenges occurred in Belize, Jamaica, Kenya, Singapore, Dominica, and SVG (Table 1; Table A, available as a supplement to the online version of this article at http://www.ajph.org).[10–15] All are former British colonies, and their criminalization laws were based on Section 377. Case filing dates range from 2010 (Belize) to 2019 (SVG and Dominica). Arguments were heard from 2013 (Belize) to 2023 (Jamaica and SVG). The latest judgment (SVG) is from 2024. In all cases except Singapore, churches and other Christian groups participated as interested parties for the defendant state. In 2 cases—Belize and Dominica—the laws were overturned. Three cases—Jamaica, SVG, and Singapore—resulted in dismissals, although Singapore's criminalization law was later overturned. The Kenya case resulted in no change to the existing statutes. In Belize and Dominica, where criminalization laws were successfully overturned, the courts specifically cited the rights to liberty, privacy and home life, freedom of expression, and equality as key in their decision-making. In challenges that failed, 2 courts—Kenya and Singapore—ruled that decriminalizing same-sex sexual intimacy would thwart the country's societal moral values. In the unsuccessful challenges, the courts ruled that only parliament could

TABLE 1— Descriptions of the Challenges to Same-Sex Sexual Intimacy Criminalization Laws by Country: 2010–2024

	Belize	Jamaica	Kenya	Singapore	Dominica	Saint Vincent and the Grenadines
Case name	*Caleb Orozco v Attorney General of Belize et al.*	*Tomlinson, Maurice Arnold v the Attorney General of Jamaica*	*Eric Gitari v Attorney General & another*	*Ong Ming Johnson v Attorney General of Singapore*	*B.G. v the Attorney General of the Commonwealth of Dominica*	*Javin Kevin Vinc Johnson & Sean Macleish v the Attorney General of Saint Vincent and the Grenadines*
Region	Central America	Caribbean	Africa	Asia	Caribbean	Caribbean
Claimant	Caleb Orozco, then-president of United Belize Advocacy Movement	Maurice Tomlinson, lawyer, law professor, and activist	Eric Gitari, executive director of the Kenyan National Gay and Lesbian Rights Commission	Ong Ming Johnson, Singaporean DJ; Choong Chee Hong, gay rights activist; Tan Seng Kee, gay activist and retired doctor	B. G. (anonymous)	Javin Johnson and Sean Macleish, Vincentian nationals residing abroad
Statute	Criminal Code Act 1888, § 53, Chapter 101	Offenses Against the Person Act, §§ 76, 77, 79	Penal Code (Cap 63), §§ 162 (a) and (c) and 165	Penal Code, § 377A and Rules of Court, Order 15 Rule 16	Sexual Offenses Act 1998, §§ 14 and 16	Criminal Code 1988, §§ 146 and 148
Filed	September 2010	November 2015	April 2016	September 2018	2019	July 2019
Start of arguments	May 2013	June 2023	October 2018	November 2019	April 2022	May 2023
Judgment delivered	August 2016	October 2023	May 2019	March 2020	April 2024	February 2024
Judgment	Overturned	Dismissed	Not overturned	Dismissed, but overturned November 2022	Overturned	Dismissed
Health considered in decision	Yes	NA	No	No	Yes	Yes

Note. NA = not available.

legislate (Jamaica) or the claimants had no legal standing because they currently lived overseas (SVG). Public health was a relevant issue for the court and was discussed in the judgments for Belize, Dominica, and SVG.

When we wrote them, we updated each testimony, containing arguments and supporting evidence, with the latest research (Table 2). Early testimonies highlighted that these laws violate the Yogyakarta Principles, whereas later ones discussed the potential loss of international aid should the laws remain, and they included more country- or region-specific evidence. The later testimonies also drew on research showing a positive correlation between criminalization and HIV burden among gay, bisexual, and other men who have sex with men (GBMSM), as well as decreases in HIV testing, increases in poor mental health, and decreases in condom use for anal intercourse.[18–25] Key arguments across the testimonies focused on the profound impact of criminalization and GBMSM stigmatization on the effectiveness of HIV prevention and treatment efforts.

Criminalization, coupled with widespread social stigmatization, is a formidable barrier to public health initiatives—owing to anticipated or

TABLE 2— Health-Related Arguments Included in the Expert Reports Written by the Center for Public Health and Human Rights by Country: 2012–2022

	Belize	Jamaica	Kenya	Singapore	Dominica	Saint Vincent and the Grenadines
Violates the Yogyakarta Principles	X	X				
Positive correlation between criminalization and HIV prevalence in GBMSM					X	X
Increases stigmatization and discrimination against GBMSM	X	X	X	X	X	X
Increases violence against GBMSM	X	X	X		X	X
Increases HIV transmission in GBMSM	X	X	X	X	X	X
Increases HIV transmission in the general population	X	X		X	X	X
Increases minority stress for GBMSM	X	X	X		X	X
Increases poor mental health for GBMSM				X	X	X
Increases health care costs					X	X
Decreases likelihood of HIV testing					X	X
Decreases likelihood of knowing own HIV status					X	X
Limits condom use for anal intercourse for GBMSM					X	X
Limits health care access, including ART, PrEP, HIV testing, and condoms by GBMSM	X	X	X	X	X	X
Increase health care worker bias against GBMSM	X	X	X		X	X
Limits education access for GBMSM	X	X	X	X		
Limits income access and economic well-being for GBMSM	X	X	X	X	X	X
Limits knowledge of HIV, HIV risk, and risk reduction among GBMSM	X	X	X		X	X
Limits data and research on HIV among GBMSM	X	X	X	X	X	X
Limits health care worker GBMSM cultural competency	X	X	X	X	X	X
Limits access to and participation in HIV prevention programs and interventions by GBMSM		X	X	X	X	X
Limits the allocation of appropriate resources for GBMSM health					X	X
Jeopardizes international aid	X		X		X	X
Country-specific evidence		X			X	X

Note. ART = antiretroviral therapy; GBMSM = gay, bisexual, and other men who have sex with men; PrEP = preexposure prophylaxis for HIV prevention.

realized discrimination, violence, and legal penalties—severely limiting GBMSM's access to essential health care services and impeding the delivery of life-saving HIV treatment and prevention interventions.[19,21–23,26–35] The lack of culturally and clinically competent health care coupled with the fear of legal and social repercussions create an environment where GBMSM are particularly in need of, yet systematically excluded from, effective HIV prevention services.[19,26,36–38]

The intersection of criminalization with other structural risk factors—such as lower education levels, income disparities, and inadequate health care infrastructure—further exacerbates GBMSM's HIV vulnerability.[19,36,37,39,40] This is not a theoretical concern but a lived reality for GBMSM in multiple countries and contexts. These structural barriers limit broader HIV epidemic control, contributing to sustained HIV transmission and hindering the achievement of global HIV control targets, such as the Joint United Nations Programme on HIV and AIDS 95–95–95 goals.[41] Indeed, we cannot meet these ambitious goals with these laws in place.[42]

The testimonies collectively advocated a comprehensive approach to HIV prevention and treatment that integrates both behavioral and biomedical interventions and is supported by the decriminalization of same-sex sexual intimacy and stigma mitigation. However, they stressed that decriminalization alone is insufficient: it must be part of a broader strategy that includes respecting, protecting, and fulfilling GBMSM human rights and ensuring their access to culturally and clinically competent health care services.

The global movement toward decriminalization is thus framed by an emphasis on human rights treaties as a moral imperative and as a public health necessity, given the clear link between criminalization, poorer health outcomes, and HIV burden.

HEALTH IN JUDGMENTS

In the first case, an openly gay man, Caleb Orozco, challenged Belize's sodomy law. In the High Court, Chief Justice Kenneth Benjamin concluded that interference with the right to privacy was not justified on the grounds of public health on the evidence before him. He cited with approval the expert report of the Belize Family Life Association, which stated that the "climate of hostility toward MSM [men who have sex with men] driv[es] their sexual behaviour underground thus hampering efforts by BFLA [Belize Family Life Association] to promote safer sex, promote health education and roll out health care."[10] He was also influenced by evidence that criminalization is a barrier to the HIV response because it perpetuates GBMSM stigma, discrimination, and violence, limiting research on GBMSM's HIV risks and restricting GBMSM's ability to access, and providers' abilities to give, care.[10]

In Dominica's High Court, Justice Kimberly Cenac-Phulgence summarized the criminalization laws "as a barrier to LGBT [lesbian, gay, bisexual, or transgender] persons seeking and receiving effective health care, particularly HIV prevention and treatment, and has exacerbated the public health challenge of eliminating the spread of HIV."[14] She observed that whereas the state may legitimately limit the enjoyment of rights for public interests, such as public health, the claimant provided evidence demonstrating that criminalization "cannot be justified on the grounds of public health"[14] and that it is harmful to the physical and mental well-being of LGBTQ+ persons and the realization of their fundamental rights. However, based on her written judgment, she did not rely on this argument because the defendant state did not argue that criminalization laws were immune from challenge on the grounds of public health.

By contrast, the defendant state in the SVG case claimed that same-sex sexual intimacy criminalization was reasonably justifiable on the grounds of public health. In her judgment, Justice Esco Lorene Henry cited our evidence that found a correlation between HIV prevalence and criminalization in 10 countries in sub-Saharan Africa, as well as evidence for a correlation between the severity of anti-LGBT legislation and HIV prevalence and health care utilization.[18,23] She also referred to our opinions that criminalization is associated with higher health care costs, because of increased HIV incidence and prevalence, and with losses in gross domestic product that lead to decreased quality of life for all citizens.[15]

Notwithstanding, Henry did not accept this evidence. In her judgment dismissing the claims, she stated that (1) there are high rates of HIV in jurisdictions without criminalization, and (2) there is no direct causal relationship between criminalization laws and reduced HIV infections. She also said that the evidence we adduced was not specific to SVG, and she was not prepared to make findings about SVG by extrapolating from other jurisdictions' data. Henry stated that, unlike in the Dominica case, a "public health crisis occasioned by an unstemmed deluge of new HIV cases is a real and serious concern which reasonably justifies a public health response of the kind embedded in the [existing laws]."[15] She said that overturning the laws would lead to increased HIV incidence because this would allow increased instances of anal intercourse; however, there is no evidence for this proposition.

The Dominica and SVG cases are interesting because our testimonies relied on nearly identical health arguments and evidence, but the outcomes differed. Furthermore, in both testimonies, we cited country-specific, albeit extremely limited, evidence. Our evidence for Dominica concerned the status of the country's HIV epidemic, behavioral risk factors for HIV among adolescent girls, and stigma and discrimination against people with HIV (PWH) by health care workers.[43,44] No evidence was presented relevant to GBMSM or the causal effects of criminalization on health and HIV in Dominica, as none existed; yet, Cenac-Phulgence said that the evidence adduced concerning the Caribbean and elsewhere was sufficient. For SVG, we cited research on HIV risks and behavior specifically in SVG, including evidence of low condom use; low GBMSM utilization of HIV testing because of confidentiality concerns; and stigma, discrimination, and harassment of GBMSM. The evidence explicitly mentioned the effects of criminalization on GBMSM in SVG, although it was in a small sample.[45]

Nonetheless, Henry concluded that the testimony lacked SVG-specific evidence and found that the provisions criminalizing same-sex sexual intimacy were reasonably justifiable on the grounds of public health, in terms of both the risk of HIV transmission and the cost to the country in treating and managing PWH. Henry noted that this latter argument on the cost of treating PWH was not raised in any of the cases previously decided in the Commonwealth Caribbean and relied on by the claimants, essentially using this as a point of distinction.

There are several takeaways from these judgments and our experiences. First, these cases are highly fact- and jurisdiction-specific: Henry's critique underscores the need for country-specific evidence.

Second, outcomes turn on how defendants present their cases. Despite similar expert evidence, the Dominica challenge appears to have succeeded where the SVG challenge did not because the state conceded that criminalization was not immune from challenge on the grounds of public health.

Third, to maximize the prospect of successfully challenging criminalization laws through strategic litigation, researchers and epidemiologists should continue to strengthen their studies and methods to be able to reasonably claim there is a causal relationship between the criminalization of same-sex sexual intimacy and negative health outcomes, such as HIV. Special attention should be paid to designing studies and analyses to meet identifiability assumptions of exchangeability, consistency, and positivity and to employing quasiexperimental approaches and advanced epidemiological methods where appropriate to generate high-quality evidence. A variety of study types and analytical methods are needed to strengthen evidence. Furthermore, we must diversify the evidence base to include countries that have previously been excluded from such research. Evidence is also needed on other subgroups of the LGBTQ+ community and on the relationship between criminalization and noncommunicable diseases, mental health, substance use, and other health outcomes.

Fourth, acceptance of a defendant's arguments on the costs incurred by states in treating HIV and the disproportionate impact this may have on a state with a small economy (e.g., SVG) is a potential new front in these cases. These economic arguments may merit further studies.

Fifth, organizations focused on LGBTQ+ health and HIV prevention and care, as well as LGBTQ+ rights groups and their strategic partners, play an important role in describing the health situation on the ground for LGBTQ+ communities. They directly observe harms and often face such harms themselves; individuals have been harassed and organizations shuttered. In the Belize case, the United Belize Advocacy Movement and Orozco testified that homophobic violence deterred LGBTQ+ individuals from pursuing HIV testing and treatment. They also testified that, as an advocacy organization, they spoke on behalf of more than 100 members who feared retaliation if named.[10] We imagine that the sheer size of Orozco's support was not insignificant to the court. Future cases should consider amplifying health organizations and rights advocacy groups' inclusion and supporting their testimonies.

Sixth, just as advocacy groups can amplify the claimants' case, churches and Christian groups can do the same for the defendants. In Belize and SVG, as we were instructed as experts for the claimants, Brendan Bain was instructed as an expert for the Coalition of Christian Churches. Bain—an infectious disease clinician, former University of the West Indies faculty member, and former Caribbean HIV/AIDS Regional Training Network director—had his employment terminated for his homophobic rhetoric.[46] In his expert evidence, he opined that GBMSM are at greater risk for HIV and sexually transmitted infections because anal intercourse is inherently harmful and that decriminalizing same-sex sexual intimacy would increase HIV transmission, erroneously suggesting that criminalization is effective HIV prevention.[10,15]

In Kenya, church groups argued that same-sex sexual intimacy was against the country's values. This was reiterated by the county's president, who stated publicly that homosexuality was not a part of Kenyan culture.[47] These arguments about anal intercourse and homosexuality as anti-Christian are insidious. In Belize, our counterargument that criminalization impedes access to health care and exacerbates HIV transmission was convincing; however, in SVG and Kenya, our evidence did little to counter such interpretations of Christian values. We must be prepared to face these homophobic arguments—arguments not grounded in evidence.

Seventh, interdisciplinary collaboration, such as that of CPHHR, Hogan Lovells, and other international law firms, is key to advancing these cases effectively. This is particularly important in cases, such as those in SVG and Jamaica, in which the interested parties spend considerable resources on advancing competing expert evidence on public health. Hogan Lovells's legal guidance and expertise in the SVG case allowed CPHHR to present digestible evidence for the court and counter the specific legal arguments that the state and the churches chose to run. The Coalition of Christian Churches raised 295 questions challenging our expert report—targeting our discussions of HIV transmission and epidemiology and our citations—likely to discredit evidence and delay proceedings. The CPHHR–Hogan Lovells partnership swiftly addressed all the issues they raised, nullifying their strategy.

Finally, importantly, parties to these cases were able to advance arguments both for and against criminalization on the grounds of public health. How these arguments are made, and how receptive judges are, can therefore result in contradictory outcomes, even if the evidence is largely the same. The Dominica and SVG cases are thus instructive, and continued cooperation between stakeholders is critical.

This analysis includes only challenges involving CPHHR. Future research should examine all cases, including other European colonial approaches to criminalization and challenges to those laws.

OPPORTUNITIES FOR FUTURE STRATEGIC LITIGATION

The importance of strategic litigation for decriminalizing same-sex sexual intimacy and for securing and safeguarding LGBTQ+ individuals' rights cannot be overstated. Future litigation must target the remaining 61 UN member states that still criminalize same-sex sexual intimacy. Furthermore, 146 countries still prohibit same-sex marriage or civil unions, and only 3 countries have national bans preventing LGBTQ+ conversion therapy.[48,49] LGBTQ+ communities face ongoing violence, inequality, and discrimination in health, education, employment, housing, adoption rights, legal gender recognition, freedom of expression, and freedom of association.

In 2024, LGBTQ+ rights suffered global setbacks. In January, Romania's National Council for Combating Discrimination issued a ruling supporting printers who cited religious reasons for not printing LGBTQ+-related posters. In February, Ghana's parliament approved the Promotion of Proper Human Sexual Rights and Ghanian Family Values Bill, which aims "to provide for proper human sexual rights and Ghanaian family values,"[1] restricting LGBTQ+ advocacy and marriage. In March, Georgia's ruling party announced constitutional reforms that banned pride marches, promotion of LGBTQ+ relationships, and more to defend "family values and minors."[1] In April, Uganda's Constitutional Court upheld the 2023 Anti-Homosexuality Act: legislation allowing discriminatory practices against LGBTQ+ people and jeopardizing their safety.[50] Although the court disapplied sections of the law limiting LGBTQ+ health care and housing access and requiring the reporting of alleged same-sex sexual acts, it maintained the death penalty for same-sex sexual intimacy.

The United States has also experienced rollbacks of LGBTQ+ rights, with significant repercussions globally. The 2022 US Supreme Court decision to overturn *Roe v Wade* (410 US 113 [1973]), combined with state-level efforts to restrict rights to same-sex marriage and for transgender individuals, has undermined previous advancements.[51] These US legal decisions are closely watched worldwide and may contribute to a broader regression in human rights. Uganda's Constitutional Court cited the US ruling in *Dobbs v Jackson Women's Health Organization* (142 S. Ct. 2228 [2022]) when upholding its 2023 Anti-Homosexuality Act.[52]

Moreover, a recent Joint United Nations Programme on HIV and AIDS report paints a dire picture for Eastern

Europe, Central Asia, the Middle East, North Africa, and Latin America, where the number of PWH is projected to nearly double by 2050.[53] Criminalization of same-sex sexual intimacy exacerbates the situation in many of these regions, heightening health risks for GBMSM and increasing barriers to care, mental health challenges, substance use, and noncommunicable diseases.[54] As global funding decreases and legal barriers remain entrenched, the potential for a resurgence of the HIV epidemic becomes increasingly likely, underscoring the need for decriminalization and increased investment in evidence-based tactics, such as strategic litigation, to address punitive laws and policies.[55]

The necessity of strategic litigation must be balanced against its potential for impact. As public health professionals, we can play a limited but impactful supporting role in strategic litigation. For those at the forefront, we want to emphasize that although the ethical imperative for litigation is clear and widespread, we must consider, given context and culture, how likely it is that our litigation will be successful. These challenges are phenomenal tools for awareness raising and conversation generating, and they often receive a lot of media attention. They may also be resource intensive and, as in Uganda, provoke significant backlash. We must ask, Will this litigation, given its likelihood of success, bring about more harm than good? With limited resources, it may be best to initiate challenges in jurisdictions where the climate is ripe for change.

Where a legal challenge is being considered, we must ask, Have other LGBTQ+ rights recently been secured in this jurisdiction? Have leaders, at the highest levels, publicly supported LGBTQ+ persons of late? Are the campaigning efforts of local LGBTQ+ advocacy organizations gaining traction? Sometimes the answer to these questions will be no, and we may still choose to challenge criminalization because of the overwhelming need. By following the lead of local community members and experts and refining our messaging and strategies based on these insights, we can better position ourselves for future legal challenges, ensuring that our approaches both remain effective and adapt to evolving circumstances.

CONCLUSIONS

Strategic litigation plays a critical role in advancing LGBTQ+ rights, particularly in the context of decriminalizing same-sex sexual intimacy. It is an important public health tool to combat the significant health risks GBMSM face in criminalized contexts, including barriers to HIV prevention, stigma, and exclusion from health care.

Cases in Belize, Dominica, and Mauritius demonstrate strategic litigation's power to uphold human rights, whereas setbacks in Jamaica, SVG, and Uganda highlight the complexities and risks involved. Our analysis underscores the importance of country-specific evidence, local public health context, and strategic partnerships between legal and public health experts in shaping outcomes. Although the outcomes of the challenges in which we were involved did not hinge on public health arguments, public health did play a role. Moreover, divergent court rulings, despite similar arguments and evidence, emphasize the need for continued refinement in litigation strategies and the importance of understanding cultural and societal attitudes.

As the cases demonstrate, challenges faced in 1 jurisdiction can ripple across borders, influencing legal, cultural, and political attitudes worldwide. Vigilance and strategic action are needed not only in individual countries but also on the international stage to safeguard and advance LGBTQ+ rights everywhere. Moving forward, the pursuit of decriminalization must be carefully balanced with the potential risks associated with the process, including backlash and exacerbating existing vulnerabilities. As public health professionals, we play a supportive role in strategic litigation. Ethical and practical considerations demand that we align our efforts with the readiness of the local context. Voices of local communities should guide these endeavors, ensuring that our actions seek to secure legal victories as well as promote long-term, positive change for LGBTQ+ individuals worldwide. AJPH

ABOUT THE AUTHORS

Sara Wallach is with the Department of Epidemiology, Mailman School of Public Health, Columbia University, New York, NY. Jirair Ratevosian and Chris Beyrer are with the Duke Global Health Institute, Duke University, Durham, NC. Tom Smith and Katie Duval are with Hogan Lovells International LLP, London, UK. Stefan Baral is with the Center for Public Health and Human Rights, Johns Hopkins Bloomberg School of Public Health, Baltimore, MD.

CORRESPONDENCE

Correspondence should be sent to Sara Wallach, 722 West 168th St, Rm 720, New York, NY 10032 (e-mail: sew2216@cumc.columbia.edu). Reprints can be ordered at https://www.ajph.org by clicking the "Reprints" link.

PUBLICATION INFORMATION

Full Citation: Wallach S, Ratevosian J, Smith T, Duval K, Baral S, Beyrer C. Strategic litigation, public health, and the decriminalization of same-sex sexual intimacy: lessons from legal challenges across former British colonies. *Am J Public Health*. 2025;115(8):1254–1263.

Acceptance Date: February 12, 2025.
DOI: https://doi.org/10.2105/AJPH.2025.308072
ORCID iDs:
Sara Wallach https://orcid.org/0000-0003-3234-1988

Jirair Ratevosian https://orcid.org/0000-0003-4451-4188

Stefan Baral https://orcid.org/0000-0002-5482-2419

Chris Beyrer https://orcid.org/0000-0003-0665-9124

CONTRIBUTORS

S. Wallach, J. Ratevosian, T. Smith, and K. Duval completed the analysis and prepared the text and tables. S. Wallach, J Ratevosian, S. Baral, and C. Beyrer conceptualized the essay. All authors reviewed the essay.

ACKNOWLEDGMENTS

S. Baral's effort was supported by the Center for HIV and Mental Health Stigma Elimination Strategies, which was funded by the National Institutes of Mental Health (NIH; P30MH136919). C. Beyrer acknowledges the Desmond M. Tutu Professorship at Johns Hopkins University.

Note. The contents of this essay are solely the responsibility of the authors and do not necessarily represent the official views of the NIH.

CONFLICTS OF INTEREST

The authors have no conflicts of interest to disclose.

HUMAN PARTICIPANT PROTECTION

No protocol approval was necessary because no human participants were involved in this study.

REFERENCES

1. ILGA World Database. Criminalisation of consensual same-sex sexual acts. Available at: https://database.ilga.org/criminalisation-consensual-same-sex-sexual-acts. Accessed March 25, 2025.
2. Cichowitz C, Rubenstein L, Beyrer C. Forced anal examinations to ascertain sexual orientation and sexual behavior: an abusive and medically unsound practice. *PLoS Med.* 2018;15(3):e1002536. https://doi.org/10.1371/journal.pmed.1002536
3. Botha K. *Our Identities Under Arrest.* 2nd ed. Geneva, Switzerland: ILGA World; 2023.
4. United Nations. Universal Declaration of Human Rights. Available at: https://www.un.org/en/about-us/universal-declaration-of-human-rights. Accessed September 6, 2024.
5. Grinspan MC, Carpenter M, Ehrt, J, et al. The Yogyakarta Principles. Available at: https://yogyakartaprinciples.org/wp-content/uploads/2017/11/A5_yogyakartaWEB-2.pdf. Accessed March 26, 2025.
6. UN General Assembly. International Covenant on Civil and Political Rights. Available at: https://www.ohchr.org/en/instruments-mechanisms/instruments/international-covenant-civil-and-political-rights. Accessed September 6, 2024.
7. Gonzalez Cabrera C. Dominica high court decriminalizes same-sex conduct. April 24, 2024. Available at: https://www.hrw.org/news/2024/04/24/dominica-high-court-decriminalizes-same-sex-conduct. Accessed September 6, 2024.
8. Anganan V. Rights groups cheer as Mauritius top court decriminalises same-sex relations. *Reuters.* October 5, 2023. Available at: https://www.reuters.com/world/africa/mauritius-supreme-court-decriminalises-same-sex-relations-2023-10-05. Accessed September 6, 2024.
9. Amnesty International. Strategic litigation. Available at: https://www.amnesty.org/en/strategic-litigation. Accessed September 6, 2024.
10. Benjamin CJKA. *Caleb Orozco v. the Attorney General of Belize* (Supreme Court of Belize; 2016). Available at: https://www.belizejudiciary.org/wp-content/uploads/2016/01/Supreme-Court-Claim-No-668-of-2010-Caleb-Orozco-v-The-Attorney-General-of-Belize-et-al1.pdf. Accessed March 25, 2025.
11. Shelly-Williams JL, Batts JD, Pettigrew-Collins JA. *Tomlinson, Maurice Arnold v. The Attorney General of Jamaica* (Supreme Court of Jamaica; 2023). Available at: https://www.supremecourt.gov.jm/sites/default/files/judgments/Tomlinson%2C%20Maurice%20Arnold%20v%20The%20Attorney%20General%20of%20Jamaica%2C%20the%20Churches%2C%20Jamaica%20Coalition%20for%20a%20Healthy%20Society%20et%20al_0.pdf. Accessed March 25, 2025.
12. Lenaola JI. *Eric Gitari v. The Honorable Attorney General* (High Court of Kenya; 2016). Available at: https://kenyalaw.org/caselaw/cases/view/122862. Accessed September 7, 2024.
13. Government of Singapore. *Ong Ming Johnson v. Attorney-General and Other Matters* (Supreme Court of Singapore; 2020). Available at: https://www.singaporelawwatch.sg/Portals/0/Docs/Judgments/2020/%5B2020%5D%20SGHC%2063.pdf. Accessed March 25, 2025.
14. Eastern Caribbean Supreme Court Commonwealth of Dominica. *Cenac Phulgence K. B.G. v. the AG of the Commonwealth of Dominica* (High Court of Justice of Dominica; 2024). Available at: https://www.humandignitytrust.org/wp-content/uploads/resources/judgment-domhcv2019.0149-bg-v-the-ag.pdf. Accessed March 25, 2025.
15. Henry EL. *Javin Kevin Vinc Johnson & Sean Macleish v. the AG of Saint Vincent and the Grenadines.* Available at: https://www.eccourts.org/judgment/javin-kevin-vinc-johnson-et-al-v-the-attorney-general-of-saint-vincent-and-the-grenadines. Accessed March 26, 2025.
16. Johns Hopkins Bloomberg School of Public Health. Center for Public Health and Human Rights. Available at: https://publichealth.jhu.edu/center-for-public-health-and-human-rights. Accessed September 6, 2024.
17. Hogan Lovells. About us. Available at: https://www.hoganlovells.com/en/about-us. Accessed September 6, 2024.
18. Lyons CE, Twahirwa Rwema JO, Makofane K, et al. Associations between punitive policies and legal barriers to consensual same-sex sexual acts and HIV among gay men and other men who have sex with men in sub-Saharan Africa: a multicountry, respondent-driven sampling survey. *Lancet HIV.* 2023;10(3):e186–e194. https://doi.org/10.1016/S2352-3018(22)00336-8
19. Beyrer C, Baral SD, Van Griensven F, et al. Global epidemiology of HIV infection in men who have sex with men. *Lancet.* 2012;380(9839):367–377. https://doi.org/10.1016/S0140-6736(12)60821-6
20. Culbert GJ, Pillai V, Bick J, et al. Confronting the HIV, tuberculosis, addiction, and incarceration syndemic in Southeast Asia: lessons learned from Malaysia. *J Neuroimmune Pharmacol.* 2016;11(3):446–455. https://doi.org/10.1007/s11481-016-9676-7
21. Tan RKJ. Internalized homophobia, HIV knowledge, and HIV/AIDS personal responsibility beliefs: correlates of HIV/AIDS discrimination among MSM in the context of institutionalized stigma. *J Homosex.* 2019;66(8):1082–1103. https://doi.org/10.1080/00918369.2018.1491249
22. Millett GA, Jeffries WL, Peterson JL, et al. Common roots: a contextual review of HIV epidemics in Black men who have sex with men across the African diaspora. *Lancet.* 2012;380(9839):411–423. https://doi.org/10.1016/S0140-6736(12)60722-3
23. Stannah J, Dale E, Elmes J, et al. HIV testing and engagement with the HIV treatment cascade among men who have sex with men in Africa: a systematic review and meta-analysis. *Lancet HIV.* 2019;6(11):e769–e787. https://doi.org/10.1016/S2352-3018(19)30239-5
24. Amola O, Grimmett MA. Sexual identity, mental health, HIV risk behaviors, and internalized homophobia among Black men who have sex with men. *J Couns Dev.* 2015;93(2):236–246. https://doi.org/10.1002/j.1556-6676.2015.00199.x
25. Mustanski B, Garofalo R, Herrick A, Donenberg G. Psychosocial health problems increase risk for HIV among urban young men who have sex with men: preliminary evidence of a syndemic in need of attention. *Ann Behav Med.* 2007;34(1):37–45. https://doi.org/10.1007/BF02879919
26. Sullivan PS, Carballo-Diéguez A, Coates T, et al. Successes and challenges of HIV prevention in men who have sex with men. *Lancet.* 2012;380(9839):388–399. https://doi.org/10.1016/S0140-6736(12)60955-6
27. United Nations Development Program. *Global Commission on HIV and the Law.* Available at: https://hivlawcommission.org/wp-content/uploads/2017/06/FinalReport-RisksRightsHealth-EN.pdf. Accessed September 6, 2024.
28. Kyomya M, Todyrs KW, Amon JJ. Laws against sodomy and the HIV epidemic in African prisons. *Lancet.* 2012;380(9839):310–312. https://doi.org/10.1016/S0140-6736(12)60682-5
29. Poteat T, Diouf D, Drame FM, et al. HIV risk among MSM in Senegal: a qualitative rapid assessment of the impact of enforcing laws that criminalize same sex practices. *PLoS One.* 2011;6(12):e28760. https://doi.org/10.1371/journal.pone.0028760
30. African Commission on Human & Peoples' Rights. *HIV, The Law and Human Rights in the African Human Rights System: Key Challenges and Opportunities for Rights-Based Responses.* Available at: https://www.unaids.org/sites/default/files/media_asset/HIV_Law_AfricanHumanRightsSystem_en.pdf. Accessed March 25, 2025.
31. Baral S, Adams D, Lebona J, et al. A cross-sectional assessment of population demographics, HIV risks and human rights contexts

among men who have sex with men in Lesotho. *J Int AIDS Soc.* 2011;14(1):36. https://doi.org/10.1186/1758-2652-14-36

32. Baral S, Trapence G, Motimedi F, et al. HIV prevalence, risks for HIV infection, and human rights among men who have sex with men (MSM) in Malawi, Namibia, and Botswana. *PLoS One.* 2009;4(3):e4997. https://doi.org/10.1371/journal.pone.0004997
33. Hamilton A, Shin S, Taggart T, et al. HIV testing barriers and intervention strategies among men, transgender women, female sex workers and incarcerated persons in the Caribbean: a systematic review. *Sex Transm Infect.* 2020;96(3):189–196. https://doi.org/10.1136/sextrans-2018-053932
34. World Health Organization. *Guidelines on HIV Self-Testing and Partner Notification: Supplement to Consolidated Guidelines on HIV Testing Services.* 2016. Available at: https://iris.who.int/handle/10665/251655. Accessed August 14, 2024.
35. Ramasubban R. Political intersections between HIV/AIDS, sexuality and human rights: a history of resistance to the anti-sodomy law in India. *Glob Public Health.* 2008;3(suppl 2):22–38. https://doi.org/10.1080/17441690801990655
36. Beyrer C, Baral SD, Collins C, et al. The global response to HIV in men who have sex with men. *Lancet.* 2016;388(10040):198–206. https://doi.org/10.1016/S0140-6736(16)30781-4
37. Philbin MM, Hirsch JS, Wilson PA, Ly AT, Giang LM, Parker RG. Structural barriers to HIV prevention among men who have sex with men (MSM) in Vietnam: diversity, stigma, and healthcare access. *PLoS One.* 2018;13(4):e0195000. https://doi.org/10.1371/journal.pone.0195000
38. Earnshaw VA, Jin H, Wickersham JA, et al. Stigma toward men who have sex with men among future healthcare providers in Malaysia: would more interpersonal contact reduce prejudice? *AIDS Behav.* 2016;20(1):98–106. https://doi.org/10.1007/s10461-015-1168-x
39. Beyrer C, Wirtz AL, Johns B, Sifakis F, Baral SD. *The Global HIV Epidemics Among Men Who Have Sex With Men.* Washington, DC: World Bank; 2011.
40. Lamontagne E, d'Elbée M, Ross MW, Carroll A, Plessis AD, Loures L. A socioecological measurement of homophobia for all countries and its public health impact. *Eur J Public Health.* 2018;28(5):967–972. https://doi.org/10.1093/eurpub/cky023
41. Joint United Nations Programme on HIV/AIDS. AIDS targets. 2025. Available at: https://aidstargets2025.unaids.org/#section-about. Accessed August 12, 2024.
42. Baral S, Millett G, Syarif O, Turpin N, Schwartz S. There is no path to ending AIDS by 2030 without improving human rights. *J Int AIDS Soc.* 2023;26(12):e26197. https://doi.org/10.1002/jia2.26197
43. George C, Alary M, Otis J. Correlates of sexual activity and inconsistent condom use among high-school girls in Dominica. *West Indian Med J.* 2007;56(5):433–438.
44. Nyblade L, Jain A, Benkirane M, et al. A brief, standardized tool for measuring HIV-related stigma among health facility staff: results of field testing in China, Dominica, Egypt, Kenya, Puerto Rico and St. Christopher & Nevis. *J Int AIDS Soc.* 2013;16(suppl 2):18718. https://doi.org/10.7448/IAS.16.3.18718
45. Myers JJ, Maiorana A, Chapman K, Lall R, Kassie N, Persaud N. How the illicit drug economy contributes to HIV risk in St Vincent and the Grenadines. *J Int Assoc Physicians AIDS Care (Chic).* 2011;10(6):396–406. https://doi.org/10.1177/1545109711418508
46. UWI fires professor amid gay lobby outrage. *Jamaica Gleaner.* May 20, 2014. Available at: https://jamaica-gleaner.com/power/52999. Accessed September 12, 2024.
47. Kiplagat S. Kenya high court declines to decriminalise anti-gay sex law. *The East African.* May 24, 2019. Available at: https://www.theeastafrican.co.ke/tea/news/east-africa/kenya-high-court-declines-to-decriminalise-anti-gay-sex-law-1418756. Accessed September 12, 2024.
48. ILGA World Database. Same-sex marriage and civil unions. Available at: https://database.ilga.org/same-sex-marriage-civil-unions. Accessed September 12, 2024.
49. Ramon Mendos L. *Curbing Deception: A World Survey on Legal Regulation of So-Called "Conversion Therapies."* Geneva, Switzerland: ILGA World; 2020. Available at: https://ilga.org/wp-content/uploads/2023/11/ILGA_World_Curbing_Deception_world_survey_legal_restrictions_conversion_therapy.pdf. Accessed March 25, 2025.
50. Human Rights Watch. Uganda: court upholds Anti-Homosexuality Act. April 4, 2024. Available at: https://www.hrw.org/news/2024/04/04/uganda-court-upholds-anti-homosexuality-act. Accessed September 12, 2024.
51. Human Rights Campaign. Map: attacks on gender affirming care by state. Available at: https://www.hrc.org/resources/attacks-on-gender-affirming-care-by-state-map. Accessed September 12, 2024.
52. Slisco A. US Supreme Court ruling cited as Uganda upholds anti-gay death penalty. *Newsweek.* April 4, 2024. Available at: https://www.newsweek.com/us-supreme-court-ruling-cited-uganda-upholds-anti-gay-death-penalty-1887085. Accessed September 12, 2024.
53. Joint United Nations Programme on HIV/AIDS. *The Urgency of Now: AIDS at a Crossroads.* Geneva, Switzerland; 2024. Available at: https://www.unaids.org/sites/default/files/media_asset/2024-unaids-global-aids-update_en.pdf. Accessed March 25, 2025.
54. Nkengasong J, Ratevosian J. Legal and policy barriers for an effective HIV/AIDS response. *Lancet.* 2023;401(10386):1405–1407. https://doi.org/10.1016/S0140-6736(23)00729-8
55. United Nations Development Programme. Pathways to achieving the global 10-10-10 HIV targets: a review of the evidence on key population and community-led interventions to address punitive and discriminatory laws and HIV-related discrimination. May 31, 2024. Available at: https://www.undp.org/publications/pathways-achieving-global-10-10-10-hiv-targets. Accessed March 25, 2025.

US Right-Wing, Pro-Family Movements in East Africa: Furthering Legislation That Fuels Health Inequities Among Sexual and Gender Minority Persons Assigned Female Sex at Birth in Western Kenya

Heather M. Tucker, PhD, MA, Anita Mbanda, Rebecca Odhiambo, BA, and Gary W. Harper, PhD, MPH

See also Global LGBTQ+ Public Health in the Face of Legal Persecution, pp. 1229–1263.

AJPH August 2025, Vol. 115, No. 8

Neocolonial US right-wing actors have targeted sexual and reproductive health and rights and sexual and gender minority rights in Kenya, influencing support for the Family Protection Bill, which is currently sitting in the Kenyan parliament and, if enacted, would further criminalize sexual and gender minority persons.

We focus on how sexual and gender minority persons assigned female sex at birth in Kenya are at the intersection of these assaults on sexual and reproductive health and sexual and gender minority rights and already experience negative health outcomes because of discrimination, barriers to sexual and reproductive health care, and other effects owing to criminalization. (*Am J Public Health*. 2025;115(8): 1264–1270. https://doi.org/10.2105/AJPH.2025.308099)

Since the 1980s, US Christian right-wing actors have been active throughout the African continent seeking to create new frontiers to promote their ideologies of the family and campaign against gender justice and sexual rights of sexual and gender minorities (SGM), with a focus on, and some success in, sub-Saharan Africa.[1] The growing political and financial influence of these actors has numerous consequences for public health in sub-Saharan Africa, including access to health care for already stigmatized groups previously affected by colonial legislation.[2] Recently, researchers have identified the US Christian right's "spending boom" on the continent in an effort to affect policy and legislation.[3]

Both the 1994 International Conference on Population and Development and the 1996 Beijing Conference developed crucial sexual and reproductive health (SRH) and rights policies to be implemented by states, with many African countries signing on in support. US right-wing conservatives responded to this progress with a renewed movement to combat SRH and rights and the rights of SGM globally, with specific interest in sub-Saharan Africa.[4]

Two organizations joining in this movement are Family Watch International (FWI) and the World Congress of Families, both declared hate groups by the Southern Poverty Law Center and both headed by Sharon Slater.[5,6] Slater promotes anti-SGM ideologies and policies and is a self-described "internationally recognized leader in the effort to promote and protect the family and family values,"[5] core values of the US Christian right wing. Slater and her organizations have had an intense international focus on Africa and the United Nations and present their work as protecting the "natural" family and family values, as well as children, whereas their policy and legal focus is on dismantling protections for SGM persons and access to SRH care and rights.[5,6]

FWI is a notorious US-led right-wing organization founded in the United States in 1999 and is currently considered a nonprofit international educational organization in consultative status with the Economic and Social Council of the United Nations. FWI has been linked directly to the sponsorship of Uganda's Anti-Homosexuality Act (Act No. 6 of 2023), which criminalizes consensual same-sex conduct "with penalties of up to life imprisonment, attempted homosexual acts with penalties of 10 years in prison, and the death penalty for those convicted of 'aggravated homosexuality.'"[7] The organization is known for its anti-SGM stance and hosts an annual training program for African leaders to oppose both SGM rights and comprehensive sexuality education as well as to negotiate at the United Nations.[8] Emerging from the US Christian right in 2000, the World Congress of Families serves as a global network of anti-SGM organizations and has considerable influence at the level of the United Nations. The World Congress of Families' policies focus on "anti-choice, anti-LGBTQ" agendas and promote "conservative ideologies that dictate who has rights as 'family.'"[9]

ENCROACHING ON KENYA

Like many countries in sub-Saharan Africa, Kenya has been influenced by these neocolonial right-wing actors, who have a growing interest and investment in the region and exploit colonial legacies. This exploitative approach to policy and law in the country by US actors has been identified as particularly central to US evangelicalism and its dominionist nature.[10] FWI and the World Congress of Families, as well as other US Christian right-wing organizations, have explicitly focused on Kenya as a strategic country of influence throughout sub-Saharan Africa and have exploited and supported cultural and religious norms that define specific rights issues as "un-African." In 2010, the American Center for Law and Justice, an organization founded by US televangelist Pat Robertson, opened offices in Nairobi, Kenya, as the East African Center for Law and Justice. The organization's aim at the time was to gain a foothold on the African continent.[11]

In the Kenyan context, US Christian right-wing actors have targeted SRH care and rights (e.g., access to abortion, protection from sexual violence, and access to comprehensive sexuality education) and SGM rights by advocating and lobbying Kenyan politicians and religious leaders for specific policies and legislation in the country, with devastating effects. We identify these actors and sound the alarm regarding the effects of their actions on the health and well-being of SGM persons assigned female at birth (AFAB)—a population that was already experiencing increasing violence, discrimination, and barriers to SRH care and rights in Kenya. Our research, as well as that of others, has shown that this group experiences heightened forms of discrimination, sexual and gender-based violence, and anti-SGM violence, owing to a perceived transgression of heteronormativity. In particular, they experience heightened forms of discrimination and stigma related to their gender and gender presentation and sexuality.[12–14]

As a transnational research team with researchers from the University of Michigan's Department of Health Behavior & Health Equity in the School of Public Health and from the Western Kenya community-based organization Women Empower, we have previously focused on community-based, participatory research–informed projects that seek to understand barriers to health care experienced by SGM persons AFAB in Western Kenya.

From 2021 through 2023, we worked on a community-based participatory research– informed mixed-methods study—the Empowerment for Us by Us study—with Women Empower, the Western Kenyan LBQT+ Feminism Forum, and the Western Kenyan Homa Bay LBQ Feminist Forum. Qualitative data from the study revealed that SGM persons AFAB experience intersectional oppression caused by cultural and sociolegal contexts and laws that criminalize and stigmatize them.[13] Such intersectional oppression contributes to poor health, low self-esteem, and a poor ability to cope with stress. Additionally, the study indicated that to change the effects of oppression, SGM persons AFAB require access to resources and continued social and community support.[13]

The Empowerment for Us by Us study also administered a survey to 227 SGM persons AFAB in Kisumu County, Kenya, in 2023. Results from this survey showed alarming data related to SRH for this population, including high rates of HIV positivity (13%), a high rate of those reporting they have a small or no chance of acquiring HIV (69%), and 37% reporting forced vaginal sex with men (H. M. Tucker, A. Mbanda, R. Pulliam et al., unpublished).

In addition to these data, research shows that in Kenya, SGM persons AFAB face extreme barriers to accessing SRH services; experience discrimination, harassment, and violence from health care workers; and are excluded from health care interventions aimed at HIV prevention and SRH for heterosexual and cisgender women.[13,15,16] It is crucial to examine the actions of US Christian right-wing actors and their potential role in disempowering—and thereby harming the health and well-being of—SGM persons AFAB.

Although we by no means seek to remove agency from Kenyan right-wing politicians and religious conservatives responsible for promoting discriminatory and violent policies and legislation, we find it imperative to highlight and contextualize the current US-based support for anti-SGM legislation and anti-SRH care and rights efforts in Kenya. We analyze how the recently proposed anti-SGM Family Protection Bill 2023 would further increase health inequities among SGM persons AFAB.

The bill is directly connected to the US-based organization FWI. In March 2023, just a week after the passage of Uganda's Anti-Homosexuality Law, the FWI sponsored the First African Regional Inter-Parliamentary Conference and Dialogue on the Global Challenges to the Protection of the African Child, the African Family, and African Culture and Values.[17] Kenyan member of parliament Peter Kaluma, who drafted the bill, attended the event and has referred to discussions at the conference as particularly influential in the bill's creation.[18] The bill would further criminalize those who are perceived to be SGM persons and homosexuality as a violation between a perpetrator and a victim. Furthermore, the bill would criminalize anyone who seeks to fund or sponsor SGM programs or services and those who provide direct services to persons who are perceived or identify as a SGM person. The bill also seeks to criminalize gender-affirming care and the "promotion of homosexuality."[19,20]

This new legislative attack on highly stigmatized populations is in addition to a history of criminalization of SGM persons, as well as attacks on gender equitable and SRH-related legislation in Kenya. We propose that, owing to the already existing intersectional oppression experienced by SGM persons AFAB, the proposed anti-SGM legislation may heighten existing violence against SGM persons AFAB, amplifying experiences of discrimination and stigma and affecting the ability of SGM persons AFAB to navigate an already precarious context, including barriers to accessing SRH services.

HISTORICAL INFLUENCES OF COLONIZATION AND CHRISTIANITY

US Christian right-wing organizations have exploited and supported cultural and religious norms that are the result of colonial histories of legislative and political domination. In fact, the current Kenyan sociopolitical context is deeply informed by heteropatriarchal social norms and cultural and religious fundamentalism, which often deems gender justice, SRH rights, and SGM rights as un-African.[21] This context is layered on the 70-year British occupation of Kenya, which exploited land and resources and changed norms related to gender and sexuality and culture through legislation and the attempt to control reproduction. This occupation included the removal of previous systems that allowed access to land regardless of gender and attempts to control reproduction and sex.[22]

For example, British colonial occupation included the implementation of several laws to regulate excision and abortion.[22] Colonial era penal code section 162 criminalized same-sex practices, or nonprocreative sex, or "unnatural carnal knowledge . . . against the order of nature."[23] This legislative and policy-related approach to control reproduction and gender and sexual orientation in Kenya normalized a Western, colonial, 2-gender system privileging only heterosexual marriage and reproduction and demonizing gender and sexual diversity.

Exploiting this colonial legacy, US-based organizations such as the East African Center for Law and Justice specifically lobby African politicians and parliaments to include Christian views when drafting legislation and policies and use influential evangelical African religious leaders to gain access to leadership in the country. The East African Center for Law and Justice works with groups such as Human Life International, a US-based Catholic organization that lobbies against access to abortion; the Kenya Christian Professionals Forum; the Kenyan Council of Churches; and various Kenyan lawyers.[1]

In 2010, this included work to ensure the criminalization of same-sex practices and abortion in the redrafting of the Kenyan constitution and language asserting that marriage is between a man and a woman.[1] The influence of these actors is evident. The 2010 constitution of Kenya permits access to safe abortion services only "when the life or health of a woman is in danger and in cases of emergency,"[17(p22)] continuing to limit access. Definitions of marriage and family in the constitutional discourse reflect similar influences. The constitutional language defines marriage as between those of opposite sexes: "Every adult has the right to marry a person of the opposite sex, based on the free consent of the parties."[24]

Also, the new constitution included a specific amendment to protect the family as the foundation of society in Article 45. The 2010 Kenyan constitution criminalizes same-sex practices, and penal code section 162 criminalizes "unnatural carnal knowledge against the order of nature" as a felony, with punishment of up to 21 years in prison for those committing the act without consent.[24] Through strategic efforts of the East African Center for Law and Justice and others, laws and policies that were enacted by the British during their colonial occupation continue to influence religious and cultural norms related to sexuality and gender in postcolonial Kenya and elsewhere in sub-Saharan Africa, and, despite their Christian and European origins, they are often touted monolithically as African.

Following the 2010 redrafting of the Kenyan constitution, efforts to define and institutionalize heterosexual marriage continue. In 2019, the national Family Protection and Promotion Policy, spearheaded by the Ministry of Labor and Social Protection, was put in place to recognize the "family as a fundamental social unit of society and basis of social order as enshrined in the Constitution of Kenya"[25] and defines family as a "societal group that is related by blood, adoption, foster care of the ties of marriage of 2 persons of opposite sex."[25] This emphasis on the heteronormative family occurs on top of an overburdened health care system, which struggles to provide SRH services amid misinformation or a lack of information, leading to service restrictions.

LIVING AT INTERSECTIONS OF OPPRESSION

Living at the intersection of these social inequities, SGM persons AFAB experience heightened forms of stigma and oppression owing to gender inequities as well as the diversity of their sexual desires or gendered expressions, leading to barriers to accessing SRH and other health-related services.[14,26,27] The criminalization of same-sex practices in the Kenyan context contributes to violence and human rights violations against SGM persons, including physical assault, rape, and sexual assault.[13] Discrimination, stigma, and violence related to the intersection of their social status and access to power because of their gender or gender presentation and sexuality increase vulnerabilities to violence and discrimination in comparison with cis-gay and cis-bisexual men in Kenya.[28]

The current context often contributes to increased forms of SGM-based violence and sexual and gender-based violence, in addition to violence and rejection from families (including forced marriages, removal of children, control, and coercion), discrimination and stigma, and a lack of autonomy over one's SRH for SGM persons AFAB.[13–15,29] Because of the current penal code, SGM persons AFAB are afraid to report incidences of abuse or violence to the police; consequently, violence against SGM folks is enacted with impunity. SGM persons AFAB fear accessing health care owing to health care workers' stigma against them. Given this social and cultural environment in Kenya and other parts of sub-Saharan Africa, SGM persons AFAB have access to very few resources to respond to and cope with these inequities and negative health outcomes.[14]

SGM persons AFAB experience these inequities in a context of high levels of unplanned pregnancies, high HIV prevalence among women and girls, and heightened mortality risks in accessing abortion, especially for adolescent girls.[30,31] SRH providers in Kenya have been documented as experiencing conflicts between their personal feelings and their cultural or religious values, affecting their ability to provide SRH services.[30] Efforts to legalize abortion to address a heightened maternal mortality rate in the country have been met with similar rhetoric and backlash to SGM rights. The 2020 Reproductive Healthcare Bill proposed in Kenya's senate was attacked by antiabortion and faith-based groups as potentially normalizing "underage sex," allowing "LGBT+ people to have children through surrogacy," and promoting widespread abortion.[32]

Similarly, proposed legislation to curb sexual and gender-based violence has been met with the opposition claiming that such policies are un-African. For instance, in 2006, activists proposed the Sexual Offenses Act to provide a legal framework for dealing with sexual offenses and gender-based violence.[4] The act was argued against by members of parliament as "against their culture,"[4(p156)] and the notion of criminalizing marital rape was met with extreme opposition, as was the notion of SRH care and rights becoming cultural norms in the Kenyan context. Scholars have noted that those in power use specific discourses that tout acts as un-African to challenge minoritized groups in several sub-Saharan Africa contexts.[33]

Additionally, while Kenyan SGM activists have legally challenged colonial era penal codes as unconstitutional, changes have not been made to decriminalize supposed "un-natural carnal knowledge" in the country. In 2016, the National Gay and Lesbian Human Rights Commission (NGLHRC), the Gay and Lesbian Coalition of Kenya, and the Nyaza, Rift Valley and Western Kenya Network filed a petition to challenge anti-SGM legislation.[33] Despite these coordinated efforts, the Kenya High Court chose to uphold the country's colonial era penal code. In February and September 2023, the Kenyan Supreme Court ruled that SGM organizations, including the NGLHRC, are legally able to operate without criminalization. However, the result of this ruling has prompted immense backlash against SGM persons, including a surge in violence. In March 2023, the NGLHRC documented nearly 400 reports that included assaults, threats, and discrimination, an increase from January of the same year.[34]

FUELING THE FLAMES OF OPPRESSION

Other US Christian right-wing organizations that exploit Kenya's colonial legacy include Human Life International and FWI, which have provided financial support for promoting "family values" in sub-Saharan Africa, which includes demonizing reproductive rights and SGM rights.[1] FWI indicates on its Web site its intention not only to criminalize SGM persons and nonreproductive sex but also to prevent comprehensive sexuality education in Kenya as an "agenda" that seeks to "sexualize children across Africa," with a comprehensive webinar hosted by Slater.[35]

In 2016, the World Congress of Families hosted a conference in Nairobi, at which Stephen Langa, founder and executive director of the anti-SGM Family Life Network Uganda, was a speaker. Langa has a blatant anti-SGM agenda and has hosted meetings in Uganda titled Seminar on Exposing the Homosexuals' Agenda, which were attended by US Christian right pastor Scott Lively, who has been directly linked to the Uganda Anti-Homosexuality Act.[11] As mentioned previously, the Family Protection Bill in 2023 was proposed by Peter Kaluma shortly after his attendance at an FWI-sponsored event.[20]

The Family Protection Bill would further criminalize and stigmatize populations that are already experiencing heightened forms of violence and would strengthen several barriers to accessing SRH care. The bill would further criminalize those perceived to be SGM persons and homosexuality as a violation between a perpetrator and a victim, anyone who seeks to fund or sponsor SGM programs or services, and anyone who provides direct services to those who are perceived or identify as a SGM person.[22] The bill also seeks to criminalize gender-affirming care and the promotion of homosexuality.[22] Through this renewed criminalization, the bill would encourage discrimination and stigma against SGM persons, including reporting individuals, organizations, and health care providers serving this population as criminal. Hence, the bill would create further difficulty for health care providers and community-based networks in providing critical SRH information and services, leading to extreme difficulties for SGM persons AFAB in accessing SRH services and living lives free of stigmatization and violence.

ACCOUNTABILITY

The US Christian right-wing actors' exploiting colonial legacies in multiple sub-Saharan Africa countries has had devastating effects. Kenya and Uganda are just 2 of the countries affected by this movement, with Burundi, Senegal, and Tanzania considering legislation similar to Uganda's Anti-Homosexuality Law. In 2023, Ghana's parliament approved the 2021 Promotion of Appropriate Sexual Rights and Family Values Bill, and in 2024 its parliament passed it.[36]

Research in sub-Saharan Africa has highlighted that criminalization of same-sex behaviors leads to higher HIV prevalence, reverses gains made in the control of HIV and sexually transmitted infections, creates barriers in conducting public health research, and increases negative mental health outcomes.[2] The International AIDS Society and the Joint United Nations Programme on HIV and AIDS have acknowledged that anti-SGM legislation in Uganda and Ghana have stalled progress toward health equity, especially in regard to ending HIV.[34] Research has indicated that the Anti-Homosexuality Act in Uganda has already affected health outcomes, including creating barriers to HIV prevention and treatment through temporary clinic closures and changes to service delivery.

Furthermore, interest in research on HIV risk in the Ugandan context has diminished owing to researchers' safety concerns, and barriers to maintaining international research ethics have increased.[2] A Ugandan-based organization, Convening for Equality, has reported more than 180 evictions, 18 cases of forced anal examinations, 176 cases of violations of torture, 159 cases of violations of the right to equality and freedom from discrimination, and 102 hospitalizations directly linked to violations against SGM persons since the law was put into effect.[34]

The neocolonial actions of US Christian right-wing actors and organizations such as the East African Center for Law and Justice, Human Life International, and FWI must be held accountable for the devastation they cause in the everyday reality of SGM persons in sub-Saharan Africa. These deeply troubling actions should be of concern to policymakers at local, national, and international levels. Although US-based allies and leaders such as former president Joe Biden have issued statements against the Anti-Homosexuality Act in Uganda and have withheld the US President's Emergency Plan for AIDS Relief funds from the country, there has been no acknowledgment of the extent to which US citizens are fueling the support and creation of such laws, and there has been no direct action toward holding these actors accountable.[37]

Governments, institutions, and organizations must work on following the guidance of SGM people and communities in accountability efforts, especially those at the intersection of right-wing interests: SGM persons AFAB, activists, and allies from sub-Saharan Africa. In 2012, Sexual Minorities Uganda sued Scott Lively, a US pastor and anti-SGM supporter of the Anti-Homosexuality Law in Uganda, for violating international law. In 2017 a US federal court affirmed charges brought against Lively; however, the court ruled that they lacked extraterritorial reach.[38] Although this attempt was unsuccessful, Ugandan activists had no support from the US government during the case. Strategically aligning with activists on the ground through legal and financial support to hold US citizens such as Slater and her organization, FWI, legally accountable for the violence and politicized homophobia they import to the continent would be a step in the right direction.

Funding and resources for organizations advocating for and providing resources to SGM communities and activists working toward accessing SRH care and rights in sub-Saharan Africa that have been diligently fighting for decades are critically underresourced and must be sustained. Guidance from policymakers in response to the effects of the Anti-Homosexuality Act in Uganda highlight the need to redistribute US institutional support, such as the US President's Emergency Plan for AIDS Relief, and global support from institutions such as the Global Fund through community-based organizations able to reach SGM communities to provide health services.[39] There must be increased support for SRH care and rights information, education, and services in sub-Saharan Africa, including political support and increased funding to provide safe services. Additionally, funding and resources must be allocated for community-based health research in sub-Saharan Africa, including health research on how criminalization and legislation contribute to oppression and negative health outcomes for underresourced populations, research that highlights the implicit effects of neocolonial US Christian right-wing actors in underresourced contexts, and research that shows the explicit connection and intersection of anti-SGM legislation and anti-SRH efforts. AJPH

ABOUT THE AUTHORS

Heather M. Tucker is with the Center for Global Health Equity, School of Medicine, University of Michigan, Ann Arbor. Anita Mbanda and Rebecca Odhiambo are with Women Empower and Mentor All, Kisumu, Kenya. Gary W. Harper is with the Department of Health Behavior & Health Equity, School of Public Health, University of Michigan, Ann Arbor.

CORRESPONDENCE

Correspondence should be sent to Heather M. Tucker, PhD, MA, Center for AIDS Prevention Studies, University of California, San Francisco, 16th St, 3rd Floor, San Francisco, CA 94158 (e-mail: heather.tucker@ucsf.edu). Reprints can be ordered at https://www.ajph.org by clicking the "Reprints" link.

PUBLICATION INFORMATION

Full Citation: Tucker HM, Mbanda A, Odhiambo R, Harper GW. US right-wing, pro-family movements in East Africa: furthering legislation that fuels health inequities among sexual and gender minority persons assigned female sex at birth in Western Kenya. *Am J Public Health*. 2025;115(8):1264–1270.

Acceptance Date: February 24, 2025.

DOI: https://doi.org/10.2105/AJPH.2025.308099

ORCID iDs:
Heather M. Tucker https://orcid.org/0000-0003-2565-1996

Gary W. Harper https://orcid.org/0000-0003-1011-1751

CONTRIBUTORS

H. M. Tucker outlined and wrote the initial draft of the essay. H. M. Tucker and G. W. Harper conceptualized the essay. All authors provided critical review and edited versions of the essay.

ACKNOWLEDGMENTS

The Empowerment for Us by Us study was supported by the Center for Global Health Equity, School of Medicine, University of Michigan.

The authors would like to thank the sexual and gender minority and lesbian, gay, bisexual, or transgender/-sexual, plus other identities (LBQT+) persons who participated in the Empowerment for Us by Us (E4UBU) study for their time and for sharing their lived experiences. We would also like to thank Caroline Rucah from the Western Kenya LBQT Feminist Forum and Cynthia Akoth Ouko from the Homa Bay LBQT Womxn's Network for their work on the original data collection. We would also like to thank other E4UBU research team members vital to the research success, including Ini-Abasi Ubong and Myla Lyons from the School of Public Health and Ashley Lacombe Duncan from the School of Social Work, University of Michigan. A thank you goes to Wilson Odero at Maseno University for his guidance with the original research project.

CONFLICTS OF INTEREST

The authors have no known conflicts of interest to declare.

HUMAN PARTICIPANT PROTECTION

The University of Michigan institutional review board provided initial approval for the Empowerment for Us by Us study (HUM002115753). Human participants ethics approval was also obtained through the Maseno University Ethics Review Committee, and a research license was obtained from the National Commission for Science, Technology and Innovation in Kenya (NACOSTI/P/22/17643).

REFERENCES

1. Kaoma KJ. *Colonizing African Values: How the US Christian Right Is Transforming Sexual Politics in Africa.* Somerville, MA: Political Research Associates; 2012.
2. Mujugira A, Muwonge T, Aliganyira B, Okoboi S. Uganda's anti-homosexuality act undermines public health. *J Int AIDS Soc*. 2024;27(5):e26259. https://doi.org/10.1002/jia2.26259
3. Institute for Journalism and Social Change. Following the money: inside the US Christian right's spending boom in Africa. October 23, 2024. Available at: https://static1.squarespace.

com/static/67b73a68e16b30181e91bfb9/t/67bc4dbe09b20d50d7c78f16/1740393927962/Inside+The+U.S.+Christian+Right%27s+Spending+Boom+in+Africa+-+IJSC.pdf. Accessed March 13, 2025.

4. Oronje RN. The Kenyan national response to internationally agreed sexual and reproductive health and rights goals: a case study of three policies. *Reprod Health Matters*. 2013;21(42):151–160. https://doi.org/10.1016/S0968-8080(13)42749-0
5. Southern Poverty Law Center. Family Watch International. Available at: https://www.splcenter.org/resources/extremist-files/family-watch-international. Accessed March 13, 2025.
6. Southern Poverty Law Center. World Congress of Families. Available at: https://www.splcenter.org/resources/extremist-files/world-congress-families. Accessed January 5, 2025.
7. Human Rights Watch. Uganda: court upholds anti-homosexuality act. April 4, 2024. Available at: https://www.hrw.org/news/2024/04/04/uganda-court-upholds-anti-homosexuality-act. Accessed January 5, 2025.
8. Cullinan K, Geloo Z, Haidula T. US Christian right group hosts anti-LGBT training for African politicians. October 27, 2020. Available at: https://www.opendemocracy.net/en/5050/us-christian-right-group-hosts-anti-lgbt-training-african-politicians. Accessed June 28, 2024.
9. Parke C. Seventeen years of tracking the World Congress of Families. May 22, 2017. Available at: https://politicalresearch.org/2017/05/22/seventeen-years-of-tracking-the-world-congress-of-families. Accessed January 2, 2025.
10. Klinken AV. Culture wars, race, and sexuality: a nascent pan-African LGBT-affirming Christian movement and the future of Christianity. *J Africana Religions*. 2017;5(2):217–238. https://doi.org/10.5325/jafrireli.5.2.0217
11. Parke C. World Congress of Families descends on Africa. September 15, 2016. Available at: https://politicalresearch.org/2016/09/15/world-congress-of-families-descends-on-africa. Accessed January 2, 2025.
12. Gay and Lesbian Coalition of Kenya. Research on the lived experiences of lesbian, bisexual, and queer women in Kenya. Available at: https://galck.org/articles/research-on-the-lived-experiences-of-lbq-women-in-kenya. Accessed March 13, 2025.
13. Tucker HM, Odhiambo R, Jadwin-Cakmak L, et al. "Empowerment for us by us (E4UBU)": developing a model of empowerment using feminist participatory methods with LBQT+ persons assigned female at birth in Western Kenya. *Int J Environ Res Public Health*. 2024;21(7):948. https://doi.org/10.3390/ijerph21070948
14. Wilson BDM, Neubauer LC, Park A, Abuor P, Harper GW. The sexual health needs of sexual minority women in Western Kenya: an exploratory community assessment and public policy analysis. *Glob Public Health*. 2019;14(10):1495–1508. https://doi.org/10.1080/17441692.2019.1611895
15. Haase S, Zweigenthal V, Müller A. Barriers in access to healthcare for Kenyan queer womxn and trans men: findings of a cross-sectional online survey and interviews. [Preprint December 1, 2021]. https://doi.org/10.21203/rs.3.rs-1076697/v1
16. Awuor ODC. Neglected or unaffected! Investigating the exclusions and silences around lesbians, bisexuals, and queer (LBQ) women and HIV in Kisumu, Kenya. December 17, 2021. Available at: https://thesis.eur.nl/pub/61055. Accessed April 23, 2024.
17. Ipas; Empower. Pulling back the cover: the roots, relationships, and rise of Family Watch International. 2023. Available at: https://www.ipas.org/wp-content/uploads/2023/07/Pulling-Back-the-Cover-OPPPBCE23b.pdf. Accessed March 13, 2025.
18. Kenya could follow Uganda as East African nations wage war on LGBT rights. News24. June 25, 2023. Available at: https://www.news24.com/news24/africa/news/kenya-could-follow-uganda-as-east-african-nations-wage-war-on-lgbt-rights-20230625. Accessed January 5, 2025.
19. Family Protection Bill. National Assembly (Kenya, 2023). Arrangement of Clauses.
20. Walimbwa J, Macharia P, Wambua S, Lazarus L, Lorway R. Political homophobia and the effect on GBMSM programmes in Kenya: the significance of a community-led rapid agency assessment. *Glob Public Health*. 2023;18(1):2271989. https://doi.org/10.1080/17441692.2023.2271989
21. Otieno PE, Makabira AM. Gender equality vs "morality": the erosion of gender agendas in Kenya. *IDS Bull*. 2024;55(1):117–128. https://doi.org/10.19088/1968-2024.110
22. Thomas LM. *Politics of the Womb: Women, Reproduction, and the State in Kenya*. Berkeley: University of California Press; 2003.
23. Gupta A. This alien legacy: the origins of "sodomy" laws in British colonialism. December 17, 2008. Available at: https://www.hrw.org/report/2008/12/17/alien-legacy/origins-sodomy-laws-british-colonialism. Accessed March 14, 2025.
24. Kenya Law: The National Council for Law Reporting. The constitution of Kenya. Available at: https://kenyalaw.org/kl/index.php?id=398. Accessed September 10, 2024.
25. Kenya Ministry of Labour and Social Protection. National policy on family promotion and protection. December 2019. Available at: https://www.socialprotection.go.ke/sites/default/files/Downloads/FINAL-Family-policy-Dec-2019.pdf. Accessed March 13, 2025.
26. Zaidi SS, Ocholla AM, Otieno RA, Sandfort TGM. Women who have sex with women in Kenya and their sexual and reproductive health. *LGBT Health*. 2016;3(2):139–145. https://doi.org/10.1089/lgbt.2014.0121
27. Haase S. Sexual health decision-making and service utilisation among Kenyan queer womxn and trans men. 2022. Available at: http://hdl.handle.net/11427/37213. Accessed June 25, 2024.
28. Jauregui JC, Mwochi CR, Crawford J, et al. Experiences of violence and mental health concerns among sexual and gender minority adults in Western Kenya. *LGBT Health*. 2021;8(7):494–501. https://doi.org/10.1089/lgbt.2020.0495
29. Kilbride E. "This is why we became activists." Violence against lesbian, bisexual, and queer women and non-binary people. February 14, 2023. Available at: https://www.hrw.org/report/2023/02/14/why-we-became-activists/violence-against-lesbian-bisexual-and-queer-women-and-non. Accessed April 16, 2024.
30. Both R, Kageha E, Kloosterman J, Chung SW, Both J, Simenel F. Gender transformative approaches to improving the sexual and reproductive health and rights of young people in Kenya. Available at: https://www.researchgate.net/publication/354223734. Accessed March 13, 2025.
31. Ajayi AI, Otukpa EO, Mwoka M, Kabiru CW, Ushie BA. Adolescent sexual and reproductive health research in sub-Saharan Africa: a scoping review of substantive focus, research volume, geographic distribution and Africa-led inquiry. *BMJ Glob Health*. 2021;6(2):e004129. https://doi.org/10.1136/bmjgh-2020-004129
32. Bhalla N. Church, anti-abortion groups seen threatening women's health bill in Kenya. Reuters. September 18, 2020. Available at: https://www.reuters.com/article/us-kenya-women-health-idUSKBN2692O8. Accessed March 13, 2025.
33. Mutua-Mambo CN. Living in a liminal space: feminist and LGBT alliances in Kenya. *Womens Stud Commun*. 2020;43(2):125–130. https://doi.org/10.1080/07491409.2020.1745598
34. Nakweya G. Anti-LGBTQ+ laws in Africa harming health and research. *Lancet*. 2024;403(10434):1323–1324. https://doi.org/10.1016/S0140-6736(24)00681-0
35. Family Watch International. Protecting children from the SRHR/CSE agenda in Kenya. 2025. Available at: https://familywatch.org/2020/05/26/kenya-cse-exposed-resources. Accessed April 13, 2024.
36. United Nations. Ghana: Türk alarmed as parliament passes deeply harmful anti-gay bill. February 28, 2024. Available at: https://www.ohchr.org/en/press-releases/2024/02/ghana-turk-alarmed-parliament-passes-deeply-harmful-anti-gay-bill. Accessed December 19, 2024.
37. Wepukhulu SK. The West harms queer Africans by failing to hold its own people accountable. July 27, 2023. Available at: https://www.opendemocracy.net/en/5050/africa-queer-rights-lgbtiq-western-anti-rights-groups-accountable. Accessed January 6, 2025.
38. Human Rights Campaign. Judge affirms charges against Scott Lively, but dismisses case on jurisdictional grounds. June 7, 2017. Available at: https://www.hrc.org/news/judge-affirms-charges-against-scott-lively-but-dismisses-case-on-jurisdicti. Accessed January 6, 2025.
39. Russell A, Burnett ME. Discrimination in public health: how funders should fight laws like Uganda's Anti-Homosexuality Act. May 28, 2024. Available at: https://www.csis.org/analysis/discrimination-public-health-how-funders-should-fight-laws-ugandas-anti-homosexuality-act. Accessed August 27, 2024.

Sustainability of the Growth of the Local Public Health Workforce During the COVID-19 Pandemic, 2019–2022

Krishna Patel, DrPH, MPH, Timothy C. McCall, PhD, Margaret Cunningham, RN, MPH, Chloe Garofalini, MPH, Joi Lee, MPA, and Aaron A. Alford, PhD, MPH, PMP

See also Castrucci, p. 1184.

Objectives. To explore whether and how the local health department (LHD) workforce shifted during the COVID-19 pandemic given the large influx of supplemental funding to public health.

Methods. We used data from the National Association of County and City Health Officials National Profile of Local Health Departments, the main source of comprehensive data collected from LHDs across the United States. Total numbers of employees, total numbers of full-time equivalents (FTEs), and employee types (full time, part time, contractual, and seasonal) were used to estimate the total LHD workforce in 2022, changes in the LHD workforce from 2019 to 2022, and changes in the LHD workforce from 2019 to 2022 by employee type.

Results. In 2022, the estimated LHD workforce consisted of 182 100 employees or 163 200 FTEs. Between 2019 and 2022, there was a 19% increase in the total LHD workforce, but the size of the workforce varied according to jurisdiction size and rurality. The largest increase was among contract workers (175%), whereas the full-time workforce grew by approximately 7%, indicating that the permanent workforce was predominantly unchanged.

Conclusions. With the surge in temporary and contract workers in 2022, there are concerns regarding the sustainability of the LHD workforce. Without continued strategic and sustained funding across jurisdiction types, the workforce may be in jeopardy. (*Am J Public Health*. 2025;115(8):1271–1277. https://doi.org/10.2105/AJPH.2025.308096)

AJPH August 2025, Vol. 115, No. 8

Underinvestment in state and local public health in the United States after the Great Recession of 2008 has been well documented,[1] as has its contemporary effects on the governmental public health workforce.[2] A recent analysis of survey data from state and local public health departments nationwide indicated that the combined labor force of these agencies declined by 16% between 2008 and 2019.[3] Employee turnover and churn remain common in this sector; in the 2021 Public Health Workforce and Needs Survey, more than half of respondents indicated plans to retire, change positions, or leave the workforce within the following year.[4]

Although funding to state and local public health has been stagnant and not commensurate with population growth,[5] the overall quantity of funds is not the only factor negatively affecting the workforce's readiness to address population health threats. Federal funding streams and hiring mechanisms in governmental public health tend to be highly vertical,[6,7] directed to specific diseases and program categories rather than to foundational public health services. State- and local-level funding streams have historically varied widely in their flexibility as well as their quantity.[8] Vertically oriented funding mechanisms frequently restrict staff scope of work, thus limiting agencies' flexibility to adapt to changing needs.

This trend toward workforce reductions in the context of ongoing verticality left many state and local health departments inadequately prepared for the COVID-19 pandemic. Recognizing the need for increased epidemiology, surveillance, laboratory, clinical, infection prevention, and communications capacity in communities across the United States, the federal government allotted surge funding to be distributed to state and local health departments through legislative activity in 2020 and 2021.

Early in March 2020, the Coronavirus Preparedness and Response Supplemental Appropriations Act[9] authorized the US Department of Health and Human Services to distribute $950 million rapidly to state and local health departments for response activities, including workforce scale-up. This was followed in late March 2020 by the Coronavirus Aid, Relief, and Economic Security Act,[10] which authorized additional funding for state and local workforce support; in April 2020 by the Paycheck Protection Program and Health Care Enhancement Act,[11] which released funds from the Public Health Social Services Emergency Fund for pandemic response activities; and in December 2020 by the Coronavirus Response and Relief Supplemental Appropriations Act.[12] In March 2021, the American Rescue Plan Act[13] allocated an additional $4.4 billion for workforce support in states and localities.

Measuring the impact of this legislative support on the local public health workforce during the COVID-19 pandemic is challenging because of the complex nature of the funding streams and the different pathways by which funds were allotted to localities (i.e., directly or via state pass throughs). Similar challenges exist in enumerating the workforce impact of programs supported by philanthropies, foundations, and other private funding sources.[14] One analysis of data from the 2021 Public Health Workforce Interests and Needs Survey, fielded in September 2021 through January 2022, indicated that most pandemic-associated surge hiring had occurred before March 2021.[14,15]

Overall, as of 2019, the National Association of County and City Health Officials (NACCHO) estimated that the local public health workforce consisted of 153 000 employees or 136 000 full-time equivalents (FTEs), as compared with the 2008 total of 184 000 employees or 162 000 FTEs.[16] In addition, before the COVID-19 pandemic, it was estimated that LHDs require approximately 54 000 more FTEs to provide the core foundational public health services.[3] There are no reliable estimates of the local governmental public health workforce during the pandemic.

Although it is difficult to understand the true effect of supplemental funding on the local governmental workforce, it is possible to observe how workforce trends have shifted from before the pandemic to indirectly gauge its importance. Therefore, our objectives in this study were to describe the overall local public health workforce in 2022 during the pandemic and characterize any shifts from 2019, including possible increases in the workforce. To address these objectives, we used the NACCHO National Profile of Local Health Departments study to examine LHD workforce data in the context of pandemic legislative trends and expand on different workforce indicators to showcase trends beyond NACCHO's previous survey work.

METHODS

The triennial National Profile of Local Health Departments is the only nationally representative survey of LHDs across the United States; it provides the most reliable estimates of LHD workforce, infrastructure, practice, services, and capacity. The survey questionnaire was developed and revised through consultation with internal and external subject matter experts including academics, public health officials, and members of government and nonprofit organizations. For the purposes of the survey, an LHD is defined as an administrative or service unit of local or state government that is concerned with health and carries some responsibility for the health of a jurisdiction smaller than the state.

The survey has been fielded every 3 years since 1989 to describe how LHD staffing, governance, funding, and activities have varied across the United States over time. It is administered to LHDs identified for surveying purposes (without duplicating US residents served); it typically includes 2 module questionnaires to survey LHDs on additional topics at random as a means of reducing survey fatigue while providing further vital information on public health infrastructure and practices. Modules are sampled via nationally representative random stratified sampling (according to population size served).

Between June and September 2022, the survey was distributed online via Qualtrics to a total of 2512 LHDs; 942 LHDs responded (37.5% response rate). Rhode Island was excluded from the study because the state has no LHDs. Additional details regarding the 2022 survey and its methodology can be found elsewhere.[17] Here we reference 2019 survey data to assess longitudinal trends in the workforce. The same methodology was used for fielding and analyzing the 2 separate 2019 and 2022 surveys. A total of 2459 LHDs were included in the 2019 study population, with a final response rate of 60.8%.[16]

Workforce Measures

For each responding agency, the research organization used the US Census Bureau classification system to compile information on jurisdiction size (defined in terms of population served, categorized as small [less than 50 000], medium [50 000–499 999], or large [500 000 or above]) and rurality (urban/rural status). LHDs were classified as urban or rural on the basis of whether the majority of the people they served were from urban settings (i.e., departments serving more than a 50% urban population were classified as urban).

In this study, we focused on 2 survey workforce items requested from all LHD respondents: the numbers of individuals and FTEs currently working and the numbers in specific job categories (full time, part time, contractual, and seasonal). Because data on these items were gathered separately, individual responses for job categories may not sum to the total.

Data Analysis

Analyses were conducted in Stata 18 (StataCorp LP, College Station, TX) via post-stratification weighting; a 7-category measure of LHD size based on population served (less than 25 000, 25 000–49 999, 50 000–99 999, 100 000–249 999, 250 000–499 999, 500 000–999 999, 1 000 000 or more) was used to adjust for nonresponses. Results obtained in this manner can be interpreted as national estimates for the survey year based on the size of the population served. We initially calculated descriptive statistics across workforce items, specifically total numbers of employees and FTEs overall and within each job category, to obtain national LHD workforce estimates. Cross tabulations with the 3-category size of jurisdiction measure and the location measure based on rurality (urban or rural) were also calculated for 2022. Workforce trends from 2019 to 2022 were based on calculations of the weighted workforce totals (employees and FTEs) for each of the 2 data sets separately.

RESULTS

Table 1 outlines the LHD workforce in terms of employees and FTEs according to size of population served and rurality. In 2022, the total estimated LHD workforce in the United States consisted of 182 100 employees (95% confidence interval [CI] = 160 200, 204 100) or 163 200 FTEs (95% CI = 144 600, 181 800). LHDs serving larger populations tended to have a larger total workforce (96 100 employees vs 63 900 for medium and 22 100 for small LHDs). Furthermore, the total workforce across urban LHDs consisted of 153 400 employees or 138 100 FTEs, much larger than the workforce across rural LHDs (28 700 employees or 25 100 FTEs).

Figure 1 illustrates trends in the overall LHD workforce from 2019 to 2022. Over this period, the LHD workforce expanded by approximately 19% to 20% for employees and FTEs. Before this upward trend, the LHD workforce had been steadily declining since 2008.[17] Further examination of these trends by jurisdiction size showed that there was limited to no increase in the total workforce between 2019 and 2022 among small LHDs, as compared with an upward trend for both total employees and FTEs among large LHDs.

Table 2 provides an overview of the LHD workforce across 4 job categories: full time, part time, contractual, and seasonal. Overall, in 2022, the LHD workforce primarily consisted of full-time employees (137 500), followed by contractual employees (22 000). As expected, LHDs serving larger jurisdictions tended to have greater numbers of employees across the 4 categories. In addition, the total estimate for employees among urban LHDs was much greater across all job categories than the estimate among rural LHDs.

An examination of job categories within the LHD workforce across time showed that the greatest relative difference was in contractual employees between 2019 and 2022 (a 175% increase; Table 3). The number of part-time employees declined from 2019 to 2022, whereas full-time employees increased by 7% between these years. The permanent workforce declined or saw modest gains, and the largest increases were among temporary and contract staff positions added after the introduction of emergency supplemental COVID-19 funding. In addition, workforce gains were not universal across jurisdiction sizes; instead, the increases in workforce job types seen were within medium and large LHDs as opposed to

TABLE 1— Size and Rurality Breakdowns of the Local Public Health Department Workforce: United States, 2022

	Total Employees, No. (95% CI)	Total FTEs, No. (95% CI)
Overall	182 100 (160 200, 204 100)	163 200 (144 600, 181 800)
Size		
Small	22 100 (20 500, 23 700)	19 000 (17 500, 20 500)
Medium	63 900 (57 600, 70 300)	55 100 (49 800, 60 500)
Large	96 100 (75 100, 117 100)	89 000 (71 200, 106 800)
Rurality		
Rural	28 700 (25 700, 31 800)	25 100 (22 400, 27 800)
Urban	153 400 (131 500, 175 400)	138 100 (119 500, 156 600)

Note. FTE = full-time equivalent; CI = confidence interval. Data are weighted and rounded to the nearest hundreds. Sample sizes were 929 (employees) and 924 (FTEs).

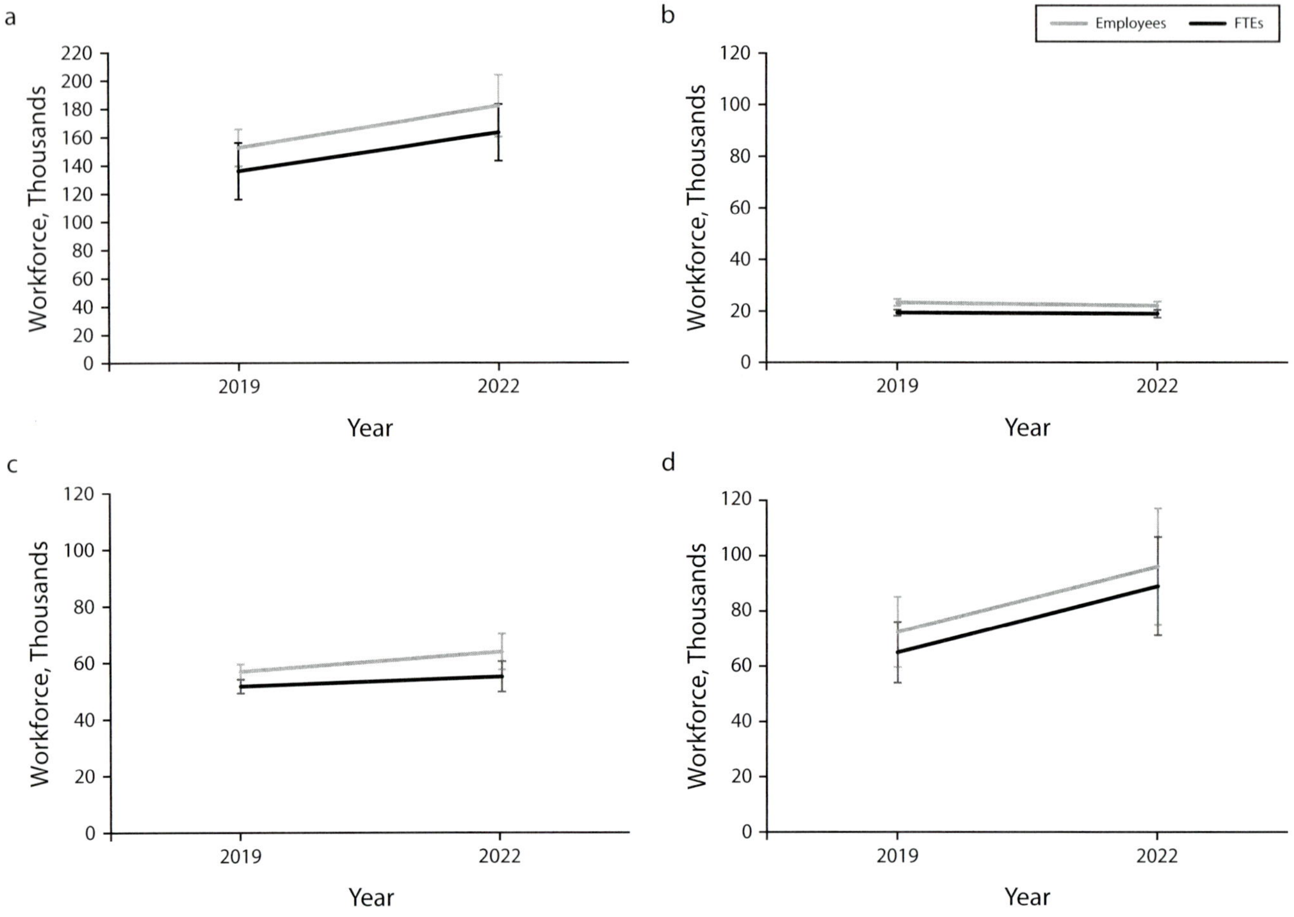

FIGURE 1— Local Public Health Workforce for (a) All Local Health Departments (LHDs), (b) Small LHDs Only, (c) Medium LHDs Only, and (d) Large LHDs Only: United States, 2019–2022

Note. The 95% confidence intervals for employee and full-time equivalent (FTE) estimates are provided for each survey year, rounded to the nearest hundreds. Lines represent changes in the weighted total number of employees or FTE estimates from the 2019 to 2022 surveys. Sample sizes were 1467 (employees) and 1468 (FTEs) for 2019 and 929 (employees) and 924 (FTEs) for 2022; however, the data were weighted for each year to allow national estimates. There is a different y-axis for all LHDs to account for total numbers and 95% confidence intervals.

TABLE 2— Local Public Health Department Employees Across Job Categories With Size and Rurality Breakdowns: United States, 2022

	Full Time, No.	Part Time, No.	Contractual, No.	Seasonal, No.
Overall	137 500	14 700	22 000	3 400
Size				
Small	17 400	3 000	1 400	100
Medium	49 500	5 900	4 900	1 300
Large	70 500	5 900	15 700	1 900
Rurality				
Rural	22 900	3 300	2 200	100
Urban	114 600	11 400	19 800	3 300

Note. Data are weighted and rounded to the nearest hundreds. Sample sizes were 892 (full time), 882 (part time), 882 (contractual), and 885 (seasonal).

small LHDs. Specifically, across jurisdiction sizes, small LHDs saw practically no growth or even workforce declines.

Contract employees increased by 123% and 249% in medium and large LHDs, respectively, with no change observed among small LHDs. The same general trend was observed among full-time and seasonal employees, with larger increases among medium and large LHDs than among small LHDs. For example, there was a 36% increase in the total seasonal workforce for large LHDs, in contrast to a 50% decline among small LHDs. The total number

TABLE 3— Local Public Health Department Job Categories by Department Size: United States, 2019–2022

	Full Time	Part Time	Contractual	Seasonal
Overall				
2019, no.	128 500	17 600	8 000	2 300
2022, no.	137 500	14 700	22 000	3 400
Difference, %	7	−16	175	48
Small LHDs				
2019, no.	17 000	4 300	1 400	200
2022, no.	17 400	3 000	1 400	100
Difference, %	2	−30	0	−50
Medium LHDs				
2019, no.	46 500	5 600	2 200	600
2022, no.	49 500	5 900	4 900	1 300
Difference, %	6	5	123	117
Large LHDs				
2019, no.	65 100	7 700	4 500	1 400
2022, no.	70 500	5 900	15 700	1 900
Difference, %	8	−23	249	36

Note. LHD = local health department. Data are weighted for each year separately and rounded to nearest hundreds. Sample sizes for 2019 were 1092 (full time), 1087 (part time), 1090 (contractual), and 1088 (seasonal). Sample sizes for 2022 were 892 (full time), 882 (part time), 882 (contractual), and 885 (seasonal).

of part-time employees declined overall; however, medium LHDs exhibited a slight increase of 5%, as compared with a 30% decrease among small LHDs and a 23% decrease among large LHDs.

DISCUSSION

The local public health workforce steadily declined from 2008 to 2019. During the COVID-19 pandemic, emergency funds allocated to public health agencies for the response likely led to the 19% increase in the total LHD workforce. Gains in staffing were primarily observed among medium and large jurisdictions, and most of this increase occurred among contractual (175% increase) and seasonal (48% increase) workers; the part-time workforce shrank, and the full-time workforce grew marginally by 7%.

Public Health and Policy Implications

A larger public health workforce after decades of decline is at first glance a welcome sign given that the workforce has been insufficient thus far to deliver necessary core and fundamental services across the country.[18] There are important implications and considerations in relation to our findings. First, gains between 2019 and 2022 were largely among contractual and seasonal workers in medium and large health departments; the workforce in small local health departments remained relatively stable or decreased. Previous work has shown that LHD hiring faced challenges in filling workforce gaps during the COVID-19 response ranging from external funding restrictions to a lack of authorizations for new staff positions.[19]

Our findings appear to indicate that LHDs were able to flex around these many limitations by bringing in temporary, contractual, and seasonal labor in response to the explosive needs driven by the COVID-19 response. Because contractual workers may not be able to transition to full-time positions or programmatic areas in need outside of COVID-19 given the expiration of pandemic supplemental funding in 2024, it is possible that the workforce will decline again. Also, despite this growth since 2019 in the local public health workforce, it falls far short of the workforce needed to provide infrastructure and public health services, estimated to be 80 000 or more FTEs.[18]

In addition, these gains occurred after an influx of funding to public health that will soon expire.[20] Without unrestricted and disease-agnostic funding, it is not possible to sustain staffing levels specifically aimed at the COVID-19-related emergency response. Although the need for a larger local public health workforce to meet the demands of the nation's public has been suggested by previous research, it cannot be sustained through COVID-19-specific continuing or expiring funds from the federal government. One reason that disease-agnostic funding is likely necessary is that small and rural jurisdictions, which experienced almost no workforce growth during COVID-19, also face higher rates of threats to public health such as heart disease, stroke, cancer, accidental injuries, suicide, and COVID-19.[21,22]

Although medium and large jurisdictions may have experienced increases in staffing during the pandemic, there remain threats to public health that COVID-19 emergency funding was not intended to address. Nearly 80% of LHDs in 2020 reported having to reassign staff from existing roles, departments, and duties to respond to the pandemic.[23] In addition, many jurisdictions reported both anecdotally and through nationally representative data collection that other critical activities that may reduce the impact of future public health crises (e.g., data modernization) either were on hold or involved no plans for implementation.[24] Funding a right-sized, permanent, and appropriately staffed local public health workforce that can meet the need for essential services must also include consideration of existing threats and the needs of jurisdictions that are typically not supported through emergency funding.

The Public Health Infrastructure Grant (awarded in December 2022)[25,26] may provide temporary mitigation of some of the losses in staffing in the absence of future growth. This funding mechanism provides disease-agnostic funding to state health departments and a variety of LHDs, both directly and indirectly, for recruitment, retention, support, and workforce training[25]; these funds may include support for the transition of temporary workers to full-time positions before they are removed from the LHD workforce. But only 21% of the $3 billion in workforce funding is allocated for staff hiring and recruitment,[27] and there is no indication that this funding will be renewed in perpetuity (or past 2027[25]) to support the future workforce long term. Future research should evaluate whether the Public Health Infrastructure Grant helps to sustain the public health workforce (including aspects such as the transition of temporary and contract positions to full-time positions) after the COVID-19 pandemic.

Finally, other incentives to support the natural growth of the local public health workforce are still likely necessary. For example, the Public Health Workforce Loan Repayment Plan included in the Consolidated Appropriations Act, which passed Congress with bipartisan support in 2022, would provide recent graduates who earned degrees in fields such as public health, epidemiology, data systems, informatics, and statistics with student loan repayments of up to $50 000 per year for 3 years of service. However, this plan has not yet been funded to implement the program. Programs such as this are just one recruitment and retention tool LHDs could use to build a stronger and larger workforce. Overall, without appropriate funding to grow and sustain the local public health workforce long term, the United States may be unprepared to respond to future public health emergencies.

Limitations

This study is not without limitations. For example, the data were self-reported by LHDs and could not be independently verified by NACCHO. For a variety of reasons, in addition to survey nonresponse, LHDs may have provided incomplete workforce information; to account for differential nonresponse among jurisdictions of different sizes, we used poststratification weighting based on jurisdiction size to produce national estimates of the LHD workforce. Although poststratification weighting helps minimize the effects of differential nonresponse, response rates for national surveys across public health were low during the COVID-19 pandemic (including the National Profile of Local Health Departments); therefore, such biases are still possible limitations of our study.

In addition, caution should be taken when attempting to sum individual categories of position types or FTEs to estimate the workforce; the survey collected total estimates from LHDs and subsequently individual category estimates (without summing them) because although these categories were defined for respondents, there was the potential for nonmutual exclusivity between categories (for example, workers on a contract may have been working full time at the agency during their contract). These data have been collected consistently over several iterations of the survey so that within-category changes and trends can be monitored, along with changes among the full workforce.

Conclusion

The growth of the local public health workforce since 2019 is potentially promising with respect to supporting consistent and sufficient delivery of public health services in the United States; however, such gains have primarily been driven by medium and large jurisdictions. In addition, there have been large relative increases in seasonal and contract staffing . Without sustained and disease-agnostic funding in future years, these increases are likely temporary. Moreover, the declines in the public health workforce that began in 2008 and continued until 2019 will likely occur again or future growth will not occur, especially in jurisdictions that did not exhibit workforce growth during this increased period of public health funding. AJPH

ABOUT THE AUTHORS

At the time of this study, all of the authors were with the National Association of County and City Health Officials, Washington, DC. Timothy C. McCall is also with the Department of Clinical Research and Leadership, The George Washington University, Washington, DC.

CORRESPONDENCE

Correspondence should be sent to Krishna Patel, DrPH, MPH, 1201 I St NW, 4th Floor, Washington, DC 20005 (e-mail: kpatel@naccho.org). Reprints can be ordered at https://www.ajph.org by clicking the "Reprints" link.

PUBLICATION INFORMATION

Full Citation: Patel K, McCall TC, Cunningham M, Garofalini C, Lee J, Alford AA. Sustainability of the growth of the local public health workforce during the COVID-19 pandemic, 2019–2022. *Am J Public Health*. 2025;115(8):1271–1277.

Acceptance Date: February 24, 2025.

DOI: https://doi.org/10.2105/AJPH.2025.308096

ORCID iDs:

Krishna Patel https://orcid.org/0009-0009-7963-0518

Timothy C. McCall https://orcid.org/0000-0002-9275-1842

Chloe Garofalini https://orcid.org/0000-0002-5246-3811

Aaron A. Alford https://orcid.org/0000-0001-5910-6174

CONTRIBUTORS

K. Patel, T. C. McCall, and M. Cunningham made substantial contributions to the conception or design of the work; acquisition, analysis, or interpretation of data; and drafting the work or revising it critically for important intellectual content. C. Garofalini, J. Lee, and A. A. Alford made substantial contributions to drafting the work or revising it critically for important intellectual content.

ACKNOWLEDGMENTS

Funding for this research was provided by the Centers for Disease Control and Prevention (grant 6NU38OT000306-03-06) and the Robert Wood Johnson Foundation (grant 78802).

We acknowledge the local health departments and their staff that completed the National Association of County and City Health Officials (NACCHO) National Profile of Local Health Departments survey in 2019 and 2022 and all of the local health departments working to support local public health before, during, and since the COVID-19 pandemic. In addition, we thank former and current NACCHO staff including David Okereke and Kellie Perkins, who reviewed and provided feedback for this article.

Note. The funders were not involved in the research for or writing of this article, and the views expressed are those of the authors only.

CONFLICTS OF INTEREST

The authors have no conflicts of interest to disclose.

HUMAN PARTICIPANT PROTECTION

No protocol approval was needed for this study because no human participants were involved.

REFERENCES

1. DeSalvo K, Parekh A, Hoagland GW, et al. Developing a financing system to support public health infrastructure. *Am J Public Health*. 2019;109(10):1358–1361. https://doi.org/10.2105/AJPH.2019.305214
2. Alfonso YN, Leider JP, Resnick B, McCullough JM, Bishai D. US public health neglected: flat or declining spending left states ill equipped to respond to COVID-19. *Health Aff (Millwood)*. 2021;40(4):664–671. https://doi.org/10.1377/hlthaff.2020.01084
3. Leider JP, McCullough JM, Singh SR, et al. Staffing up and sustaining the public health workforce. *J Public Health Manag Pract*. 2023;29(3):E100–E107. https://doi.org/10.1097/PHH.0000000000001614
4. de Beaumont Foundation, Association of State and Territorial Health Officials. Public Health Workforce Interests and Needs Survey: 2021 dashboard. Available at: https://www.phwins.org/national. Accessed December 20, 2024.
5. Beck AJ, Boulton ML. Trends and characteristics of the state and local public health workforce, 2010–2013. *Am J Public Health*. 2015;105(suppl 2):S303–S310. https://doi.org/10.2105/AJPH.2014.302353
6. Mays GP, Scutchfield FD, Bhandari MW, Smith SA. Understanding the organization of public health delivery systems: an empirical typology. *Milbank Q*. 2010;88(1):81–111. https://doi.org/10.1111/j.1468-0009.2010.00590.x
7. Bishai DM, Resnick B, Lamba S, et al. Being accountable for capability—getting public health reform right this time. *Am J Public Health*. 2022;112(10):1374–1378. https://doi.org/10.2105/AJPH.2022.306975
8. United Health Foundation. America's health rankings: public health funding in the United States. Available at: https://www.americashealthrankings.org/explore/measures/PH_funding. Accessed December 20, 2024.
9. US Congress. Coronavirus Preparedness and Response Supplemental Appropriations Act (Pub L No. 116-123). Available at: https://www.govinfo.gov/app/details/PLAW-116publ123. Accessed December 20, 2024.
10. US Congress. Coronavirus Aid, Relief, and Economic Security Act (Pub L No. 116-136). Available at: https://www.congress.gov/116/plaws/publ136/PLAW-116publ136.pdf. Accessed December 20, 2024.
11. US Congress. Paycheck Protection Program and Health Care Enhancement Act (Pub L No. 116-139). Available at: https://www.congress.gov/116/plaws/publ139/PLAW-116publ139.pdf. Accessed December 20, 2024.
12. US Congress. Consolidated Appropriations Act (Pub L No. 116-260). Available at: https://www.govinfo.gov/content/pkg/PLAW-116publ260/pdf/PLAW-116publ260.pdf. Accessed December 20, 2024.
13. American Rescue Plan Act (Pub L 117-2). Available at: https://www.govinfo.gov/content/pkg/PLAW-117publ2/pdf/PLAW-117publ2.pdf. Accessed December 20, 2024.
14. Lee KM, Bosold A, Alvarez C, et al. Surging the public health workforce: lessons learned from the COVID-19 response at state, tribal, local, and territorial public health agencies. Available at: https://aspe.hhs.gov/sites/default/files/documents/da3419d752f6f8c0359a126a9045fefb/surging-the-ph-workforce.pdf. Accessed December 20, 2024.
15. McCullough JM, Robins M. The opportunity cost of COVID for public health practice: COVID-19 pandemic response work and lost foundational areas of public health work. *J Public Health Manag Pract*. 2023;29(suppl 1):S64–S72. https://doi.org/10.1097/PHH.0000000000001656
16. National Association of County and City Health Officials. 2019 National Profile of Local Health Departments. Available at: https://www.naccho.org/uploads/downloadable-resources/Programs/Public-Health-Infrastructure/NACCHO_2019_Profile_final.pdf. Accessed December 20, 2024.
17. Cunningham M, Patel K, McCall TC, et al. 2022 National Profile of Local Health Departments. Available at: https://www.naccho.org/resources/lhd-research/national-profile-of-local-health-departments. Accessed December 20, 2024.
18. de Beaumont Foundation, Public Health National Center for Innovations. Staffing up: workforce levels needed to provide basic public health services for all Americans. Available at: https://debeaumont.org/wp-content/uploads/2021/10/Staffing-Up-FINAL.pdf. Accessed December 20, 2024.
19. Kirkland C, Oldfield-Tabbert K, Karnik H, Orr J, Martin S, Leider JP. Public health workforce gaps, impacts, and improvement strategies from COVID-19. *Int J Environ Res Public Health*. 2022;19(20):13084. https://doi.org/10.3390/ijerph192013084
20. US Department of the Treasury. Coronavirus state and local fiscal recovery funds. Available at: https://home.treasury.gov/system/files/136/2023-Interim-Final-Rule.pdf. Accessed December 20, 2024.
21. NIHCM Foundation. Rural health during the pandemic: challenges and solutions to accessing care. Available at: https://nihcm.org/publications/rural-health-during-the-pandemic. Accessed December 20, 2024.
22. Seshamani M, Jacobs D, Moody-Williams J, Fleisher L. Addressing rural health inequities in Medicare. Available at: https://www.cms.gov/blog/addressing-rural-health-inequities-medicare. Accessed December 20, 2024.
23. Hall K, Brees K, McCall TC, et al. 2020 Forces of Change: the COVID-19 edition. Available at: https://www.naccho.org/uploads/downloadable-resources/2020-Forces-of-Change-The-COVID-19-Edition.pdf. Accessed December 20, 2024.
24. Cunningham MC, Patel K, Garofalini C, et al. 2023 Forces of Change Survey. Available at: https://www.naccho.org/resources/lhd-research/forces-of-change. Accessed December 20, 2024.
25. Centers for Disease Control and Prevention. Public Health Infrastructure Grant. Available at: https://www.cdc.gov/infrastructure-phig/about/index.html. Accessed December 20, 2024.
26. US Government. Grant opportunity: strengthening US public health infrastructure, workforce, and data systems. Available at: https://www.grants.gov/search-results-detail/340034. Accessed December 20, 2024.
27. Centers for Disease Control and Prevention. Public Health Infrastructure Grant: health department profiles. Available at: https://www.cdc.gov/infrastructure-phig/php/data-research/profiles/index.html. Accessed December 20, 2024.

Identification of Transgender and Gender-Diverse Individuals in the All of Us Research Program, 2017–2022

Fanghui Shi, PhD, Xueying Yang, PhD, Ruilie Cai, MS, Jiajia Zhang, PhD, Sayward E. Harrison, PhD, Shan Qiao, PhD, Sarah Grace Frary, MA, and Xiaoming Li, PhD

See also Tordoff et al., p. 1192.

Objectives. To develop computable phenotype algorithms to identify a transgender and gender-diverse (TGD) cohort by using diverse data sources in All of Us, a national community-engaged program to facilitate health equity in the United States by partnering with 1 million participants.

Methods. We identified TGD individuals in All of Us by applying inclusion criteria based on conditions, laboratory measurements, or medications related to being TGD in electronic health record data or confirmed survey responses, using participant data collected between May 31, 2017, and July 1, 2022.

Results. Of 413 457 participants, we identified 4781 (1.2%) as TGD. Participants aged 18 to 29 years (26.1% vs 8.2%), who were bisexual (20.7% vs 3.5%), with annual income of less than $25 000 (35.9% vs 24.7%), and with housing security concerns (31.9% vs 16.0%) accounted for a larger proportion of TGD individuals than non-TGD individuals.

Conclusions. Combining survey and electronic health record data enables the identification of TGD individuals who have been missed by previous studies that used survey data alone in All of Us to explore health disparities in TGD people. (*Am J Public Health*. 2025;115(8):1278–1287. https://doi.org/10.2105/AJPH.2025.308129)

AJPH August 2025, Vol. 115, No. 8

In the latest *Standards of Care for the Health of Transgender and Gender-Diverse People*, version 8, "transgender and gender-diverse" (TGD) is used as a broad term to describe people whose gender identity or expression differs from the gender typically associated with their sex assigned at birth.[1,2] This term was chosen to be as inclusive as possible and highlight the diversity of gender identities, expressions, and experiences of TGD people. Currently, 0.4% to 1.3% of the US general population is estimated to be TGD, although the number may change considerably based on how the term is defined.[3] The expansion of TGD categories beyond transgender male and transgender female, such as nonbinary and gender fluid, has contributed to variations in estimates across studies and data sets.[1,2] Additionally, changes in social acceptance and political climate (e.g., freedom of gender expression and access to gender-affirming care) can affect how many individuals disclose their TGD identity.[4]

Studies have consistently reported a high prevalence of a range of negative health indicators among TGD individuals, such as mental health distress and HIV and other sexually transmitted infections.[5,6] Despite such health disparities, there is a lack of gender identity data collected in large population-based health systems, limiting quantitative research about TGD individuals.[7–9] There is a compelling need to integrate multiple data sources to generate more diverse and larger TGD samples, which is important for identifying health inequities, understanding the drivers of these disparities, and designing health care interventions and tailored services for TGD people.[10]

The National Institutes of Health's (NIH's) All of Us (AoU) research program is a national community-engaged program aiming to improve health by partnering with 1 million participants, more than 80% of whom are from historically underrepresented communities in biomedical research in the United States.[11,12] The AoU program integrates self-reported survey data (including gender identity, sexual orientation, and sex assigned at birth) with electronic health record (EHR) data (including *International Classification of Diseases* [*ICD*] codes for gender dysphoria, medication information, and gender-affirming surgery records), physical measurements, and biospecimens to create a data repository.[12] This allows researchers to identify diverse and large volunteer TGD cohorts from different sources.

However, there is a lack of standardization regarding the classification of TGD individuals on the AoU platform.[13] Studies using AoU research program data have relied predominantly on survey questions alone to identify TGD individuals, and have defined gender-diverse people as anyone who answered the gender identity item by endorsing at least 1 of the following responses: nonbinary, transgender, or "none of these describe me."[14–17] Relying solely on survey data is limited by social desirability bias, as participants may be unwilling to disclose their gender minority status. This may lead to underestimation of the proportion of TGD individuals in AoU. Other health measures, such as prescription data and clinical diagnoses from EHRs, are additional sources of population-level data that could help identify TGD persons and describe their health and well-being.[18]

Using diverse data sources available from the AoU research program, we aimed to develop computable phenotype algorithms to identify TGD people on the AoU platform and examine the prevalence of TGD persons in populations with different sociodemographic characteristics, such as sex assigned at birth, race/ethnicity, age, sexual orientation, and social determinants of health (e.g., insurance coverage, income, education, and housing insecurity).

METHODS

Sponsored by the NIH, the AoU research program was launched in 2015 as part of the Precision Medicine Initiative, which aims to revolutionize biomedical research and health care delivery by using comprehensive health data from diverse populations across the United States. All US adults (aged ≥ 18 years) who are not in prison and can provide consent to participate are eligible to participate in AoU. This program opened for enrollment in May 2018 and seeks to recruit at least 1 million participants to provide large-scale population health data.

More than 100 funded partner organizations and more than 860 institutional sites have joined AoU and have been helping recruit participants and collect measurements or samples. As of February 4, 2024, more than 762 000 participants have consented to join the program, and more than 523 000 of them have completed the initial steps of the program, including taking the first 3 surveys, donating 1 or more biospecimens to the biobank, and providing physical measurements. The AoU's Data and Research Center has collected various data types, including survey responses, EHRs, physical measurements, whole genome sequences, genotyping arrays, Fitbit records, structural variants, and long-read sequences. All registered researchers can access the data easily with a secure Internet connection.[12]

We conducted all analyses on a secure NIH-provided informatics platform that enables users to access and analyze AoU data. In our analyses, we included participants from the most recent version of the AoU controlled tier data (version 7), which contains individual-level data from participants enrolled in the AoU research program between May 31, 2017, and July 1, 2022.

Cohort Identification

We identified inferred TGD individuals using a 3-tier hierarchical strategy that integrated self-reported AoU survey and EHR data (e.g., procedure, drug exposure, and condition; Figure 1).

We based tier 1 on responses to 2 survey questions: 1 question for sex at birth, "What was your biological sex assigned at birth?" (response options included "male," "female," "prefer not to answer," "none of these," and "intersex"), and 1 question for gender identity, "What terms best express how you describe your gender identity?" (response options included "woman," "man," "nonbinary," "transgender," "prefer not to answer," and "additional options"). When participants selected "additional options" for the gender identity question, they were presented with further response options, including "specified gender," "gender fluid," "gender queer," "unsure," "gender variant," "two spirit," "trans woman," and "trans man."

We coded participants as inferred TGD if they met any of the following criteria:

1. responded "intersex" (concept code: 1585848) or "none of these" (concept code: 1585849) for the sex at birth question;
2. responded "nonbinary" (concept code: 1585841), "transgender" (concept code: 1585842), or "additional options" (concept code: 903079; excluding individuals skipped [concept code: 903096]) to the gender identity question;
3. were assigned "male" (concept code: 1585846) at birth and had a

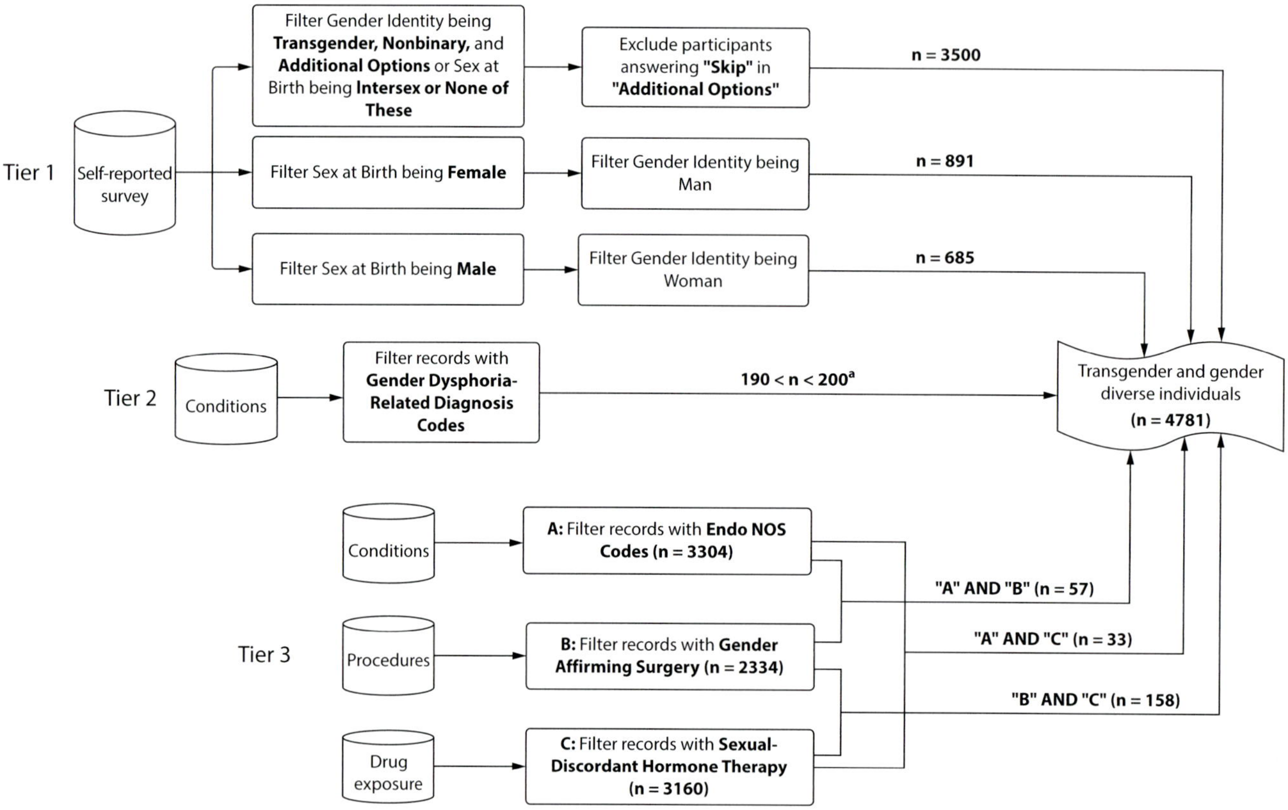

FIGURE 1— Pipeline for Cohort Construction and the Counts of Individuals Identified at Each Step: United States, All of Us Research Program, May 31, 2017–July 1, 2022

[a]Counts < 20 cannot be displayed because of the National Institutes of Health's All of Us research program data and statistics dissemination policy. To prevent secondary calculation, tier 2 individual counts are presented as ranges instead of exact numbers.

gender identity of "woman" (concept code: 1585840); or

4. were assigned "female" (concept code: 1585847) at birth and had a gender identity of "man" (concept code: 1585839).

In the survey responses, "prefer not to answer" is an intentional nonresponse, which may indicate sensitivity or discomfort with the question; "skip" means the participant did not answer the question at all, which could have been unintentional (e.g., they missed it).

Tier 2 was based on gender dysphoria diagnosis codes from the "condition occurrence" table. Previous studies using Medicare claims or commercial insurance data primarily identified TGD individuals with gender dysphoria–related *ICD-9*/*ICD-10* (*International Classification of Diseases, Ninth Revision, Clinical Modification*. Hyattsville, MD: National Center for Health Statistics; 1980/*International Classification of Diseases, 10th Revision*. Geneva, Switzerland: World Health Organization; 1992) codes, a method shown to have an acceptable positive predictive value.[19] We identified participants as "suspected TGD" if they had at least 1 record of gender dysphoria diagnosis based on *ICD-9/10* codes (Table A, available as a supplement to the online version of this article at http://www.ajph.org) in the "condition occurrence" table of the EHR data.

We based tier 3 on a combination of 3 additional data categories, including (1) endocrine disorder not otherwise specified (Endo NOS) codes (Table B, available as a supplement to the online version of this article at http://www.ajph.org), which are often used for billing transgender services to avoid potential disclosure or stigmatization of individuals' gender identity[20]; (2) *ICD-9/10* or common procedure terminology codes for gender-affirming surgery (e.g., genital reconstructive surgery; Table C, available as a supplement to the online version of this article at http://www.ajph.org); and (3) RxNorm medication codes for sex-discordant hormone therapy (Table D, available as a supplement to the online version of this article at http://www.ajph.org).

To enhance positive predictive value, we excluded participants who had a specific nondiabetic endocrine code (e.g., adrenal or thyroid disorders) within 1 year of the record of Endo NOS codes (Table B). Given that some gender-affirming surgery might be because of a cancer diagnosis, we excluded individuals with documentation of both the specific gender-affirming surgery code and the specific cancer diagnosis code to increase the specificity of this strategy. For example, we did not consider patients who were diagnosed with vaginal cancer and had a record of vaginectomy.[18] The list of cancer diagnoses that should be considered for some gender-affirming surgery is listed in Table C.

To increase positive predictive value, we defined a minimum dose threshold for certain hormone therapies that may also be prescribed at lower doses for nontransgender conditions. Specifically, we classified individuals assigned female at birth as receiving sex-discordant hormone therapy if they had an average daily dose of at least 7 milligrams of intramuscular testosterone or 2 milligrams of testosterone in gel or transdermal patch form. We considered individuals assigned male at birth to be receiving sex-discordant hormone therapy if they had a minimum daily dose of 50 milligrams of spironolactone. Consistent with published guidelines, we filtered a list of exclusionary diagnoses for masculinizing hormone prescriptions for women and a list of exclusionary diagnoses for spironolactone prescriptions for men to increase the specificity of using sex hormones to identify gender minorities[18] (Table E, available as a supplement to the online version of this article at http://www.ajph.org).

In AoU, we identified Endo NOS diagnosis codes, gender-affirming surgery–related procedure codes, and sex-discordant hormone therapy in the "condition occurrence" domain, "procedure" domain, and "drug exposure" domain, respectively. We categorized participants into inferred TGD cases if they had records of (1) at least 1 Endo NOS diagnosis code and 1 trans-related procedure code, (2) at least 1 Endo NOS code and 1 sex-discordant hormone therapy, or (3) at least 1 gender-affirming surgery–related procedure code and 1 sex-discordant hormone therapy.

Other Sociodemographic Characteristics

We derived 7 other sociodemographic variables from the AoU database, and we further categorized their responses for analysis: age at enrollment (18–29, 30–44, 45–64, and ≥ 65 years), race/ethnicity (non-Hispanic White, non-Hispanic Black, Hispanic, and other/unknown), highest education attainment (less than high school, high school or higher, and unknown), insurance coverage (covered by health insurance, not covered by health insurance, and unknown), annual household income (< $25 000, $25 000–$50 000, ≥ $50 000, and unknown), housing insecurity (yes, no, and unknown), and sexual orientation (straight, bisexual, gay, none, lesbian, and skip/unknown).

Data Analysis

We conducted descriptive statistics (e.g., count number and percentage) to compare sociodemographic characteristics of AoU participants by TGD status (TGD and non-TGD individuals) and to compare TGD individuals exclusively identified through survey-based criteria (tier 1) and EHR-based criteria (tiers 2 and 3). We calculated *P* values using the χ^2 test to assess whether differences in descriptive characteristics were significant ($P < .05$). We employed a Venn diagram to display the counts and overlap of TGD individuals identified in 3 distinct tiers of cohort identification in AoU. We conducted all analyses in R (RStudio, Boston, MA).

RESULTS

Using survey data and different domains in EHR data, we identified 4781 of the 413 457 participants (1.2%) as TGD individuals (Table 1). Among all TGD individuals, we identified 3500 based on a single question about sex at birth or gender identity. Of these, 891 were assigned female at birth with a gender identity of man, and 685 were assigned male at birth with a gender identity of woman. Between 190 and 200 participants had at least 1 record of a gender dysphoria–related *ICD-9/10* code. Additionally, 57 had records of both an Endo NOS–related code and a gender-affirming surgery–related code; 33 had both an Endo NOS–related code and sex-discordant hormone therapy; and 158 had records of both gender-affirming surgery and sex-discordant hormone therapy (Figure 1).

According to the Venn diagram (Figure 2), TGD individuals were mostly identified by survey question alone (> 4570) and a combination of Endo NOS codes, gender-affirming surgery, and sex-discordant hormone therapy (236; 4.9%) and less commonly identified by gender dysphoria–related diagnosis codes (> 190 and < 200). We identified 34 participants as TGD in all 3 tiers, 149 in tiers 1 and 2, more than 69 and less than 74 in tiers 1 and 3, and less than 54 in tiers 2 and 3.

Among TGD people, 2903 (60.7%) were assigned female at birth, 1717 (35.9%) were male at birth, and 82 (1.7%) were intersex or none of these

TABLE 1— Sociodemographic Characteristics of All of Us Participants by Transgender and Gender-Diverse Status (Yes/No): United States, May 31, 2017–July 1, 2022

Characteristic	Total, No. (%)	Transgender and Gender-Diverse Individuals		P[a]
		No, No. (%)	Yes, No. (%)	
Total	413 457	408 676	4 781	
Sex at birth				<.001
Female	249 565 (60.4)	246 662 (60.4)	2 903 (60.7)	
Male	155 169 (37.5)	153 452 (37.6)	1 717 (35.9)	
Intersex/none of these	238 (0.1)	156 (0.0)	82 (1.7)	
Unknown[b]	8 485 (2.0)	8 406 (2.1)	79 (1.7)	
Age at enrollment, y				<.001
18–29	34 561 (8.4)	33 314 (8.2)	1 247 (26.1)	
30–44	95 452 (23.1)	93 612 (22.9)	1 840 (38.5)	
45–64	145 333 (35.1)	144 232 (35.3)	1 101 (23.0)	
≥ 65	138 111 (33.4)	137 518 (33.6)	593 (12.4)	
Race/ethnicity				<.001
Non-Hispanic Black	77 069 (18.6)	76 467 (18.7)	602 (12.6)	
Non-Hispanic White	222 646 (53.9)	219 914 (53.8)	2 732 (57.1)	
Hispanic	64 672 (15.6)	63 983 (15.7)	689 (14.4)	
Other/unknown[c]	49 070 (11.9)	48 312 (11.8)	758 (15.9)	
Sexual orientation				<.001
Bisexual	15 191 (3.7)	14 201 (3.5)	990 (20.7)	
Gay	9 451 (2.3)	9 054 (2.2)	397 (8.3)	
Lesbian	5 144 (1.2)	4 709 (1.2)	435 (9.1)	
None[d]	8 692 (2.1)	7 268 (1.8)	1 424 (29.8)	
Straight	359 648 (87.0)	358 410 (87.7)	1 238 (25.9)	
Unknown[b]	15 331 (3.7)	15 034 (3.7)	297 (6.2)	
Education				.8
High school degree or more	387 253 (93.7)	367 395 (89.9)	4 238 (88.6)	
Less than a high school degree	12 674 (3.1)	26 433 (6.5)	346 (7.2)	
Unknown[b]	13 530 (3.3)	14 848 (3.6)	197 (4.1)	
Insurance coverage				.016
Yes	371 633 (89.9)	367 289 (89.9)	4 344 (88.7)	
No	26 779 (6.5)	26 426 (6.5)	353 (7.2)	
Unknown[b]	15 045 (3.6)	14 843 (3.6)	202 (4.1)	
Income, $				
< 25 000	102 719 (24.8)	101 002 (24.7)	1 717 (35.9)	
25 000–50 000	61 819 (15.0)	60 947 (14.9)	872 (18.2)	
> 50 000	165 811 (40.1)	164 400 (40.2)	1 411 (29.5)	
Unknown[b]	83 108 (20.1)	82 327 (20.1)	781 (16.3)	
Housing security concern				<.001
No	336 772 (81.5)	333 590 (81.6)	3 182 (66.6)	
Yes	66 649 (16.1)	65 124 (15.9)	1 525 (31.9)	
Unknown[b]	10 036 (2.4)	9 962 (2.4)	74 (1.5)	

[a]Pearson χ^2 test.
[b]Including skip, prefer not to answer, and don't know.
[c]Including > 1 race/ethnicity, skip, other, and prefer not to answer.
[d]Including "queer," "polysexual, omnisexual, sapiosexual, or pansexual," "asexual," "two spirit," "mostly straight, but sometimes attracted to people of your own sex," and "have not figured out or are in the process of figuring out your sexuality."

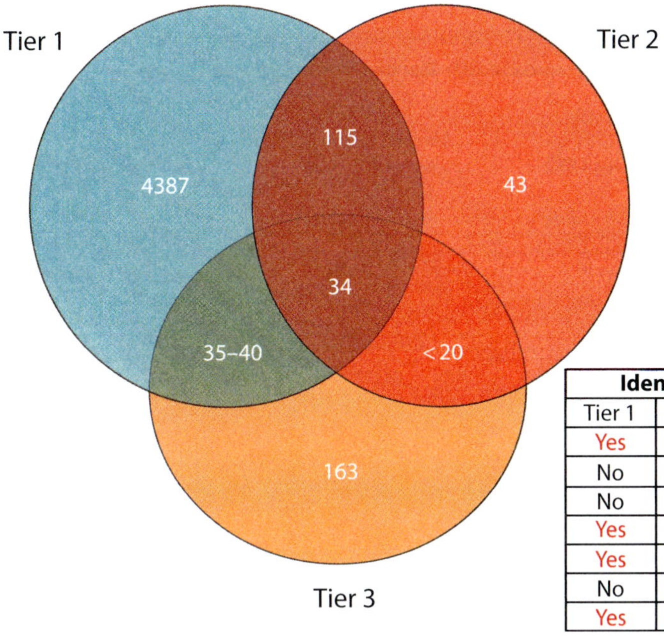

Identification in Each Tier			
Tier 1	Tier 2	Tier 3	Count
Yes	No	No	4387
No	Yes	No	43
No	No	Yes	163
Yes	Yes	No	115
Yes	No	Yes	35–40
No	Yes	Yes	< 20
Yes	Yes	Yes	34

FIGURE 2— Venn Diagram Displaying the Counts of Transgender and Gender-Diverse Individuals Based on 3 Tiers of Identification: United States, All of Us Research Program, May 31, 2017–July 1, 2022

Note. More detailed information about the number of transgender and gender-diverse individuals identified in each tier can be found in Figure 1. Counts smaller than 20 cannot be displayed because of the National Institutes of Health's All of Us research program data and statistics dissemination policy. To prevent secondary calculation, the intersection between tier 1 and tier 2 is presented as a range.

at birth. At enrollment, most of the TGD individuals were aged 30 to 44 years (38.5%) and were non-Hispanic White (57.1%). Regarding sexual orientation, most TGD individuals responded "none" (29.8%), followed by "straight" (25.9%), "bisexual" (20.7%), "lesbian" (9.1%), and "gay" (8.3%). For socioeconomic status–related characteristics, 88.6% of the TGD participants had a high school degree or more, 88.7% were covered by health insurance, and 35.91% had an annual household income of less than $25 000 (Table 1).

Most of the sociodemographic distributions between TGD and non-TGD individuals were significantly different. For example, participants who were aged 18 to 29 years (26.1% vs 8.2%), were bisexual (20.7% vs 3.5%), had an annual income of less than $25 000 (35.9% vs 24.7%), and had housing security concerns (31.9% vs 16.0%) accounted for a larger proportion among TGD individuals than non-TGD individuals ($P < .001$ for all characteristics; Table 1).

Regarding TGD individuals exclusively identified in the survey (tier 1) and by EHR (tiers 2 and 3) data, most demographic characteristics were also statistically different. For example, TGD individuals who we identified by EHR data were more likely to born as male (65.6% vs 33.8%), have no housing security concerns (83.3% vs 66.0%), have insurance coverage (95.7% vs 88.1%), and be heterosexual (75.6% vs 23.9%) than those who were identified in survey data ($P < .05$ for all characteristics; Table 2).

DISCUSSION

Using a comprehensive computable phenotyping algorithm based on multiple types of data, including self-reported surveys, diagnosis and procedure codes, and therapy records, we identified 4781 unique TGD individuals among participants enrolled in AoU from May 31, 2017, to July 1, 2022. Combining both survey and EHR data enabled us to identify TGD individuals who have been missed by previous studies that used survey data only in AoU to explore health disparities in TGD people. A higher proportion of the TGD participants than the non-TGD participants was younger, had a sexual orientation as a sexual minority, and reported socioeconomic deprivation. Compared with TGD individuals exclusively identified based on EHR data, those identified in survey data were younger, were a sexual minority, had housing security concerns, and had no health insurance coverage.

The computable phenotyping algorithm we developed was an expansion

TABLE 2— Demographic Characteristics of Transgender and Gender-Diverse Individuals Exclusively Identified Through Survey Data and Electronic Health Record Data: United States, May 31, 2017–July 1, 2022

Characteristic	Overall, n = 4 632	Electronic Health Record, n = 209	Survey, n = 4423	P[a]
Sex at birth				<.001
Female	2 845 (61.4)	. . .[b]	. . .[b]	
Male	1 634 (35.3)	137 (65.6)	1 497 (33.8)	
Unknown[c]	153 (3.3)	. . .[b]	. . .[b]	
Age at enrollment, y				<.001
18–44	3 007 (64.9)	44 (21.1)	2 963 (67.0)	
45–64	1 054 (22.8)	73 (34.9)	981 (22.2)	
≥ 65	571 (12.3)	92 (44.0)	479 (10.8)	
Sexual orientation				<.001
Heterosexual	1 215 (26.2)	158 (75.6)	1 057 (23.9)	
Sexual minority	3 130 (67.6)	. . .[b]	. . .[b]	
Unknown[c]	287 (6.2)	. . .[b]	. . .[b]	
Race/Ethnicity				.06
Hispanic	677 (14.6)	25 (12.0)	652 (14.7)	
Non-Hispanic Black	584 (12.6)	30 (14.4)	554 (12.5)	
Non-Hispanic White	2 630 (56.8)	132 (63.2)	2 498 (56.5)	
Other/unknown[d]	741 (16.0)	22 (10.5)	719 (16.3)	
Education				.6
Less than a high school degree	152 (3.3)	. . .[b]	. . .[b]	
High school degree or more	4 333 (93.5)	198 (94.7)	4 135 (93.5)	
Unknown[c]	147 (3.2)	. . .[b]	. . .[b]	
Insurance coverage				.002
Yes	4 095 (88.4)	200 (95.7)	3 895 (88.1)	
No	342 (7.4)	. . .[b]	. . .[b]	
Unknown[c]	195 (4.2)	. . .[b]	. . .[b]	
Income				.019
< 25 000	1 662 (35.9)	68 (32.5)	1 594 (36.0)	
25 000–50 000	839 (18.1)	28 (13.4)	811 (18.3)	
> 50 000	1 367 (29.5)	81 (38.8)	1 286 (29.1)	
Unknown[c]	764 (16.5)	32 (15.3)	732 (16.6)	
Housing security concern				<.001
No	3 093 (66.8)	174 (83.3)	2 919 (66.0)	
Yes	1 467 (31.7)	. . .[b]	. . .[b]	
Unknown[c]	72 (1.5)	. . .[b]	. . .[b]	

[a]Pearson χ^2 test.
[b]Counts < 20 (and corresponding percentages) cannot be displayed because of the National Institutes of Health's All of Us research program data and statistics dissemination policy. Some additional data were collapsed or obscured to prevent secondary calculation of these values.
[c]Including skip, prefer not to answer, and don't know.
[d]Including > 1 race/ethnicity, skip, other, and prefer not to answer.

of multiple previously validated algorithms, which enabled the capture of participants who would have been missed by 1 algorithm alone and can improve the performance of case identification.[17] Tier 1 consisted of a single-item measure, which asked about participants' gender identity directly, and a 2-step measure, which explored the consistency between sex assigned at birth and gender identity. The single-item measure had the limitation of misleading information because some TGD people may identify themselves as only male or female, and the 2-step measure had the advantage of recognizing a wider spectrum of TGD identities.[21]

In tier 2, at least 1 gender dysphoria diagnosis code from the "condition occurrence" domain was required, but this method was limited because not all TGD people experience gender dysphoria,[22] and clinicians may underuse the gender dysphoria code to avoid labeling a patient as transgender.[23] The use of a combination of transgender-related procedure codes, Endo NOS diagnosis codes, and prescriptions in tier 3 went beyond the gender dysphoria codes. It improved the generalizability by promoting the identification of additional potential TGD people missed by tier 2.[18]

We identified 209 TGD individuals as being under tier 2 or 3 but not tier 1, which may indicate inconsistencies between survey-based and EHR-based identification methods. The observed inconsistency underscores the limitations of relying solely on either data source for accurate classification. Social desirability bias may contribute to underreporting in survey responses, as some TGD individuals may be reluctant to disclose their gender identity or intentionally choose "man" or "woman" owing to concerns about potential stigmatization and privacy.[18] However, these individuals may still be identified through EHR data if they have documented gender-affirming care or gender dysphoria–related diagnoses, leading to discrepancies across classification tiers.

We found that TGD individuals identified exclusively by survey data were more likely to be younger, report housing insecurity, lack health insurance, identify as a sexual minority, and have been assigned female at birth compared with those identified in EHR data. Younger individuals and those willing to disclose their sexual minority identities may feel more comfortable disclosing their gender identity in surveys. Furthermore, individuals with significant financial challenges, such as housing insecurity or lack of health insurance, were less likely to seek medical care, reducing their likelihood of being identified as TGD in EHR data.[24] These findings further underscore the importance of integrating multiple data sources to enhance the comprehensiveness of TGD phenotyping algorithms in research and health care settings.

The overall proportion of TGD people found in AoU was 1.16%, which is higher than the 0.52% prevalence proportion in a report based on the 2017 to 2020 Behavioral Risk Factors Surveillance System (BRFSS) data.[25] One explanation for this is that the AoU research program emphasizes recruiting more participants from groups that have been historically underrepresented in biomedical research.[12] We considered individuals with a low household income, limited access to medical care, or low education attainment as well as those who were sexual and gender or racial minorities "historically underrepresented."[12] Consequently, we observed TGD individuals, who were more likely to belong to these underrepresented groups, in higher proportions in this study group. Another explanation is that we estimated the number of TGD individuals reported using the BRFSS data based solely on survey questions. This method failed to identify those who could be captured only by EHR data, leading to an underrepresentation of the TGD population.

The younger age distribution of TGD individuals observed in our study is consistent with previous research and may reflect generational differences in societal acceptance, access to health care resources, and the inclusion of more comprehensive gender identity measures in surveys.[26] Older TGD individuals may have greater concerns about gender identity disclosure owing to the experience of social discrimination and difficulty accessing health care, potentially resulting in underrepresentation in both survey and EHR data.[27] Additionally, older TGD adults may face greater financial insecurity than their younger counterparts, which may increase their reliance on social services.[28] However, many social service programs, such as Social Security and veterans' benefits, require identity documents that match the gender in which applicants present themselves. This requirement may discourage older TGD adults from changing the gender marker on official documents, further complicating their access to essential resources.[29]

In addition, this study provides consistent evidence that TGD-identified individuals face a higher risk of low socioeconomic status, as indicated by factors such as lower household income and increased housing insecurity.[30,31] Using data from BRFSS, Conron et al. found that transgender adults are more likely to be in poverty (31% vs 9%) and unemployed (33% vs 12%) than are their nontransgender peers.[32] However, in terms of race/ethnicity, TGD-identified adults in this study were more likely to report being non-Hispanic White and less likely to report being non-Hispanic Black or Hispanic. This trend contrasts with previous research using population-based samples, which have indicated that Hispanic and Latinx people of any race are more likely to identify as transgender than are non-Hispanic White people.[33] This may be because communities with better access to supportive environments and health care services have higher self-reporting rates of TGD identities. Studies like AoU that primarily include individuals already engaged with health care systems may reflect different demographic patterns than population-based surveys that include individuals with a broader range of health care access.

Limitations

The novelty of this study lies in its integration of self-reported survey data and EHRs to identify TGD individuals, offering a more comprehensive approach that captures individuals who might be missed by methods relying solely on survey data. However, some limitations need to be acknowledged. First, the findings of this study cannot be generalized to the entire TGD population in AoU because not all TGD people disclose their gender identity in the survey or have a TGD-related diagnosis and because the AoU cohort does not include TGD individuals younger than 18 years. Additionally, if the TGD individuals did not seek health care or receive a diagnosis outside the institutions included in AoU, false negative results may have occurred.

Second, the differences in underlying populations in each data source may bias results. For example, non-Hispanic White TGD individuals are more likely to be privately insured and have fewer barriers to receiving gender-affirming care than non-Hispanic Black or Hispanic individuals.[34,35] This could partially explain the large proportion of non-Hispanic individuals among TGD people identified.

Third, we did not include algorithms described in previous literature owing to data accessibility. More natural language processing methods and gender identity terminology algorithms based on unstructured clinical notes are needed. Lastly, individuals with greater health care access and financial stability may be overrepresented in AoU. This selection bias may lead to the underrepresentation of TGD individuals who face greater socioeconomic challenges.

Public Health Implications

By accurately identifying TGD individuals in integrated diverse data sets in AoU, registered researchers can analyze health care utilization patterns, health outcomes, and treatment responses specific to TGD populations. This approach holds promise for using AoU as a rich resource to enhance our understanding of the health disparities among TGD individuals and inform the development of targeted interventions and support services. AJPH

ABOUT THE AUTHORS

Fanghui Shi, Xueying Yang, Shan Qiao, and Xiaoming Li are with the Department of Health Promotion, Education, and Behavior, Arnold School of Public Health, University of South Carolina, Columbia. Ruilie Cai and Jiajia Zhang are with the Department of Epidemiology and Biostatistics, Arnold School of Public Health, University of South Carolina, Columbia. Sayward E. Harrison and Sarah Grace Frary are with the Department of Psychology, University of South Carolina College of Arts and Sciences, Columbia.

CORRESPONDENCE

Correspondence should be sent to Fanghui Shi, Room 529, 915 Greene St, Columbia, SC 29208 (e-mail: FSHI@e-mail.sc.edu). Reprints can be ordered at https://www.ajph.org by clicking the "Reprints" link.

PUBLICATION INFORMATION

Full Citation: Shi F, Yang X, Cai R, et al. Identification of transgender and gender-diverse individuals in the All of Us research program, 2017–2022. *Am J Public Health*. 2025;115(8):1278–1287.

Acceptance Date: March 17, 2025.

DOI: https://doi.org/10.2105/AJPH.2025.308129

ORCID iDs:

Fanghui Shi https://orcid.org/0000-0002-5603-5398

Xueying Yang https://orcid.org/0000-0001-6788-0688

Ruilie Cai https://orcid.org/0000-0003-2218-8000

Shan Qiao https://orcid.org/0000-0003-1834-1834

Sarah Grace Frary https://orcid.org/0000-0003-1405-5603

Xiaoming Li https://orcid.org/0000-0002-5555-9034

CONTRIBUTORS

F. Shi conceptualized and wrote the first draft and critically revised the article. F. Shi, X. Yang, and J. Zhang set up the statistical test design. F. Shi and R. Cai conducted the data analysis, which was reviewed and verified by J. Zhang. All authors reviewed and edited the article and had final responsibility for the decision to submit for publication.

ACKNOWLEDGMENTS

We gratefully acknowledge All of Us (AoU) participants for their contributions, without whom this research would not have been possible. We also thank the National Institutes of Health's AoU research program for making available the participant and cohort data examined in this study.

CONFLICTS OF INTEREST

The authors have no conflicts of interest to declare.

HUMAN PARTICIPANT PROTECTION

This study used de-identified data from the All of Us Researcher Workbench and was exempt from institutional review board approval under program policy, as it did not constitute human participants research.

REFERENCES

1. Coleman E, Radix AE, Bouman WP, et al. *Standards of Care for the Health of Transgender and Gender Diverse People*, version 8. *Int J Transgend Health*. 2022;23(suppl1):S1–S259. [Erratum in: *Int J Transgend Health*. 2022;23(suppl 1):S259–S261. https://doi.org/10.1080/26895269.2022.2125695]. https://doi.org/10.1080/26895269.2022.2100644
2. Tan KK, Treharne GJ, Ellis SJ, Schmidt JM, Veale JF. Gender minority stress: a critical review. *J Homosex*. 2020;67(10):1471–1489. https://doi.org/10.1080/00918369.2019.1591789
3. Warrier V, Greenberg DM, Weir E, et al. Elevated rates of autism, other neurodevelopmental and psychiatric diagnoses, and autistic traits in transgender and gender-diverse individuals. *Nat Commun*. 2020;11(1):3959. https://doi.org/10.1038/s41467-020-17794-1
4. Thompson HM, Wang TM, Talan AJ, Baker KE, Restar AJ. First they came for us all—responding to anti-transgender structural violence with collective, community-engaged, and intersectional health equity research and advocacy. *Health Educ*

Behav. 2024;51(1):5–9. https://doi.org/10.1177/10901981231201146

5. Reisner SL, Poteat T, Keatley J, et al. Global health burden and needs of transgender populations: a review. *Lancet*. 2016;388(10042):412–436. https://doi.org/10.1016/S0140-6736(16)00684-X
6. Delozier AM, Kamody RC, Rodgers S, Chen D. Health disparities in transgender and gender expansive adolescents: a topical review from a minority stress framework. *J Pediatr Psychol*. 2020;45(8):842–847. https://doi.org/10.1093/jpepsy/jsaa040
7. Reisner SL, Conron KJ. "Counting" transgender and gender-nonconforming adults in health research: recommendations from the gender identity in US surveillance group. *Transgend Stud Q*. 2015;2(1):34–57. https://doi.org/10.1215/23289252-2848877
8. Tordoff DM, Minalga B, Gross BB, et al. Erasure and health equity implications of using binary male/female categories in sexual health research and human immunodeficiency virus/sexually transmitted infection surveillance: recommendations for transgender-inclusive data collection and reporting. *Sex Transm Dis*. 2022;49(2):e45–e49. https://doi.org/10.1097/OLQ.0000000000001533
9. Graham R, Berkowitz B, Blum R, Bockting W, Bradford J, de Vries B. *The Health of Lesbian, Gay, Bisexual, and Transgender People: Building a Foundation for Better Understanding*. Washington, DC: Institute of Medicine of the National Academies; 2011.
10. Shover CL, DeVost MA, Beymer MR, Gorbach PM, Flynn RP, Bolan RK. Using sexual orientation and gender identity to monitor disparities in HIV, sexually transmitted infections, and viral hepatitis. *Am J Public Health*. 2018;108(suppl4):S277–S283. https://doi.org/10.2105/AJPH.2018.304751
11. Sankar PL, Parker LS. The Precision Medicine Initiative's All of Us research program: an agenda for research on its ethical, legal, and social issues. *Genet Med*. 2017;19(7):743–750. https://doi.org/10.1038/gim.2016.183
12. Denny JC, Rutter JL, Goldstein DB, et al. The "All of Us" research program. *N Engl J Med*. 2019;381(7):668–676. https://doi.org/10.1056/NEJMsr1809937
13. Barr PB, Bigdeli TB, Meyers JL. Prevalence, comorbidity, and sociodemographic correlates of psychiatric disorders reported in the All of Us research program. *JAMA Psychiatry*. 2022;79(6):622–628. https://doi.org/10.1001/jamapsychiatry.2022.0685
14. Tran NK, Lunn MR, Schulkey CE, et al. Prevalence of 12 common health conditions in sexual and gender minority participants in the All of Us research program. *JAMA Netw Open*. 2023;6(7):e2324969. https://doi.org/10.1001/jamanetworkopen.2023.24969
15. Wong CN, Wilczek MP, Smith LH, et al. Frailty among sexual and gender minority older adults: the All of Us database. *J Gerontol A Biol Sci Med Sci*. 2023;78(11):2111–2118. https://doi.org/10.1093/gerona/glad149
16. Kamal K, Young K, Ly S, et al. Investigating the association between gender minority identity and skin cancer prevalence: a cohort study in the United States All of Us research program. *J Eur Acad Dermatol Venereol*. 2023;37(9):e1151–e1153. https://doi.org/10.1111/jdv.19156
17. Nock MR, Kamal K, Zampella JG, Roberson ML, Cohen JM, Barbieri JS. Barriers to care among sexual and gender minority individuals with chronic inflammatory skin diseases in the US. *JAMA Dermatol*. 2023;159(12):1323–1331. https://doi.org/10.1001/jamadermatol.2023.3328
18. Jasuja GK, de Groot A, Quinn EK, et al. Beyond gender identity disorder diagnoses codes: an examination of additional methods to identify transgender individuals in administrative databases. *Med Care*. 2020;58(10):903–911. https://doi.org/10.1097/MLR.0000000000001362
19. Proctor K, Haffer SC, Ewald E, Hodge C, James CV. Identifying the transgender population in the Medicare program. *Transgend Health*. 2016;1(1):250–265. https://doi.org/10.1089/trgh.2016.0031
20. Wolfe HL, Reisman JI, Yoon SS, et al. Validating data-driven methods for identifying transgender individuals in the Veterans Health Administration of the US Department of Veterans Affairs. *Am J Epidemiol*. 2021;190(9):1928–1934. https://doi.org/10.1093/aje/kwab102
21. Costa AB, Rosa LO, Fontanari AMV. Sampling bias in Brazilian studies on transgender and gender diverse populations: the two-step measure for assessing gender identity in surveys. *Cad Saude Publica*. 2022;38(1):e00180420. https://doi.org/10.1590/0102-311x00180420
22. Davy Z, Toze M. What is gender dysphoria? A critical systematic narrative review. *Transgend Health*. 2018;3(1):159–169. https://doi.org/10.1089/trgh.2018.0014
23. Rowniak S, Bolt L. The effects of cross-gender hormones on the quality of life of transgender individuals: a systematic review protocol. *JBI Database System Rev Implement Rep*. 2015;13(7):93–103. https://doi.org/10.11124/jbisrir-2015-2228
24. Kattari SK, Hasche L. Differences across age groups in transgender and gender non-conforming people's experiences of health care discrimination, harassment, and victimization. *J Aging Health*. 2016;28(2):285–306. https://doi.org/10.1177/0898264315590228
25. Herman JL, Flores AR, O'Neill KK. *How Many Adults and Youth Identify as Transgender in the United States?* Los Angeles, CA: Williams Institute, UCLA School of Law; 2022.
26. Porter KE, Brennan-Ing M, Chang SC, et al. Providing competent and affirming services for transgender and gender nonconforming older adults. *Clin Gerontol*. 2016;39(5):366–388. https://doi.org/10.1080/07317115.2016.1203383
27. Siverskog A. "They just don't have a clue": transgender aging and implications for social work. In: Westwood S, ed. *Lesbian, Gay, Bisexual, and Transgender Aging*. New York, NY: Routledge; 2017:312–332.
28. Hartzell E, Frazer M, Wertz K, Davis M. *The State of Transgender California: Results From the 2008 California Transgender Economic Health Survey*. San Francisco, CA: Transgender Law Center; 2009.
29. Campbell LF, Arkles G. Ethical and legal concerns for mental health professionals. In Singh A, Dickey LM, eds. *Affirmative Counseling and Psychological Practice With Transgender and Gender Nonconforming Clients*. Washington, DC: American Psychological Association; 2017:95–118. https://doi.org/10.1037/14957-005
30. Koch JM, McLachlan CT, Victor CJ, Westcott J, Yager C. The cost of being transgender: where socio-economic status, global health care systems, and gender identity intersect. *Psychol Sex*. 2020;11(1–2):103–119. https://doi.org/10.1080/19419899.2019.1660705
31. Carpenter CS, Lee MJ, Nettuno L. Economic outcomes for transgender people and other gender minorities in the United States: first estimates from a nationally representative sample. *South Econ J*. 2022;89(2):280–304. https://doi.org/10.1002/soej.12594
32. Conron KJ, Scott G, Stowell GS, Landers SJ. Transgender health in Massachusetts: results from a household probability sample of adults. *Am J Public Health*. 2012;102(1):118–122. https://doi.org/10.2105/AJPH.2011.300315
33. Feldman JL, Luhur WE, Herman JL, Poteat T, Meyer IH. Health and health care access in the US transgender population health (TransPop) survey. *Andrology*. 2021;9(6):1707–1718. https://doi.org/10.1111/andr.13052
34. Beltran TG, Lett E, Poteat T, Hincapie-Castillo JM. Computational phenotyping within electronic healthcare data to identify transgender people in the United States: a narrative review. *Pharmacoepidemiol Drug Saf*. 2024;33(3):e5732. https://doi.org/10.1002/pds.5732
35. Chyten-Brennan J, Patel VV, Ginsberg MS, Hanna DB. Algorithm to identify transgender and gender nonbinary individuals among people living with HIV performs differently by age and ethnicity. *Ann Epidemiol*. 2021;54:73–78. https://doi.org/10.1016/j.annepidem.2020.09.013

Trends in AIDS Drug Assistance Program Support for People With HIV, by Age, Sex, Race, and US Region, 2008–2021

Kathleen A. McManus, MD, MSCR, Amy Killelea, JD, Tim Horn, MS, Amber Steen, MA, Brian Sun, MD, Jessica Keim-Malpass, RN, PhD, CPNP-AC, Auntré Hamp, MEd, MPH, LPC, Andrew Strumpf, MPH, and Elizabeth T. Rogawski McQuade, PhD, MPH

See also Dombrowski et al. p. 1187.

Objectives. To evaluate trends in AIDS Drug Assistance Program (ADAP) utilization among demographic subpopulations.

Methods. For 2008 to 2021, we collected US state-level data regarding ADAP client utilization and estimated HIV prevalence data. We used descriptive statistics to describe state ADAP utilization by geography, demographics (age, sex, race), and programmatic characteristics.

Results. ADAP utilization proportion increased from 14.0% of all people with HIV (PWH) in 2008 to 22.3% in 2021. The proportion of female PWH supported by ADAP was lower in both 2008 (12.2%) and 2021 (18.3%) compared with the proportion of male PWH supported (2008: 14.5%; 2021: 22.9%). In 2008, the utilization proportion was lower for Black PWH at 11.7% compared with 16.0% for White PWH. In 2021, the utilization proportion for Black PWH was 25.2% compared with 28.4% for White PWH.

Conclusions. ADAP enrollment and utilization have increased substantially. Despite equity gains, Black PWH and women were served at lower proportions by ADAP.

Public Health Implications. National and state partners of ADAPs should examine ways to ensure that ADAP utilization is equitable in terms of age, sex, race/ethnicity, and other sociodemographic factors. (*Am J Public Health*. 2025;115(8):1288–1298. https://doi.org/10.2105/AJPH.2025.308101)

AJPH August 2025, Vol. 115, No. 8

The Ryan White HIV/AIDS Program (RWHAP) has been a vital safety net for low-income people with HIV (PWH) for more than 40 years. AIDS Drug Assistance Programs (ADAPs) are a key component of RWHAP. ADAPs receive federal funding to provide HIV and other essential medications to uninsured, low-income PWH and assistance to cover premiums and HIV-related cost-sharing for insured, low-income PWH. In 2022, ADAPs served more than 235 000 clients, representing 20% of the 1.1 million PWH in the United States.[1] Unlike private insurance and Medicaid, ADAP does not provide major medical coverage.

Because ADAPs are run at the state level, each state may approach ADAP programmatic and policy decisions differently, as long as they meet a federal floor of requirements (e.g., minimum formulary standards and eligibility limited to "low-income" individuals).[2–4] This means that the specific drugs on each ADAP's formulary, the extent to which an ADAP provides insurance premium and cost-sharing assistance, and even the income eligibility threshold vary by state. External factors—like whether a state has expanded its Medicaid program under the Affordable Care Act (ACA) and whether the state allocates state funding to ADAP—may have an impact on the choices ADAPs make to structure services and the income thresholds for eligibility.[1]

Since their inception, ADAPs have evolved to meet the changing needs of clients. As more antiretroviral therapies (ARTs) have been approved by the US Food and Drug Administration, ADAPs have expanded their formularies to include new medications, such as single-tablet and long-acting injectable regimens.[5] In response to comorbidities and the need to address holistic needs, almost all ADAPs have expanded their formularies to include non-ART medications, including hepatitis C virus direct-acting antivirals and medication-assisted therapy for substance use disorders. Many ADAPs have expanded their insurance assistance programs, developing sophisticated premium and cost-sharing support operations to assist the growing number of ADAP clients who need help affording, or gaining access to, insurance that provides prescription drug coverage. In 2021, 44% of all ADAP clients received financial assistance from ADAPs toward insurance coverage.[6]

To date, to our knowledge, there have been no longitudinal studies examining ADAP utilization and demographic changes of clients over time. Such studies are necessary to understand how ADAPs have evolved and responded to the changing needs of clients and to the rapidly evolving health care landscape outside of ADAP. Longitudinal studies may inform funding and programmatic changes needed to strengthen programs, considering emerging challenges. Understanding client utilization and demographic patterns can help identify gaps in communities being served by ADAP. We evaluated trends in ADAP utilization among key demographic subpopulations using national, regional, and state-level longitudinal data.

METHODS

This longitudinal, descriptive study examined state ADAPs of 51 jurisdictions (the 50 US states and the District of Columbia [DC]) with jurisdiction-level aggregate data for each year. Data on ADAP clients were collected from the National Alliance of State and Territorial AIDS Directors National RWHAP Part B and ADAP Monitoring Project Annual Reports for 2008 through 2021.[5,7–18]

For the 51 jurisdictions, we collected publicly available data on the number of PWH by different demographic subgroups from the Centers for Disease Control and Prevention's AtlasPlus.[19] In the 2017 ADAP Monitoring Project report[14] (which reported calendar year 2015) and in subsequent reports, race and ethnicity were reported separately, making comparisons to AtlasPlus data incompatible. Given this, we collected ADAP client data by race subgroup from the Ryan White Compass Dashboard when assessing trends in utilization by race for years 2016 through 2021.[20]

Variables

We collected 3 categories of ADAP characteristics: state-level policy, utilization, and client demographics. State-level policy included the states' annual Medicaid expansion status, defined as whether they had implemented the program by January 1.[21]

Utilization data included the number of ADAP clients supported. Thirty-eight state-years were missing annual ADAP utilization data at the demographic level in the ADAP Monitoring Project Annual Reports. For 31 state-years, we collected and imputed utilization data from the ADAP Data Report.[22] Seven state-years' data were not available (Table A, available as a supplement to the online version of this article at https://ajph.org).

Client demographics included age, sex, and race. Age categories were 13 to 24 years, 25 to 44 years, and 45 years or older. Sex categories were male and female because AtlasPlus was limited to biological sex at birth at the state level. The only race categories included were Black or White. Other racial groups were excluded because of AtlasPlus's data suppression at the state level.

Statistical Analyses

We used descriptive statistics to summarize and describe longitudinal trends in state ADAP utilization by geography, demographics, and programmatic characteristics. We calculated the ADAP utilization proportion as the number of clients supported by ADAP divided by the total number of PWH for each calendar year. We calculated the absolute change in utilization by subtracting the utilization proportion in 2008 from the utilization proportion in 2021. We calculated relative change by dividing the absolute change in proportions by the 2008 proportion multiplied by 100. We analyzed all characteristics at the national and regional levels. We defined regions according to the US Census Bureau as Northeast, Midwest, West, and South.[23] We performed analysis using R (R Foundation for Statistical Computing, Vienna, Austria) and RStudio (RStudio Inc, Boston, MA).

RESULTS

Of 714 possible state-years of data, 707 state-years (99%) had complete data and were analyzed. We removed 7 state-years (1%) with incomplete data.

National Program Utilization

The utilization of ADAP service increased for PWH from 2008 to 2021. Of 764 312 PWH in 2008, 106 747 were served by ADAP (14.0%), and by 2021, 238 585 PWH of the 1 071 005 PWH were served by ADAP (22.3%), resulting in a relative increase of 59.3% (Table 1). In 2015, ADAPs experienced the largest jump in utilization; 15.1% of PWH were served by ADAP in 2014, which increased to 23.7% in 2015 (Table B, available as a supplement to the online version of this article at https://ajph.org). The utilization proportion remained stable at 23.0% to 23.2% between 2016 and 2018, before rising to 23.9% in 2019 and peaking at 24.4% in 2020 with more than 250 000 PWH served by ADAP (Figure A, available as a supplement to the online version of this article at https://ajph.org).

Regional Program Utilization

Consistent with national trends, ADAP utilization increased in each region. States in the South account for the highest number of PWH with 326 052 in 2008 (42.7%). For 2008, while the 39 926 ADAP clients in the South constituted 37.4% of the ADAP client population, the utilization proportion relative to their regional PWH population was the lowest of all the regions (12.2%; Figure 1). In the West, ADAP utilization relative to their regional PWH population was the highest of any region in 2008 (18.7%), while the Midwest and Northeast were lower (13.6% and 13.4%, respectively). Similar to the national trends, all regions experienced the largest increase in utilization proportion from 2014 to 2015; however, the highest increase was observed in the Midwest (15.8% to 24.6%) followed by the West (17.7% to 25.9%), South (15.8% to 24.0%), and Northeast (14.8% to 21.0%). By 2021, the number of PWH served by ADAP in the South increased to 114 493 (23.2%), equivalent to a relative change of 90.2%, and accounted for nearly half of the population of ADAP clients (48.0%). Both the Northeast and West regions had lower relative change in ADAP utilization (29.1% and 29.9%,

TABLE 1— Demographic Characteristics of People With HIV (PWH) and PWH Who Were Served by AIDS Drug Assistance Programs (ADAPs) in the United States for 2008, 2014, and 2021

	2008		2014		2021		Absolute Change Served by ADAP, Δ%	Relative Change Served by ADAP, %
	No. of PWH	Served by ADAP, No. (Row %)	No. of PWH	Served by ADAP, No. (Row %)	No. of PWH	Served by ADAP, No. (Row %)		
Total	764 312	106 747 (14.0)	920 107	146 623 (15.9)	1 071 005	238 585 (22.3)	8.3	59.3
Age, y								
13–24	32 860	2 961 (9.0)	37 638	5 564 (14.8)	28 056	6 706 (23.9)	14.9	165.6
25–44	345 279	53 779 (15.6)	325 847	59 304 (18.2)	366 625	96 431 (26.3)	10.7	68.6
≥ 45	386 173	50 110 (13.0)	556 622	79 884 (14.4)	676 324	133 437 (19.7)	6.7	51.5
Sex								
Female	193 615	23 645 (12.2)	222 409	30 617 (13.8)	234 597	45 065 (18.3)	6.1	50.0
Male	570 697	82 857 (14.5)	697 698	113 520 (16.3)	802 941	189 170 (22.9)	8.4	57.9
Race								
Black	308 543	36 088 (11.7)	371 957	53 655 (14.4)	432 227	108 817 (25.2)	13.5	127.4
White	242 640	38 873 (16.0)	278 259	48 195 (17.3)	306 428	85 765 (28.0)	12.4	77.5
Region								
Northeast	202 313	27 164 (13.4)	222 887	32 928 (14.8)	234 977	40 751 (17.3)	3.9	29.1
Midwest	88 820	12 078 (13.5)	108 882	17 191 (15.8)	128 839	31 266 (24.3)	10.8	80.0
South	326 052	39 926 (12.2)	410 494	65 005 (15.8)	492 922	114 493 (23.2)	11.0	90.2
West	147 127	27 579 (18.7)	177 844	31 499 (17.7)	214 267	52 075 (24.3)	5.6	29.9
Medicaid expansion								
Expanded Medicaid	...	...	498 389	76 062 (15.2)	659 820	131 336 (21.0)	5.8	38.2
Did not expand Medicaid	...	...	421 718	70 561 (16.7)	411 185	107 249 (26.1)	9.4	56.3

Note. Because of missing data, the values in each column may not sum to the column total.

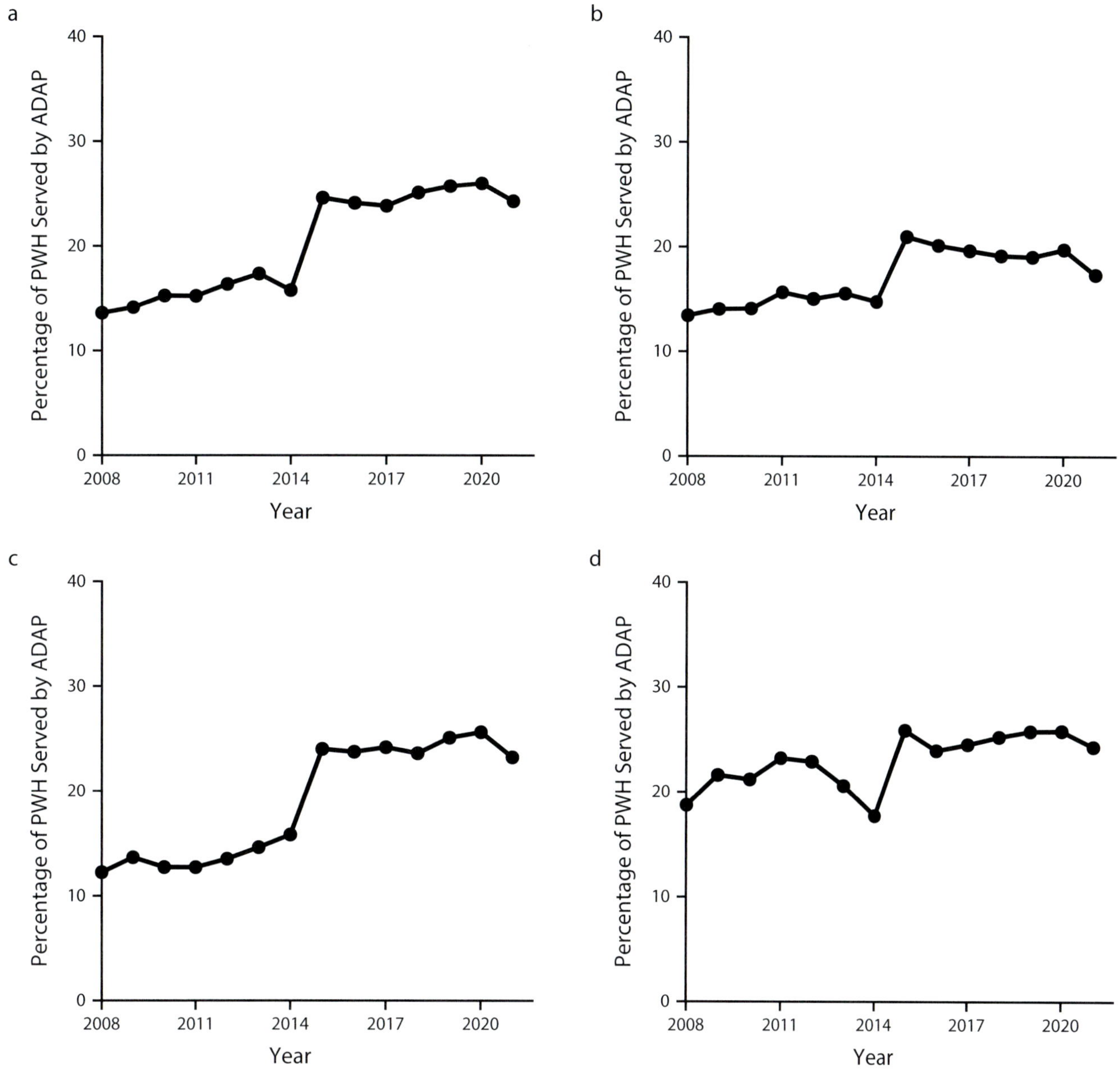

FIGURE 1— **Proportion of People With HIV (PWH) Served by AIDS Drug Assistance Programs (ADAPs) in (a) the Midwest, (b) the Northeast, (c) the South, and (d) the West: United States, 2008–2021**

respectively) compared with their cohorts in the South and Midwest (90.2% and 80.0%, respectively). Furthermore, in 2021, the ADAP utilization proportion was lowest in the Northeast (17.3%) compared with the other regions, despite the 234 977 PWH in the Northeast accounting for 21.9% of all PWH.

Client Demographics

From 2008 to 2021, ADAP utilization increased for every demographic subgroup of PWH, but at variable rates. In 2008, 2961 PWH aged 13 to 24 years were served by ADAP, which accounted for the lowest utilization proportion (9.0%) compared with PWH aged 25 to 44 years and 45 years or older (15.6% and 13.0%, respectively; Figure B, available as a supplement to the online version of this article at https://ajph.org). By 2021, 133 437 clients aged 45 years or older were served by ADAP, accounting for more than half (55.9%) of all clients. More than a quarter of PWH aged 25 to 44 years were served by

ADAP (26.3%), followed by PWH aged 13 to 24 years and 45 years or older (23.9% and 19.7%, respectively). As a result, PWH aged 13 to 24 years had the highest relative change (165.6%) compared with PWH aged 25 to 44 years and 45 years or older (68.6% and 51.5%, respectively). However, the utilization proportion was continually highest among PWH aged 25 to 44 years, a trend that did not differ by region (Figure C, available as a supplement to the online version of this article at https://ajph.org).

Utilization proportions differed by sex, with 23 645 female PWH utilizing ADAP in 2008 (12.2%) compared with 82 857 male PWH (14.5%), which increased to 45 065 (18.3%) for female PWH and 189 170 (22.9%) for male PWH by 2021 (Figure D, available as a supplement to the online version of this article at https://ajph.org). The relative change was 50.0% for female PWH and 57.9% for male PWH. Both the number of PWH served and utilization proportions were consistently higher for male PWH by region, except in 2013 in Southern ADAPs (Figure 2).

In 2008, despite Black PWH constituting 40.4% of all PWH and White PWH constituting 31.7% of all PWH, fewer Black PWH were served by ADAP than White PWH (36 088 and 38 873). In 2008, the utilization proportion was higher for White PWH at 16.0% compared with 11.7% for Black PWH. The difference in utilization proportion between Black and White PWH began to narrow in 2014 (14.4% and 17.3%, respectively), and by 2015, the increase in ADAP utilization observed in the overall population was equivalent for Black and White PWH (resulting in proportions of 22.8% and 25.7%, respectively; Figure E, available as a supplement to the online version of this article at https://ajph.org). In 2021, 108 817 Black PWH utilized ADAP (25.2%) compared with 85 765 White PWH who utilized ADAP (28.4%). From 2008 to 2021, the relative change in utilization proportion for Black PWH was 127.4% compared with 77.5% for White PWH. Regionally, utilization proportions were consistently higher for White PWH compared with Black PWH in the Northeast and West, but were closer and, in some years, higher for Black PWH in the South and Midwest (Figure 3).

Program Utilization by State Medicaid Expansion Status

Utilization varied depending on state Medicaid expansion status. Starting in 2014, 76 062 PWH were served by ADAP in jurisdictions that chose to expand Medicaid (15.2%) while 70 561 were served in jurisdictions without expansion (16.7%; Figure F, available as a supplement to the online version of this article at https://ajph.org). In 2021, the proportion of PWH served by ADAP in states with Medicaid expansion was lower compared with states that did not expand (21.0% and 26.1%). Subsequently, the relative change in clients served by ADAP increased by 38.2% among jurisdictions that expanded Medicaid, while jurisdictions that did not expand Medicaid increased by 56.3%. Overall, more PWH were served by ADAP among jurisdictions that expanded Medicaid compared with jurisdictions that did not (Table 1), while the utilization proportion was higher in jurisdictions that did not expand Medicaid (Figure F). Regionally, the gap in utilization proportion between Medicaid expansion and nonexpansion states was most notable in the Midwest (Figure G, available as a supplement to the online version of this article at https://ajph.org).

DISCUSSION

ADAP has evolved over the years, reflected by the changes in ADAP client composition over the study years. The largest ADAP utilization increase occurred in tandem with the private health insurance expansion through the ACA, suggesting that ADAP utilization was responsive to external policy changes. What is also striking are the geographic differences in both utilization and client demographics.

Program Utilization Over Time

Over the study period, ADAP enrollment and utilization have increased substantially, both in total number of ADAP clients served and the proportion of PWH in the jurisdiction served by ADAP. The ACA's massive coverage expansion beginning in 2014—which included expansion of Medicaid in many states and expanded access to individual market private health insurance—was likely a major catalyst for ADAP growth. For individual market private insurance, the ACA reforms eliminated longstanding private insurance policies that either excluded PWH from coverage altogether or based premium amounts on health status and priced PWH out of the market.[24] Even as more ADAP clients are able to access subsidized private insurance through the ACA marketplaces, many low-income PWH need ADAP assistance to cover their premiums and cost-sharing.[1]

Every geographic region saw increases in PWH served by ADAP over the study period. This was true even in

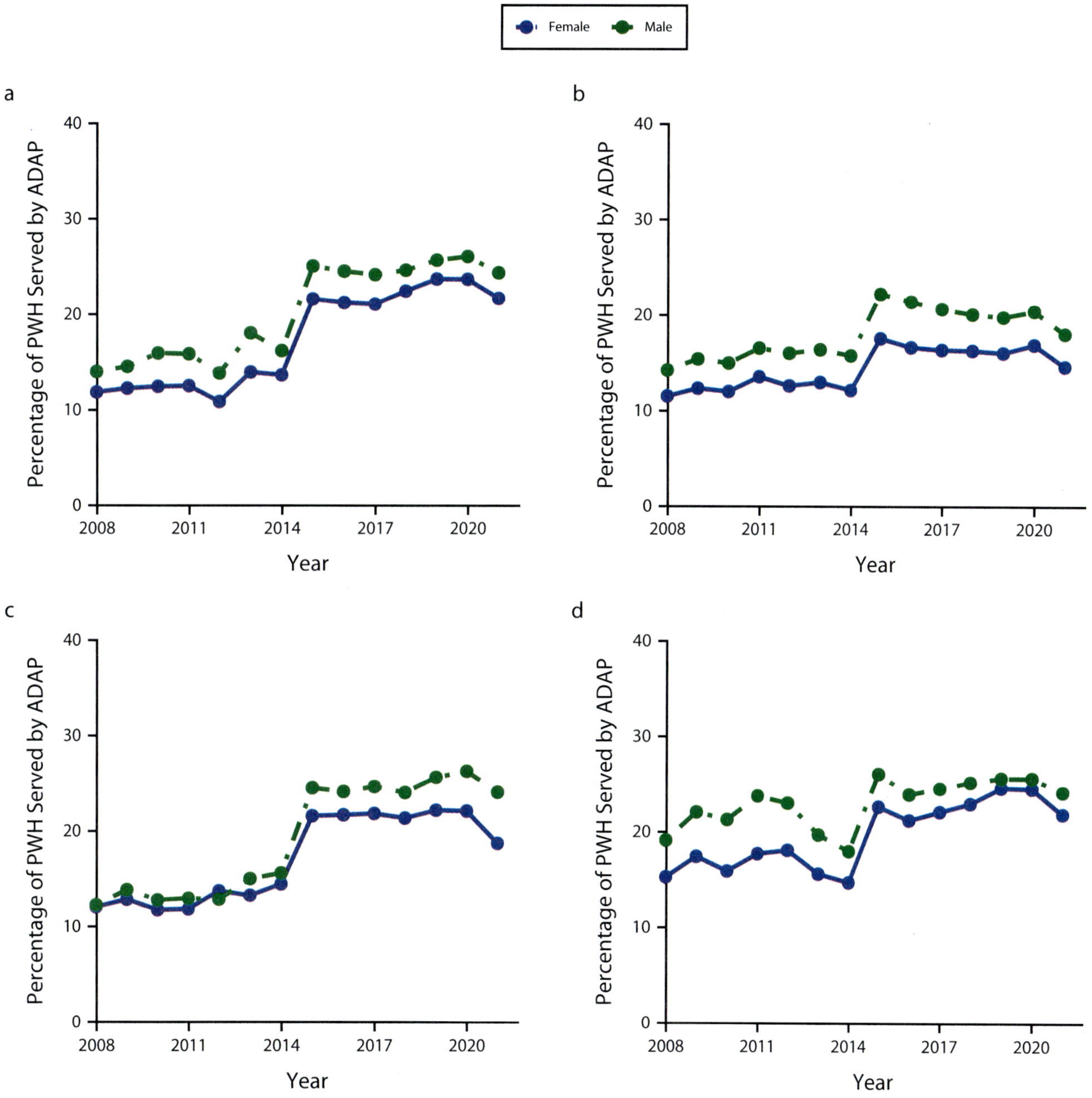

FIGURE 2— Proportion of People With HIV (PWH) Served by AIDS Drug Assistance Programs (ADAPs), by Sex in (a) the Midwest, (b) the Northeast, (c) the South, and (d) the West: United States, 2008–2021

the South, where many states have not yet expanded Medicaid, indicating that ADAP enrollment increases caused by ACA coverage expansion were likely driven in large part by the availability of marketplace coverage. In fact, even though all regions experienced increases in ADAP utilization over the study period, Medicaid expansion states experienced slightly less dramatic increases than non–Medicaid expansion states, which may demonstrate that some ADAPs disenroll people once they have Medicaid coverage and supports the theory that PWH enrolled in Medicaid may have fewer ADAP needs. However, this does not mean that PWH have reduced RWHAP wrap-around support service needs when on Medicaid.[25]

What is remarkable about the overall increase in ADAP enrollment is that it has not been accompanied by any concurrent federal funding increase

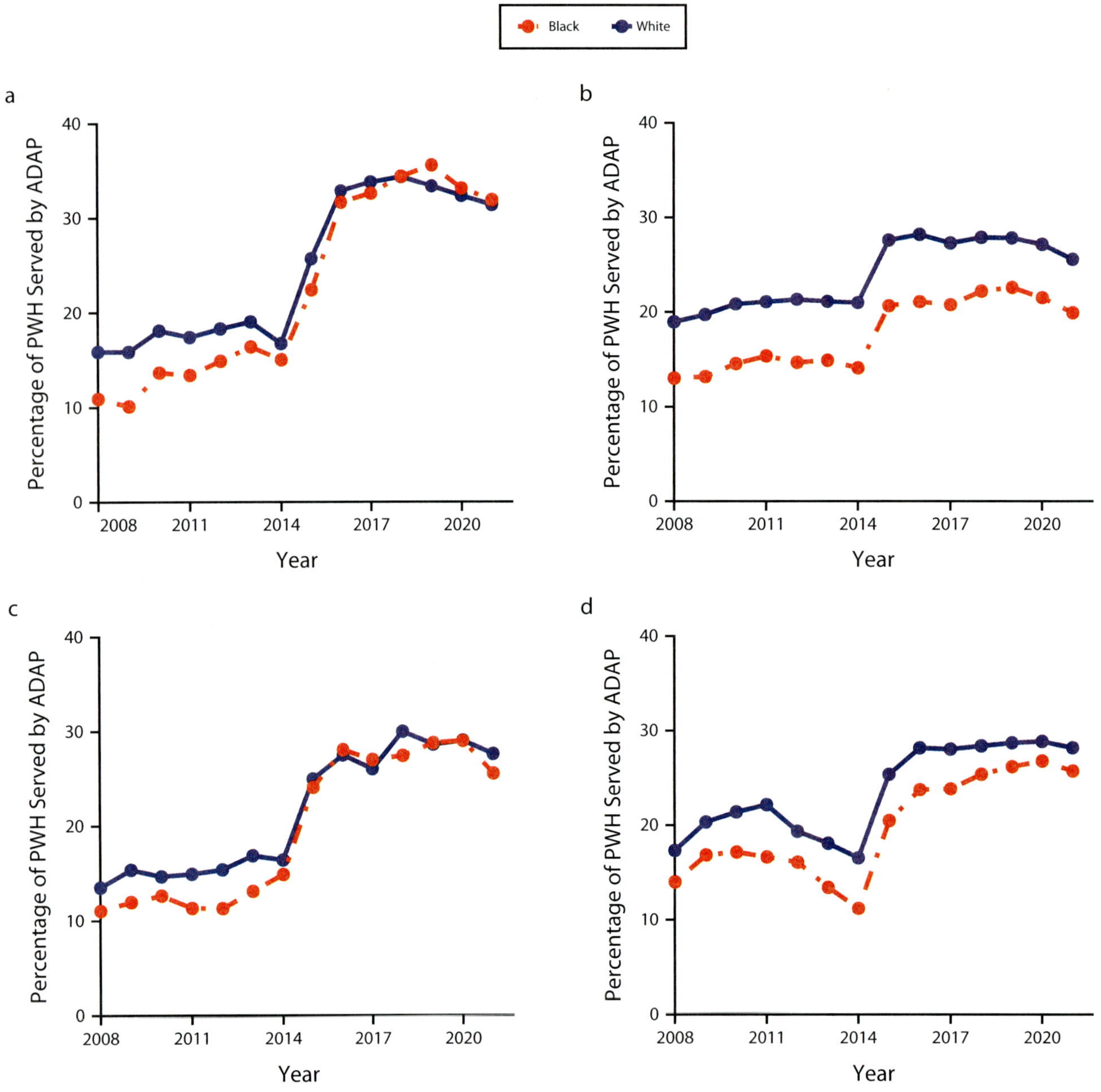

FIGURE 3— Proportion of Black and White People With HIV (PWH) Served by AIDS Drug Assistance Programs (ADAPs) in (a) the Midwest, (b) the Northeast, (c) the South, and (d) the West: United States, 2008–2021

for the program. Instead, RWHAP base funding has remained flat for more than a decade.[1,26] This may mean that ADAPs are becoming more reliant on nonfederal funding, including manufacturer rebates and 340B revenue, to ensure programs are able to grow with increasing enrollment and need.[27]

Program Inequities

Over the study period, ADAPs have closed the gap in Black PWH served by ADAPs compared with White PWH, and in 2021, the increases in ADAP utilization were consistent across Black and White PWH. However, there are still structural barriers that are preventing Black PWH from using ADAP in numbers consistent with the HIV epidemic demographic trends. A recent study that examined ADAP disenrollments in Washington State found that young, Black, and uninsured PWH were most likely to be disenrolled and that a significant proportion of eligible PWH were denied ADAP services because of a program's eligibility policy (e.g., requiring completion of recertification paperwork every 6 months) rather than documented ineligibility.[28] Since then, many states have shifted to longer periods, up to 2 years, between recertifications.[18] The Washington State study noted that the racial disparities were likely driven in part by the interconnectedness of race and other social determinants of health. This disparity underscores the need for targeted and intentional outreach efforts, including increasing funding and partnerships with Black-led community-based organizations with deep reach into communities that are not currently being served by ADAP and examination of application and recertification processes to identify barriers that can be removed.

Similarly, despite some gains over the study period, women are not being served by ADAP in proportion to the number of women with HIV in each jurisdiction. This is concerning because private health insurance and ADAP are associated with increased odds of retention in care among women with HIV.[29] Reaching women may require new partnerships with family planning clinics, domestic violence clinics, obstetrics and gynecology specialists, and other nontraditional community partners.[30]

It may be useful for federal policymakers to examine how ADAPs can support the federal Ending the HIV Epidemic (EHE) initiative and health equity within this initiative.[31] It is 1 of the 4 goals of the National HIV/AIDS Strategy to reduce HIV-related disparities and health inequities.[32] Currently, ADAP does not directly receive any EHE funding. Instead, most of the funding goes to city and county governmental public health programs. The EHE funding allocated for RWHAP recipients goes to RWHAP Part A and RWHAP Part B recipients, and while there is nothing prohibiting recipients from allocating EHE funding to ADAP, these allocations have been largely absent from EHE programming.[33]

Challenges of an Aging Clientele

In 2008, 47% of ADAP clients were aged 45 years or older compared with 56% in 2021. In addition, the proportion of PWH aged 45 years or older supported by ADAP has increased from 13% in 2008 to 20% in 2021. The aging of the ADAP population reflects the advances in HIV ART and the evolution of HIV into a manageable, lifelong, chronic condition, and as the overall number of PWH increases, both as PWH age and as new transmissions persist, ADAPs are seeing increased enrollment. Many ADAP clients are nearing eligibility for Medicare, the federal program that provides health coverage for individuals aged 65 years or older. From 2016 to 2022, the percentage of ADAP clients aged 65 years or older has almost doubled.[1,15] Health Resources and Services Administration has been making strides in encouraging the RWHAP and HIV care system to update clinical care models to be responsive to people aging with HIV.[34] However, preparing ADAPs to help clients navigate the transition to Medicare coverage and to help cover Medicare premiums and cost-sharing is essential to ensure uninterrupted care and treatment. ADAPs may need to evaluate their formularies to ensure they are comprehensive enough to meet the needs of an aging client population that may have comorbidities that impact their HIV care and treatment.

Whether and how to adapt ADAPs to changes in the ages of clients will vary by jurisdiction. The average age of clients served by ADAP varies by geography. In the South, for instance, 4% of ADAP clients are between the ages of 13 and 24 years, and 47% are between the ages of 25 and 44 years compared with ADAPs in the Northeast, which have 2% clients between the ages of 13 and 24 years and 32% between the ages of 25 and 44 years.[6] One reason for this difference could be that in states that did not expand Medicaid (predominantly in the South), ADAPs are serving a greater proportion of younger, low-income clients who would have been eligible for Medicaid had the state expanded under the ACA. This variation across geographic regions underscores the impact that a state's policy and coverage landscape has on ADAP and how important tailored funding, policy, and programmatic responses are to support ADAPs to adapt to evolving needs.

Effects of the COVID-19 Pandemic

During the COVID-19 public health emergency, ADAP and the RWHAP played a vital role in ensuring that individuals could maintain access to HIV care and treatment.[35] However, other health policy responses to COVID-19—primarily the federal requirement that state Medicaid programs suspend their normal renewal and termination processes and keep everyone on the program continuously enrolled during the emergency—took pressure off of ADAP and decreased ADAP enrollment.[36] In every geographic region, there was a significant decline in ADAP utilization from 2020 to 2021, when the Medicaid continuous coverage requirements were in effect. Because state Medicaid programs restarted their Medicaid eligibility renewal processes in April 2023, it is possible ADAPs will continue to see flux in their enrollment numbers.

Strengths and Limitations

Some strengths of this analysis include the longitudinal data and the combination of ADAP-specific data with HIV surveillance data to give a better picture of ADAP's role in the US HIV health care delivery system.

This work has limitations, including that we could not quantify the proportion of eligible PWH who are served by ADAP because income and insurance status are not reported for all PWH annually to the state or federal government. For 2022, national estimates were that 84% of PWH had income less than 400% of the federal poverty level, which would make them eligible by income for ADAP in the majority of jurisdictions if they meet other eligibility criteria.[1,37] While it is possible that the groups that are served at lower proportions had smaller proportions of PWH who were eligible, data from the American Community Survey demonstrates that the mean and median incomes of Black people are less than those of White people and that the mean and median incomes of women are less than those of men.[38] We acknowledge that income level alone is not enough to determine a PWH's eligibility for ADAP, given that PWH with low incomes may have access to comprehensive coverage through Medicaid, Medicare, or other insurance, and may have little or no need for ADAP insurance assistance, depending on how comprehensive the coverage is. Changes in ADAP enrollment and utilization vary by state and across time. For instance, whether and when a state expanded Medicaid under the ACA, and national public health and economic crises like the COVID-19 pandemic, can cause churn across programs that can make it difficult to determine an eligible ADAP PWH population.

Another limitation was that we could not conduct the analysis for all race/ethnicity groups because of data limitations. The analysis could not be conducted for Hispanic PWH because the definition of Hispanic was different between the 2 data sources.[18,19] Future work could explore (1) differences for more race/ethnicity groups and urban or rural populations, (2) ADAPs' shifting use of direct medication provision and insurance assistance programs, (3) cost implications and funding needs, and (4) the causes of disparities.

Conclusions

National and state partners of ADAPs should examine ways to ensure that, at the local and state level, ADAP enrollment, ADAP recertifications, and access to ADAP-subsidized health insurance have uptake among PWH that is equitable in terms of age, sex, race/ethnicity, and other sociodemographic factors. Further investing in ADAP, through EHE funds or other federal and state funds, may help ADAPs prioritize health equity. Equitable utilization of ADAP is essential, given that ADAP-supported health insurance has been associated with increased viral suppression,[39–41] and disenrollment from ADAP has been associated with loss of viral suppression.[42] Despite flat funding, ADAPs are ensuring lifesaving access to ART for some of the most vulnerable PWH, which is important for efforts to end the HIV epidemic. AJPH

ABOUT THE AUTHORS

Kathleen A. McManus, Amy Killelea, and Jessica Keim-Malpass are with the University of Virginia School of Medicine, Charlottesville. Tim Horn and Auntré Hamp are with National Alliance of State and Territorial AIDS Directors (NASTAD), Washington, DC. Amber Steen is with the University of Virginia School of Nursing, Charlottesville. Brian Sun and Andrew Strumpf were with the University of Virginia School of Medicine at the time of the study. Elizabeth T. Rogawski McQuade is with the Rollins School of Public Health, Emory University, Atlanta, GA.

CORRESPONDENCE

Correspondence should be sent to Kathleen A. McManus, PO Box 801379, Charlottesville, VA 22098 (e-mail: km8jr@uvahealth.org). Reprints can be ordered at https://www.ajph.org by clicking the "Reprints" link.

PUBLICATION INFORMATION

Full Citation: McManus KA, Killelea A, Horn T, et al. Trends in AIDS Drug Assistance Program support for people with HIV, by age, sex, race, and US region, 2008–2021. *Am J Public Health*. 2025;115(8):1288–1298.

Acceptance Date: February 25, 2025.

DOI: https://doi.org/10.2105/AJPH.2025.308101

ORCID iDs:

Kathleen A. McManus https://orcid.org/0000-0001-5786-0018

Amber Steen https://orcid.org/0009-0008-9258-0132

Brian Sun https://orcid.org/0009-0001-7313-0493

Jessica Keim-Malpass https://orcid.org/0000-0002-7035-8556

Elizabeth T. Rogawski McQuade https://orcid.org/0000-0002-4942-3747

CONTRIBUTORS

K. A. McManus, A. Killelea, and T. Horn contributed to the concept and design. K. A. McManus, A. Killelea, T. Horn, A. Steen, B. Sun, J. Keim-Malpass, A. Hamp, and E. T. Rogawski McQuade contributed to acquisition, analysis, or interpretation of data. K. A. McManus, A. Killelea, A. Strumpf, and E. T. Rogawski McQuade drafted the article. T. Horn, A. Steen, B. Sun, J. Keim-Malpass, and A. Hamp critically revised the article for important intellectual content. K. A. McManus, A. Killelea, T. Horn, A. Steen, J. Keim-Malpass, and E. T. Rogawski McQuade obtained funding.

ACKNOWLEDGMENTS

This work was supported by the National Institute of Allergy and Infectious Diseases at the National Institutes of Health (grant R01AI170093).

Note. The content is solely the responsibility of the authors and does not necessarily represent the official views of the National Institutes of Health.

CONFLICTS OF INTEREST

K. A. McManus reports unpaid leadership positions: member of the Ryan White Medical Providers Coalition Steering Committee and chair of the Advisory Committee to Virginia Medication Assistance Program. A. Killelea reports being a paid consultant for NASTAD and JSI. A. Steen reports stock ownership in Merck & Company.

HUMAN PARTICIPANT PROTECTION

The University of Virginia institutional review board for human participant research certified the study as non–human participant research.

REFERENCES

1. National Alliance of State and Territorial AIDS Directors. 2024 National RWHAP Part B ADAP Monitoring Project Annual Report. 2024. Available at: https://nastad.org/2024-rwhap-part-b-adap-monitoring-report. Accessed May 30, 2024.
2. Health Resources and Services Administration HIV/AIDS Bureau. Ryan White HIV/AIDS Program services: eligible individuals & allowable uses of funds. October 22, 2018. Available at: https://ryanwhite.hrsa.gov/sites/default/files/ryanwhite/grants/service-category-pcn-16-02-final.pdf. Accessed May 30, 2024.
3. HIV/AIDS Bureau Division of State HIV/AIDS Programs. *AIDS Drug Assistant Program (ADAP) Manual*. June 2023. Available at: https://targethiv.org/sites/default/files/media/documents/2023-06/adap-manual.pdf. Accessed May 30, 2024.
4. The Public Health and Welfare, 42 USC §300ff-26 (2009).
5. National Alliance of State and Territorial AIDS Directors. National ADAP Formulary Database. 2024. Available at: https://nastad.org/adap-formulary-database. Accessed May 30, 2024.
6. Horn T, McManus K, Steen A. 2021–2022 National Ryan White HIV/AIDS Program Part B and AIDS Drug Assistance Program Monitoring Project Report. National Alliance of State and Territorial AIDS Directors. 2022. Available at: https://nastad.org/partb-adap-2021-2022-report. Accessed January 25, 2022.
7. Kaiser Family Foundation. National Alliance of State and Territorial AIDS Directors. National ADAP Monitoring Project Annual Report. 2009. Available at: https://www.kff.org/wp-content/uploads/2013/01/7861.pdf. Accessed July 12, 2021.
8. National Alliance of State and Territorial AIDS Directors. National ADAP Monitoring Project Annual Report Module Two. 2011. Available at: https://www.kff.org/wp-content/uploads/sites/2/2011/05/201152_module_two_-_national_adap_monitoring_project_annual_report_-_may_2011.pdf. Accessed July 18, 2021.
9. National Alliance of State and Territorial AIDS Directors. National ADAP Monitoring Project Annual Report Module Three. 2012. Available at: https://www.yumpu.com/en/document/read/19007783/2012-national-adap-monitoring-project-annual-report-nastad. Accessed July 18, 2021.
10. National Alliance of State and Territorial AIDS Directors. National ADAP Monitoring Project Annual Report. 2013. Available at: http://nastad.org/docs/NASTAD-National-ADAP-Monitoring-Project-Report-Module-1-2013-1.pdf. Accessed July 18, 2021.
11. National Alliance of State and Territorial AIDS Directors. National ADAP Monitoring Project Annual Report. 2014. Available at: https://www.hivlawandpolicy.org/sites/default/files/NASTAD%20National%20ADAP%20Monitoring%20Project%20Annual%20Report%20-%20February%202014.pdf. Accessed July 18, 2021.
12. National Alliance of State and Territorial AIDS Directors. National ADAP Monitoring Project: 2015 Annual Report. 2015. Available at: https://www.nastad.org/sites/default/files/NASTAD-ADAP-Monitoring-Project-Annual-Report-May-2015.pdf. Accessed May 15, 2021.
13. National Alliance of State and Territorial AIDS Directors. National ADAP Monitoring Project: 2016 Annual Report. 2016. Available at: http://www.nastad.org/sites/default/files/2016-National-ADAP-Monitoring-Project-Annual-Report.pdf. Accessed February 22, 2018.
14. National Alliance of State and Territorial AIDS Directors. 2017 National ADAP Monitoring Project Annual Report. 2017. Available at: https://publications.nastad.org/adap-2017. Accessed February 22, 2018.
15. National Alliance of State and Territorial AIDS Directors. National Ryan White HIV/AIDS Program Part B and ADAP Monitoring Project: 2018 Annual Report. 2018. Available at: https://nastad.org/sites/default/files/2021-12/PDF-2018-ADAP-Report.pdf. Accessed July 18, 2021.
16. National Alliance of State and Territorial AIDS Directors. National Ryan White HIV/AIDS Program Part B and ADAP Monitoring Project: 2019 Annual Report. 2019. Available at: https://publications.partbadap-2019.nastad.org. Accessed August 27, 2019.
17. National Alliance of State and Territorial AIDS Directors. 2020 National RWHAP Part B and AIDS Drug Assistance Program Monitoring Project Annual Report. 2020. Available at: http://publications.partbadap-2020.nastad.org. Accessed July 27, 2021.
18. National Alliance of State and Territorial AIDS Directors. National ADAP Monitoring Project: 2023 Annual Report. 2023. Available at: https://nastad.org/2023-rwhap-part-b-adap-monitoring-report. Accessed May 30, 2023.
19. Centers for Disease Control and Prevention. NCHHSTP AtlasPlus. May 1, 2023. Available at: https://www.cdc.gov/nchhstp/atlas/index.htm. Accessed May 30, 2024.
20. Health Resources and Services Administration. Ryan White HIV/AIDS Program Compass Dashboard. 2024. Available at: https://web.archive.org/web/20250122145758/https://data.hrsa.gov/topics/hiv-aids/compass-dashboard. Accessed May 30, 2024.
21. Kaiser Family Foundation. Status of state action on the Medicaid expansion decision. 2024. Available at: https://www.kff.org/medicaid/issue-brief/status-of-state-medicaid-expansion-decisions-interactive-map. Accessed February 2, 2024.
22. Health Resources and Services Administration. Data reports and slide decks: archived ADAP annual data reports. 2025. Available at: https://web.archive.org/web/20250124113204/https://ryanwhite.hrsa.gov/data/reports. Accessed August 4, 2022.
23. *Geographic Areas Reference Manual*. Washington, DC: US Census Bureau; 1994.
24. Kaiser Family Foundation. The Affordable Care Act 101. 2024. Available at: https://www.kff.org/health-policy-101-the-affordable-care-act/?entry=table-of-contents-what-is-the-affordable-care-act. Accessed August 2, 2024.
25. Cahill SR, Mayer KH, Boswell SL. The Ryan White HIV/AIDS Program in the age of health care reform. *Am J Public Health*. 2015;105(6):1078–1085. https://doi.org/10.2105/AJPH.2014.302442
26. Kaiser Family Foundation. The Ryan White HIV/AIDS Program: the basics. 2020. Available at: https://www.kff.org/hivaids/fact-sheet/the-ryan-white-hivaids-program-the-basics. Accessed July 19, 2021.
27. National Alliance of State and Territorial AIDS Directors. Ryan White HIV/AIDS Program: uses of ADAP rebate and program income funds. 2024. Available at: https://web.archive.org/web/20240921055225/https://nastad.org/sites/default/files/2024-06/NASTAD-ADAP-RebateAndProgramFunds_060324-2.pdf. Accessed May 30, 2024.
28. Erly S, Khosropour CM, Hajat A, et al. Characterization of the population affected by the 6-month recertification criterion of the Ryan White HIV/AIDS Program's AIDS Drug Assistance Program in Washington State, 2017–2019. *J Acquir Immune Defic Syndr*. 2022;89(1):27–33. https://doi.org/10.1097/QAI.0000000000002824
29. Kay ES, Edmonds A, Ludema C, et al. Health insurance and AIDS Drug Assistance Program (ADAP) increases retention in care among women living with HIV in the United States. *AIDS Care*. 2021;33(8):1044–1051. https://doi.org/10.1080/09540121.2020.1849529
30. Ford N, Newman M, Malumo S, Chitembo L, Gaffield ME. Integrating sexual and reproductive health services within HIV services: WHO guidance. *Front Glob Womens Health*. 2021;2:735281. https://doi.org/10.3389/fgwh.2021.735281
31. Fauci AS, Redfield RR, Sigounas G, Weahkee MD, Giroir BP. Ending the HIV epidemic: a plan for the United States. *JAMA*. 2019;321(9):844–845. https://doi.org/10.1001/jama.2019.1343
32. The White House. National HIV/AIDS Strategy (2022–2025). 2021. Available at: https://files.hiv.gov/s3fs-public/NHAS-2022-2025.pdf. Accessed April 10, 2022.
33. National Alliance of State and Territorial AIDS Directors. Ending the HIV Epidemic. 2024. Available at: https://nastad.org/issues/ending-hiv-epidemic. Accessed May 30, 2024.
34. Health Resources and Services Administration. Emerging strategies to improve health outcomes for people aging with HIV: demonstration sites. 2021. Available at: https://www.hrsa.gov/grants/find-funding/HRSA-22-028. Accessed May 30, 2024.
35. McManus KA, Strumpf AM, Killelea A, et al. Ryan White HIV/AIDS Part B and AIDS Drug Assistance Programs during COVID-19: safety net public health programs' challenges and innovations. *Front Public Health*. 2023;11:1172009. https://doi.org/10.3389/fpubh.2023.1172009
36. Dolan R, Musumeci M, Tolbert J, Rudowitz R. Medicaid maintenance of eligibility (MOE) requirements: issues to watch. KFF. December 17, 2020. Available at: https://www.kff.org/medicaid/issue-brief/medicaid-maintenance-of-eligibility-moe-requirements-issues-to-watch. Accessed October 10, 2024.
37. Centers for Disease Control and Prevention. Individual-level social determinants of health and quality of life among persons with diagnosed HIV

infection—Medical Monitoring Project, United States, 2022 data cycle (June 2022–May 2023). November 2024. Available at: https://stacks.cdc.gov/view/cdc/168909. Accessed January 21, 2025.

38. US Census Bureau, US Department of Commerce. American Community Survey, ACS 1-year estimates subject tables, Tables S1902, S1903, S2002. 2023. Available at: https://data.census.gov/table/ACSST1Y2023.S1903?q=mean%20income%20by%20Owner%20Sex. Accessed January 21, 2025.

39. McManus KA, Rhodes A, Bailey S, et al. Affordable Care Act qualified health plan coverage: association with improved HIV viral suppression for AIDS Drug Assistance Program clients in a Medicaid nonexpansion state. *Clin Infect Dis.* 2016;63(3):396–403. https://doi.org/10.1093/cid/ciw277

40. McManus KA, Rhodes A, Yerkes L, Engelhard CL, Ingersoll KS, Dillingham R. Year 2 of Affordable Care Act qualified health plans (QHPs) in a Medicaid nonexpansion state: QHPs associated with viral suppression for Virginia AIDS Drug Assistance Program clients. *Open Forum Infect Dis.* 2018;5(12):ofy283. https://doi.org/10.1093/ofid/ofy283

41. McManus KA, Christensen B, Nagraj VP, et al. Evidence from a multistate cohort: enrollment in Affordable Care Act qualified health plans' association with viral suppression. *Clin Infect Dis.* 2020;71(10):2572–2580. https://doi.org/10.1093/cid/ciz1123

42. Erly SJ, Khosropour CM, Hajat A, Sharma M, Reuer JR, Dombrowski JC. AIDS Drug Assistance Program disenrollment is associated with loss of viral suppression beyond differences in homelessness, mental health, and substance use disorders: an evaluation in Washington State 2017–2019. *PLoS One.* 2023;18(5):e0285326. https://doi.org/10.1371/journal.pone.0285326

Youth Detention and Incarceration Facilities in the United States (2010 to February 2023): Mapping Closure Intents and Implementation

Emily J. Johnson, MPP, Hunter Pluckebaum, MPH, Karin D. Martin, PhD, MPP, MA, Benjamin Danielson, MD, Brenda Majercin, MA, Sheila Ater Capestany, MPH, MSW, and Vivian H. Lyons, PhD, MPH

See also Helmcamp, p. 1190.

Objectives. To characterize youth detention and incarceration facility closure attempts in the United States from January 2010 to February 2023 and inform ongoing attempts for facility closure.

Methods. We conducted a landscape analysis of youth facilities with stated intent to close during our study period. For each facility, we coded for jurisdiction (state vs local), year of attempt, stated reasons for closure, outcome of the facility (closed, remained open, or other), facility size, and what happened to youths after the facility closed.

Results. We identified a total of 118 facilities in 33 states that had committed to closure in our study period. The most cited reasons for the intention to close were cost (69% of facilities), declining numbers (46%), operational and facilities issues (36%), reform (33%), and conditions of confinement and abuse (30%). Sixty-two percent of identified facilities closed (n = 73).

Conclusions. Most facilities that had announced closures did close. For facilities that closed, the most commonly cited reasons were cost and decreasing numbers. Reform as a reason was more common in facilities that remained open than closed. (*Am J Public Health*. 2025;115(8):1299–1307. https://doi.org/10.2105/AJPH.2025.308118)

AJPH August 2025, Vol. 115, No. 8

The extensive detention and incarceration of youths in the United States sets it apart from most other countries, raising serious questions of morality and efficacy. With more than 240 000 youths confined in 2019, the United States has 3 times higher confinement rates than South America and 11 times higher confinement rates than Western Europe.[1] Youth behavior does not explain this disparity. Even when countries have similar rates of self-reported youth behavior like theft and assault, the US rates of incarceration are notably higher.[2,3] The American emphasis on incarceration, rooted in a racist history of slavery and discriminatory criminal legal policies and practices against Black people, makes it an extreme outlier.[4] Moreover, pretrial and preconviction detention is common in the United States—such that 60% of youths incarcerated in the United States are detained before and during the adjudication process.[5] This is the case even though fewer than one third of youths are detained for or convicted of serious violent offenses.[2] Despite the success of both pre- and postsentencing diversion programs in reducing subsequent criminal legal system involvement compared with detention and incarceration,[6,7] youth detention has continued to be used for the majority of youths adjudicated in the United States.

Youth detention and incarceration remain harmful,[2,8] ineffective,[7] and expensive,[9] and disproportionately impact youths of color.[2,10] Even a short period in detention carries serious health impacts, such as depression and self-harm, that can affect youths into adulthood.[11,12] Because of substandard educational offerings in confinement, youths in detention face additional challenges reintegrating back into schools after release, with negative impacts on education and jobs through adulthood.[2,13] Youth detention is ineffective because it fails to address the root causes of why a young person may engage in criminalized behavior in the first place and does not reduce risk of future arrests, reconvictions, or return to detention.[2] Stays in detention, including pretrial, are associated with increased risk of arrest in the following year, even after adjusting for prior cases, severity of charges, age at first offense, race, and sex.[14] Community-based alternatives are more cost-effective than youth detention.[9] The average cost of incarcerating a single youth is $214 620 per year.[15] For that cost, most states could cover tuition for nearly 20 students to a public, 4-year university.[16]

A pragmatic need to support the ongoing strategic planning process for the detention center closure in King County, Washington, was the impetus for this study. Despite growing efforts to close youth detention facilities and replace them with community-based alternatives, there have been few academic efforts examining efforts to close these facilities across the United States. By investigating previous closure attempts, we sought to identify patterns in closure, reasons for attempting closure, and whether the facilities closed, remained open, or were reopened or replaced. We aimed to describe the national landscape of youth detention and incarceration closures to identify common reasons cited in successful closures and to inform closure strategies nationally. In doing so, we address a major gap in the research on closure attempts.

METHODS

We began this effort by conducting a scoping review of evaluations of closure attempts for youth detention and incarceration centers from January 2010 to February 2023. We performed searches of PubMed, Web of Science, SSRN, EMBASE, CINAHL, and EBSCO for studies that conducted evaluations of detention and incarceration center closures in the United States. Given the relatively unsteady field, we used broad search terms including "youth prison," "juvenile detention center," "closure," closing," and "closed." The literature search resulted in 681 articles, of which 4 studies met eligibility criteria: 2 reports, 1 case study, and 1 master's thesis. See Appendix A (available as a supplement to the online version of this article at https://ajph.org) for the scoping review details.

Assessment of State and County Closure Attempts

As our next step, and to understand the scope of attempted youth detention closures in the United States, we began identifying facilities that met our eligibility criteria using existing lists of closed facilities compiled by advocacy and research groups working to close youth incarceration facilities.[17–20]

We then initiated a snowball sampling method using existing news articles and government reports to identify additional jurisdictions that had committed to closing their facilities. For this study, we did not differentiate between detention (the temporary holding of an individual, before trial or before sentencing) or incarceration (long-term confinement after sentencing), as our focus remained on facility closure and not the length of time or legal reason for individuals' confinement.[11] We identified nearly half of the additional facilities using this snowball sampling method, largely with facilities that were closed in the same state or county where other facilities were closed. Additional closures were identified through a scoping review of news articles in the EBSCO database using broad search terms including "juvenile jail"; "juvenile detention"; "juvenile incarceration"; "youth jail"; "youth prison"; "youth incarceration"; "youth detention"; "youth correctional facilities"; "juvenile correctional facilities" AND "closure"; "closing"; "closed"; or "close" to ensure we identified all relevant articles. In total, 252 news articles were screened to identify closures to include in the landscape assessment. We identified 21 additional facilities via the scoping review.

For each facility identified, we coded for jurisdiction, the name of the facility, the year of closure (if applicable), the stated reasons for the facility's intent to close (allowing multiple stated reasons for each facility), the outcome of the facility (i.e., closed, remained open, or reopened/replaced/other [hereafter "other"]), documented barriers if the facility did not close, capacity size of the facility, what happened to youths after the facility closed, and what happened to staff after the facility closed. To count as a facility closure, the facility must have shut down completely, rather than having been modified or temporarily closed. In a few cases, when the current status of the facility was unclear, we attempted to call jurisdictions directly but were not able to confirm current facility status (n = 4). We included these facilities in the analysis. See Appendix B (available as a supplement to the online version of this article at https://ajph.org) for the full data compiled in the landscape analysis.

Statistical Analysis

We used descriptive statistics to describe detention facility size and stated initial reason for closure attempt by closure process outcome—(1) closed, (2) remained open, or (3) other, including facilities that reopened or privatized, were replaced, merged, or renovated—by local and state facilities. As some closure process outcomes were rare, we subsequently combined "reopened," "replaced," "privatized," and "other" categories so that the remainder of analyses compared 3 process outcomes (closed, remained open, other). Some facilities cited multiple reasons for their stated intent to close. When comparing the distribution of stated reasons for closure by outcome (closed, remained open, other), we weighted each facility's reasons for closure by the total number of reasons cited for that facility. For example, if a facility had 4 stated reasons to close, each reason was weighted at 0.25. Using stacked bar charts, we examined weighted reasons for stated intent to close by closure attempt outcome (closed, remained open, other) for state and local facilities separately. We plotted the frequency of completed closure outcome (closed, remained open, or other) by year for state and local facilities separately. Finally, we mapped state-level variation in which states had stated intention and which states completed closures both or neither during the study period. As a sensitivity analysis, we additionally stratified our results by state versus local facilities to identify any important differences between these 2 systems.

RESULTS

We identified a total of 118 facilities that had committed to closure between January 2010 and February 2023 in the United States (Table 1). Approximately half (54%) of the facilities were found through snowball sampling, 24% through the rapid scoping review, and 22% through existing resources. Most facilities were state facilities (n = 81; 69%), while about a third were local facilities (n = 37; 31%).

Commitment to Closure

During the study period, 33 states (65%) had at least 1 facility with a stated intent to close (Figure 1). Of the 118 facilities that had committed to close, the most commonly cited reasons for the intention to close were cost (cited for 69% of facilities), declining numbers (46%), operational and facilities issues (36%), reform (33%), and conditions of confinement and abuse (30%; Figure 2). Most facilities (72%) cited multiple reasons for closure (mean = 2.1 reasons; range = 1–4; Table 1).

Closure Outcome

End result of closure intention. By February 2023, 73 facilities identified in this study had closed (62%). Among the closed facilities, nearly half (42%) were large capacity (> 100 youths) and almost one third (33%) were medium capacity (21–100 youths). During the study period, 30 states (91%) closed at least 1 facility (Table 1). The year with the most facility closures was 2011 (19 facilities closed, with 1 that later reopened), followed by 2013 (10 facilities closed, with 1 that later reopened), and then 2020 (9 facilities closed; Appendix B).

Reason for closure by end result of closure intention. Weighted reasons for closure varied by whether a facility was closed, remained open, or had another outcome (e.g., reopened, replaced, merged). Among facilities that closed, cost was cited most frequently (45%), followed by declining numbers (25%). Among facilities that remained open, reform was cited slightly more than cost (32% vs 27%, respectively). For facilities that had another outcome, the most common reasons were operational and facility issues (32%), followed by cost (20%) and conditions of confinement and abuse (18%; Figure 2).

Differences by state and local facilities. State facilities that closed were most often large capacity (55% with > 100 youths), while local facilities that closed were most often smaller and medium-sized (36% with < 20 youths, 32% with 21–100 youths). Both state and local facilities cited cost and declining numbers as the primary reasons (73% and 40% vs 60% and 60%, respectively) and had similar rates of closure (63% of state and 59% of local facilities; Table 1).

When facilities remained open, reform was cited more often than when facilities closed. For state facilities, reform tied with cost as primary reasons for attempted closure (29% weighted), while for local facilities that remained open, reform was the primary reason for attempted closure (38% weighted; Appendix C, available as a supplement to the online version of this article at https://ajph.org).

Commitment to facility closure and successful closures of state and local facilities differed by geography and time. Thirteen states committed to closing both local and state facilities. For states that committed to close only local or only state facilities, more states made commitments to close state facilities than local facilities (15 vs 3, respectively). Over the study period, 2011 was the year with the highest number of state facilities that closed (n = 15), while 2020 had the most local facilities that closed (n = 6; Appendix B).

TABLE 1— Facility Landscape Analysis Results: United States, January 2010–February 2023

	Closed, No. (%)	Remained Open, No. (%)	Other, No. (%)	Total, No. (%)
State facilities				
No. (%)	51 (63.0)	17 (21.0)	13 (16.1)	81 (100.0)
Capacity category[a]				
1: ≤ 20 youths	5 (9.8)	1 (5.9)	1 (7.7)	7 (8.6)
2: 21–100 youths	17 (33.3)	11 (64.7)	8 (61.5)	36 (44.4)
3: > 100 youths	28 (54.9)	5 (29.4)	3 (23.1)	36 (44.4)
Unknown	1 (2.0)	0 (0.0)	1 (7.7)	2 (2.5)
Stated reason for closure (categories)[b]				
Cost	41 (80.4)	11 (64.7)	7 (53.9)	59 (72.8)
Reform	13 (25.5)	11 (64.7)	5 (38.5)	29 (35.8)
Declining numbers	22 (43.1)	7 (41.2)	3 (23.1)	32 (39.5)
Conditions of confinement and abuse	15 (29.4)	5 (29.4)	5 (38.5)	25 (30.9)
Operational and facility issues	14 (27.5)	5 (29.4)	8 (61.5)	27 (33.3)
Local facilities[c]				
No. (%)	22 (59.5)	7 (18.9)	8 (21.6)	37 (100.0)
Capacity[a]				
1: ≤ 20 youths	8 (36.4)	0 (0.0)	1 (12.5)	9 (24.3)
2: 21–100 youths	7 (31.8)	2 (28.6)	6 (75.0)	15 (40.5)
3: > 100 youths	3 (13.6)	5 (71.4)	1 (12.5)	9 (24.3)
Unknown	4 (18.2)	0 (0.0)	0 (0.0)	4 (10.8)
Stated reason for closure (categories)[b]				
Cost	14 (63.6)	4 (57.1)	4 (50.0)	22 (59.5)
Reform	4 (18.2)	6 (85.7)	0 (0.0)	10 (27.1)
Declining numbers	15 (68.2)	3 (42.9)	4 (50.0)	22 (59.5)
Conditions of confinement and abuse	3 (13.6)	1 (14.3)	6 (75.0)	10 (27.1)
Operational and facilities issues	7 (31.8)	3 (42.9)	5 (62.5)	15 (40.5)

[a]The column proportions for capacity of facilities were calculated using the total number of data available.
[b]These categories for closure are non–mutually exclusive categories.
[c]Local facilities means facilities operated by counties and cities. Out of the 37 local facilities, 2 were city facilities.

See Appendix C for more details on the differences between state and local facilities.

DISCUSSION

A few important patterns emerged from our analysis. Between 2010 and 2023 and across 33 states, 81 state and 37 local facilities stated an intention to close. Ultimately, 63% of state facilities and 59% of local facilities closed. Approximately one fifth of facilities stayed open despite a stated intent to close. Some other facilities with a stated intention to close were closed initially but were replaced, reopened, privatized, or merged (13 state, 8 local). Large facilities with more than 100 youths made up the majority (55%) of closed state facilities, mirroring broader trends of the movement away from large facilities to smaller facilities.[21] Most of the completed closures at the state level took place in 2011, while most of the completed closures at the local level took place between 2015 and 2020. Although some advocates for continued youth confinement argue that secure detention is needed to deter youth crime, these closures occurred during a 74% overall decline in youth crime rates between 2010 and 2020.[22,23]

Despite the evidence that reform efforts have led to changes within the youth criminal legal system, our data show that reform was cited less often for facilities that closed than for facilities that remained open.[24] When weighted, the public factors that seem to drive decision-making in closed state and

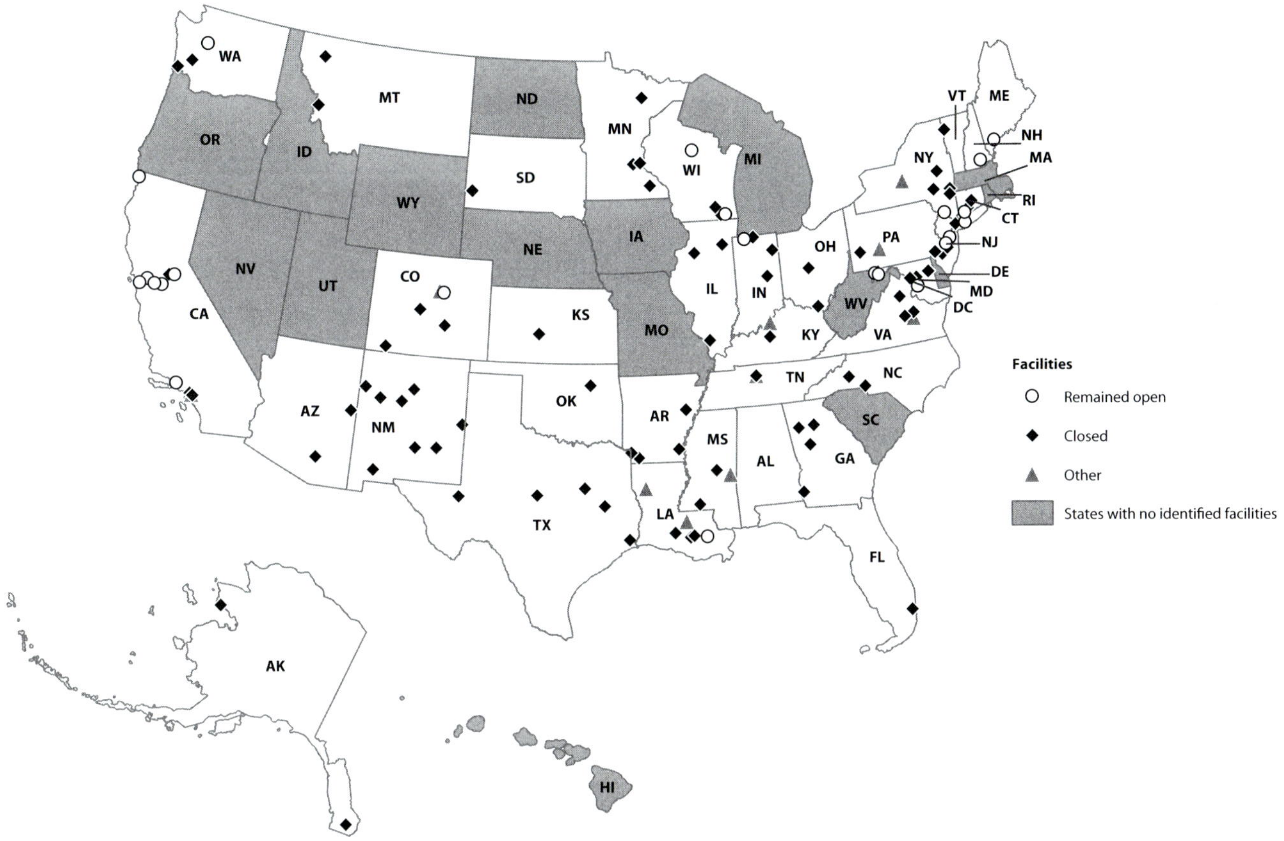

FIGURE 1— US States by Facility Outcome: January 2010–February 2023

Note. Please see Appendix B (available as a supplement to the online version of this article at https://ajph.org) for more information on the facilities included in this figure.

local facilities tended to be cost and decreasing numbers. Facilities that remained open more often cited reform as a reason for intent to close than facilities that closed. It is possible that focusing on reform by itself, without other accompanying reasons, may bring about additional political obstacles to closure despite evidence that incarceration is unnecessary and ineffective. This may be particularly true in the current political environment with its increasing focus on the criminalization of behavior as well as targeted efforts to quash reforms addressing racial inequities.

It is reasonable to assume that broader societal and economic trends likely influence closures of youth carceral facilities—both intended and completed. The high number of completed closures of state facilities (n = 16) in 2011, with a majority being large facilities (> 100 youths), was likely related to the economic recession that took place in the United States in the late aughts. Faced with budget constraints, states had difficulty justifying the high cost of youth incarceration as the incarcerated population decreased.[25] In contrast, a relatively high number of local facilities closed between 2015 and 2020. Decades of efforts by local jurisdictions, supported in part by national programming such as the Annie E. Casey Foundation's Juvenile Detention Alternatives Initiative, led to significant reductions in the number of youths incarcerated before adjudication in local facilities.[24] Like states in the Great Recession, local jurisdictions faced the challenge of continuing to justify high costs of incarceration with lower numbers of youths in detention, made possible by those reform efforts. The COVID-19 pandemic also led to an initial dramatic drop in youths held in detention—nearly 30%—as jurisdictions reduced confinement to help slow the spread of the virus, although that trend soon reversed as the numbers of youths in detention rose throughout 2021 and 2022 without political will to maintain those gains.[26]

Despite overall reductions in the number of youths in detention and incarceration, youths detained remain disproportionately Black, Indigenous, and Latinx.[27] In 2019, Black youths

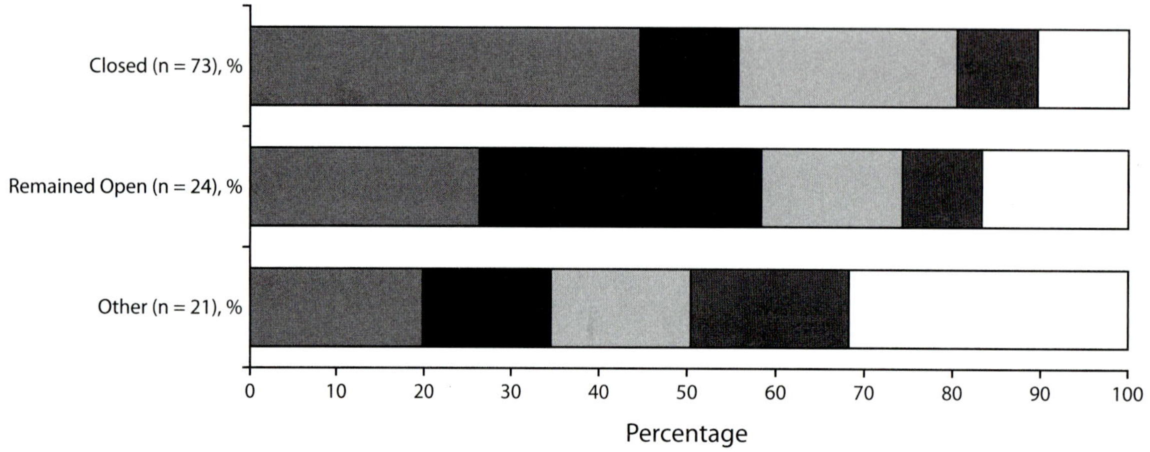

	Closed (n = 73), %	Remained Open (n = 24), %	Other (n = 21), %
Cost	44.6	26.4	19.8
Reform	11.1	31.9	14.7
Declining numbers	24.8	16.0	15.9
Conditions of confinement/abuse	9.1	9.0	17.9
Operational issues/facility issues	10.4	16.7	31.7

FIGURE 2— **Facility Outcome by Weighted Stated Reasons for Closure: United States, January 2010–February 2023**

were 41% of youths in state and local facilities, despite being only 15% of the total youth population. Meanwhile, non-Hispanic White youths made up 33% of detained youth, despite representing 52% of the total youth population.[28] White youths are more likely to shoplift and engage in violent behavior than Black youths, yet Black youths are more likely to be arrested and charged.[29] When Black and Indigenous youths are arrested or come in contact with the juvenile legal system, they are significantly less likely to be offered diversion programs[30] and are nearly 5 times more likely to be detained than White youths in the same position.[10] The racialized approach to criminalizing youths of color is evident throughout society and at every stage of the criminal legal process: school disciplinary policies, including in-school and out-of-school suspensions and expulsions, whether police confront a youth, and whether a youth is arrested, charged, taken into custody, or detained.[27,28]

Facility closures by themselves do not address this disproportionality because they do not address the underlying needs of youths and their families. Instead, additional system transformations rooted in solutions from impacted youths and communities and fundamentally different approaches are needed to improve youth experiences and outcomes. There were 8 facility closures that reportedly released some youths to community programming or to their families, in addition to transporting some youths to other facilities. In the rest of the facilities that closed, the youths were exclusively transported to other facilities (89%). The unintended negative effects of sending youths to nearby facilities when facilities close are especially pronounced when local detention centers close and arrested youths are sent to other counties for pretrial detention. In New Mexico, where 8 facilities successfully closed during our study period, the remaining local detention centers strained to fill the need—resulting in youths being sent to facilities around the state. As a result, some youths are now held in detention centers more than 120 miles away from their home counties.[31]

Moving youths from their communities, especially to facilities located far away, disrupts key connections with family and legal support, exacerbates feelings of loneliness and disconnection, requires time-intensive and costly transportation to and from court, and hinders successful reintegration of those youths back into their communities.[31] This echoes the practice of separating youths of color from their families used in both American chattel slavery and Native American boarding schools.[32] In contrast, keeping youths in the

AJPH August 2025, Vol. 115, No. 8

community with appropriate supports can maintain critical connections with their families and help address their underlying needs.[33] To achieve this, system transformation efforts could include credible messenger mentoring models, wraparound supports for youths and families, and restorative justice interventions.[33]

Limitations

This study should be considered in light of its limitations. One of the larger limitations of our analysis is data completeness. Because no comprehensive list of facility closures was available, we sought to minimize this limitation by supplementing our landscape analysis methods, including gray literature review, snowball sampling, and advocacy reports that compiled lists of facilities. This approach allowed us to identify 98% of long-term secure state facilities but only 20% of local detention facilities.[21] However, as the Office of Juvenile Justice and Delinquency Prevention aggregates closure data, we were unable to use their data to identify specific closed facilities to ensure data completeness. We assume that the missing local facilities we do not have in this study do not differ substantially from the facilities we include. Despite the high degree of missingness for local facilities, the high proportion of identified state-level facilities and agreement between local and state findings increases our confidence in our findings. Another large limitation of our analysis is that it only captures the stated reasons for intent to close facilities. It does not identify any additional underlying reasons that may have played a role or those that were not made public. Discerning any reasons for closure beyond what was publicly stated exceeds the scope of this analysis.

Public Health Implications

A national movement to end youth incarceration and detention has been gaining momentum. Advocacy organizations, such as the Youth First Justice Collaborative, launched state and local campaigns in 15 jurisdictions to close youth detention and incarceration facilities. Several local jurisdictions, including King County; San Francisco, California; and Contra Costa, California, have committed to closing their youth detention facilities and replacing them with community-based alternatives. These efforts seek to redress the harm of youth detention and incarceration, especially the disproportionately negative consequences for youths of color. It is important that these commitments to closure persist to counter an emerging wave of "tough-on-crime" policies for youths in particular.[34]

This study illuminates pathways for future research to explore facility closures. Such research should investigate the impact of specific drivers supporting completed closures of youth facilities, including the combination of stated reasons to appeal to different audiences. Notably, we only found 1 paper in our scoping review that explores the strategies used by activists to close a youth detention center.[35] As more jurisdictions rethink their approach to juvenile justice, research should examine the particulars of budgeting and processes for actually closing facilities and expanding community alternatives. Supplementing reform arguments for facility closure with cost and reducing numbers may provide broader support.

Finally, our study extends the existing research landscape of youth incarceration and highlights potential opportunities for collaboration between advocacy and academia. Most of the academic articles within the youth legal system field that we found in our scoping review focus on reform efforts, rather than on decarceration and abolition. While emerging research has focused on the impacts of individual diversion programs and evaluations of specific programming, scholarship in this domain is not fully grappling with the complexities of actually closing youth incarceration facilities. This work is fundamentally rooted in the complexities of engaging critical audiences—including local and state governmental leaders—to reimagine the current system of incarceration and envision alternatives that support youths and their families, center impacted youths and harmed parties, and foster youth healing, accountability, and true community safety. In our experience, public will and broad community support are also essential to ensure politicians stay committed to closures and fund the robust alternatives needed to better support youths. Interdisciplinary and cross-sector collaboration will be needed to promote facility closures with corresponding system transformation efforts for meaningful and sustained reductions in youth detention and incarceration. AJPH

ABOUT THE AUTHORS

Emily J. Johnson was with the King County Department of Community and Human Services, Seattle, WA, at the time of this study, and Hunter Pluckebaum was with Allies in Healthier Systems for Health & Abundance in Youth (AHSHAY), Seattle. Karin D. Martin is with the Evans School of Public Policy and Governance at the University of Washington, Seattle. Sheila Ater Capestany is with the King County Department of Community and Human Services. Benjamin Danielson is with the Department of Psychiatry and Behavioral Sciences at the University of Washington, Seattle. Brenda Majercin and Vivian H. Lyons are affiliated with the AHSHAY Center, Seattle.

CORRESPONDENCE

Correspondence should be sent to Vivian H. Lyons, 120 Lakeside Ave #310, Seattle, WA 98122 (e-mail: vivian@ahshay.org). Reprints can be ordered at https://ajph.org by clicking the "Reprints" link.

PUBLICATION INFORMATION

Full Citation: Johnson EJ, Pluckebaum H, Martin KD, et al. Youth detention and incarceration facilities in the United States (2010 to February 2023): mapping closure intents and implementation. *Am J Public Health*. 2025;115(8):1299–1307.

Acceptance Date: March 11, 2025.

DOI: https://doi.org/10.2105/AJPH.2025.308118

ORCID iDs:

Emily J. Johnson https://orcid.org/0009-0008-7441-9556

Karin D. Martin https://orcid.org/0000-0003-1094-6425

Vivian H. Lyons https://orcid.org/0000-0003-0481-5939

CONTRIBUTORS

E. J. Johnson compiled the landscape analysis, conducted data analysis, and wrote and revised the article. H. Pluckebaum contributed to the project's conceptual design, conducted the scoping review, and wrote scoping review findings. K. D. Martin contributed to the conceptual design of the project, provided feedback on initial findings, and provided feedback on article drafts. B. Danielson, B. Majercin, and S. A. Capestany contributed to the project's conceptual design and provided feedback on article drafts. V. H. Lyons contributed to the conceptual design of the project, provided feedback on initial findings, wrote and revised the article, and supervised the project. All authors approved the submitted version and agreed to be accountable for all aspects of the work in ensuring that questions related to the accuracy or integrity of any part of the work are appropriately investigated and resolved.

ACKNOWLEDGMENTS

The authors thank Emma Gause at Boston University School of Public Health for her creation of the geospatial map of the facility outcomes in the United States.

CONFLICTS OF INTEREST

The authors declare that they do not have any conflicts of interest.

HUMAN PARTICIPANT PROTECTION

This study was exempt from institutional review board review as it did not include any individual data or protected health information.

REFERENCES

1. Mendel R. *Why Youth Incarceration Fails: An Updated Review of the Evidence.* The Sentencing Project. 2022. Available at: https://www.sentencingproject.org/app/uploads/2023/03/Why-Youth-Incarceration-Fails.pdf. Accessed November 17, 2024.
2. Enzmann D, Marshall IH, Killias M, Junger-Tas J, Steketee M, Gruszczynska B. Self-reported youth delinquency in Europe and beyond: first results of the second international self-report delinquency study in the context of police and victimization data. *Eur J Criminol.* 2010;7(2):159–183. https://doi.org/10.1177/1477370809358018
3. Hazel N. Cross-national comparison of youth justice. Youth Justice Board. 2008. Available at: https://dera.ioe.ac.uk/id/eprint/7996/1/Cross_national_final.pdf. Accessed May 17, 2025.
4. Hinton E, Cook D. The mass criminalization of Black Americans: a historical overview. *Annu Rev Criminol.* 2021;4(1):261–286. https://doi.org/10.1146/annurev-criminol-060520-033306
5. Sawyer W. Youth confinement: the whole pie 2019. Prison Policy Initiative. December 19, 2019. Available at: https://www.prisonpolicy.org/reports/youth2019.html. Accessed November 17, 2024.
6. Wilson HA, Hoge RD. The effect of youth diversion programs on recidivism. *Criminal Justice Behavior.* 2013;40(5):497–518. https://doi.org/10.1177/0093854812451089
7. Shelden R. Detention diversion advocacy: an evaluation. Office of Juvenile Justice and Delinquency Prevention. 1999. Available at: https://www.ojp.gov/ncjrs/virtual-library/abstracts/detention-diversion-advocacy-evaluation. Accessed May 17, 2025.
8. Lambie I, Randell I. The impact of incarceration on juvenile offenders. *Clin Psychol Rev.* 2013;33(3):448–459. https://doi.org/10.1016/j.cpr.2013.01.007
9. Washington State Institute for Public Policy. The juvenile justice system in Washington State: recommendations to improve cost-effectiveness. Washington State Institute for Public Policy. 2002. Available at: https://www.wsipp.wa.gov/ReportFile/806/Wsipp_The-Juvenile-Justice-System-in-Washington-State-Recommendations-to-Improve-Cost-Effectiveness_Full-Report.pdf. Accessed November 17, 2024.
10. Ericson RD, Eckberg DA. Racial disparity in juvenile diversion. *Race and Justice.* 2016;6(1):35–56. https://doi.org/10.1177/2153368715594848
11. Holman B, Ziedenberg J. The dangers of detention: the impact of incarcerating youth in detention and other secure facilities. Justice Policy Institute. 2006. Available at: https://justicepolicy.org/wp-content/uploads/2022/02/06-11_rep_dangersofdetention_jj.pdf. Accessed November 17, 2024.
12. Barnert ES, Dudovitz R, Nelson BB, et al. How does incarcerating young people affect their adult health outcomes? *Pediatrics.* 2017;139(2):e20162624. https://doi.org/10.1542/peds.2016-2624
13. McCluskey M. 'What if this were your kid?' *The Atlantic.* December 24, 2017. Available at: https://www.theatlantic.com/politics/archive/2017/12/juvenile-solitary-confinement/548933. Accessed November 17, 2024.
14. Walker SC, Herting JR. The impact of pretrial juvenile detention on 12-month recidivism: a matched comparison study. *Crime & Delinquency.* 2020;66(13-14):1865–1887. https://doi.org/10.1177/0011128720926115
15. Justice Policy Institute. Sticker shock: the cost of youth incarceration. July 30, 2020. Available at: https://justicepolicy.org/research/policy-brief-2020-sticker-shock-the-cost-of-youth-incarceration. Accessed November 17, 2024.
16. Scheckel M. The average cost of college tuition. *Business Insider.* November 12, 2024. Available at: https://www.businessinsider.com/personal-finance/student-loans/average-college-tuition. Accessed May 17, 2025.
17. Love H, Harvell S, Warnberg C, Durnan J. Transforming closed youth prisons: repurposing facilities to meet community needs. Urban Institute. 2018. Available at: https://www.urban.org/sites/default/files/publication/98628/transforming_closed_youth_prisons.pdf. Accessed November 17, 2024.
18. Harvell S, Warnberg C, Matei A, Mensing E. Closing youth prisons: lessons from agency administrators. Urban Institute. March 25, 2020. Available at: https://www.urban.org/research/publication/closing-youth-prisons-lessons-agency-administrators. Accessed November 17, 2024.
19. Porter ND. Repurposing correctional facilities to strengthen communities. The Sentencing Project. August 11, 2022. Available at: https://www.sentencingproject.org/reports/repurposing-correctional-facilities-to-strengthen-communities. Accessed November 17, 2024.
20. No Kids in Prison. Youth prison & juvenile detention facility closures during COVID-19. July 9, 2020. Available at: https://www.nokidsinprison.org/youth-prison-juvenile-detention-facility-closures-during-covid19-2. Accessed November 17, 2024.
21. Puzzanchera C, Hockenberry S, Sladky TJ, Kang W. *Juvenile Residential Facility Census Databook.* Office of Juvenile Justice and Delinquency Prevention. 2022. Available at: https://www.ojjdp.gov/ojstatbb/jrfcdb. Accessed November 17, 2024.
22. Puzzanchera C. Youth arrests for violent crime in 2020 drop to new low. Office of Justice Programs. 2022. Available at: https://www.ojp.gov/files/archives/pressreleases/2022/youth-arrests-violent-crime-2020-drop-new-low. Accessed November 17, 2024.
23. Mendel R. Data reveals violence among youth under 18 has not spiked in the pandemic. The Sentencing Project. June 14, 2022. Available at: https://www.sentencingproject.org/policy-brief/data-reveals-violence-among-youth-under-18-has-not-spiked-in-the-pandemic. Accessed November 17, 2024.
24. Honeycutt T, Zweig J, Hague M, et al. Keeping youth out of the deep end of the juvenile justice system. Urban Institute. 2020. Available at: https://www.urban.org/sites/default/files/publication/102766/keeping-youth-out-of-the-deep-end-of-the-juvenile-justice-system_2.pdf. Accessed November 17, 2024.
25. National Research Council, Division of Behavioral and Social Sciences and Education, Committee on Law and Justice, Committee on Assessing Juvenile Justice Reform, Bonnie RJ, Johnson RL, Chemers BM, Schuck JA, eds. *Reforming Juvenile Justice: A Developmental Approach.* The National Academies Press. 2013. Available at: https://nap.nationalacademies.org/catalog/14685/reforming-juvenile-justice-a-developmental-approach. Accessed November 17, 2024.

26. Annie E. Casey Foundation. The number of youth in secure detention returns to pre-pandemic levels. 2022. Available at: https://www.aecf.org/blog/the-number-of-youth-in-secure-detention-returns-to-pre-pandemic-levels. Accessed November 17, 2024.

27. Development Services Group Inc. Literature review: racial and ethnic disparity in juvenile justice processing. Office of Juvenile Justice and Delinquency Prevention. March 2022. Available at: https://nationalreentryresourcecenter.org/resources/racial-and-ethnic-disparity-juvenile-justice-processing. Accessed May 17, 2025.

28. Puzzanchera C, Hockenberry S, Sickmund M. *Youth and the Juvenile Justice System: 2022 National Report*. Office of Juvenile Justice and Delinquency Prevention. 2022. Available at: https://www.ncjfcj.org/wp-content/uploads/2023/01/2022-national-report.pdf. Accessed May 17, 2025.

29. Padgaonkar NT, Baker AE, Dapretto M, et al. Exploring disproportionate minority contact in the juvenile justice system over the year following first arrest. *J Res Adolesc*. 2021;31(2):317–334. https://doi.org/10.1111/jora.12599

30. Rovner J. Black disparities in youth incarceration. The Sentencing Project. 2023. Available at: https://www.sentencingproject.org/fact-sheet/black-disparities-in-youth-incarceration. Accessed November 17, 2024.

31. Jansen S. Fewer New Mexico detention centers means problems for families, staff. *Youth Today*. March 8, 2020. Available at: https://youthtoday.org/2020/03/fewer-new-mexico-detention-centers-means-problems-for-families-staff. Accessed November 17, 2024.

32. Thampapillai R. The colourful truth: the reality of Indigenous overrepresentation in juvenile detention in Australia and the United States. *American Indian Law Journal*. 2018;7(1):12–21. Available at: https://digitalcommons.law.seattleu.edu/cgi/viewcontent.cgi?article=1193&context=ailj. Accessed November 17, 2024.

33. Mendel R. Effective alternatives to youth incarceration. The Sentencing Project. 2023. June 28, 2023. Available at: https://www.sentencingproject.org/reports/effective-alternatives-to-youth-incarceration. Accessed November 17, 2024.

34. Hernández A. 'Tough-on-crime' policies are back in some places that had reimagined criminal justice. *Stateline*. March 18, 2024. Available at: https://stateline.org/2024/03/18/tough-on-crime-policies-are-back-in-some-places-that-had-reimagined-criminal-justice. Accessed November 17, 2024.

35. Holland M. *Closing Down the Hall: San Francisco's Efforts to Redefine Juvenile Justice*. Master's Thesis. University of San Francisco. May 2021. Available at: https://repository.usfca.edu/thes/1386. Accessed November 17, 2024.

Access to Paid Sick Leave and COVID-19 Vaccination Status Among Employed Adults Aged 18–64 Years in the United States, 2021–2022

Eric W. Lundstrom, PhD, MPH, Abay Asfaw, PhD, and Rebecca Tsai, PhD

AJPH August 2025, Vol. 115, No. 8

Objectives. To measure the associations between access to paid sick leave (PSL) and COVID-19 vaccination status in the United States, both overall and stratified by occupation and industry of employment.

Methods. We extracted data on employed adults aged 18 to 64 years from the 2021 and 2022 US Medical Expenditure Panel Survey. We assessed associations between PSL and COVID-19 vaccination status using logistic regression. We used marginal effects analyses to estimate associations within occupation and industry groups.

Results. Our analytic sample (n = 15 089) represented more than 114 million employed US adults. Access to PSL was significantly associated with receipt of a COVID-19 vaccination (adjusted odds ratio = 1.33; 95% confidence interval = 1.14, 1.55). Marginal effects analyses indicated that this association was significant within most occupation and industry groups.

Conclusions. These findings suggest PSL is associated with higher COVID-19 vaccination rates among US workers. PSL remains an important tool for improving preventive health care access and reducing rates of infectious disease in the United States. (*Am J Public Health*. 2025;115(8):1308–1311. https://doi.org/10.2105/AJPH.2025.308095)

The United States remains one of the few high-income nations without a national paid sick leave (PSL) policy.[1] As a result, 1 in 5 US workers cannot take time off work to recover from illness—or to access preventive health care resources, such as vaccinations—without risking lost wages.[1] Access to PSL may increase vaccination rates by allowing workers to take time off from work to receive a vaccine and to recover from its side effects. Although previous ecological studies indicate that city-level PSL policies are associated with higher COVID-19 vaccination rates, this association has not been assessed nationally or by occupation or industry of employment.[1] This study reports associations between PSL and COVID-19 vaccination status in the United States, both overall and stratified by occupation and industry, for 2021 to 2022.

METHODS

We used data from the US Medical Expenditure Panel Survey (MEPS), a nationally representative survey of health care utilization, employment, and health outcomes in the United States.[2] Specifically, we used the 2021 and 2022 Full Year Consolidated MEPS data files, which contain information collected from 19 807 individuals employed for the entirety of the year in which they were interviewed. Approximately 20% of this initial sample was excluded because their survey information was reported by a proxy, they were aged younger than 18 years or 65 years or older, or they were missing data on variables used for analysis. Respondents employed in military occupations or industries were excluded because they likely had PSL and were required to receive a COVID-19 vaccine during the study period. Self-employed individuals were excluded because these respondents were missing information on PSL status in MEPS.

We defined respondents as having PSL if they indicated that their current main job offered PSL at any time within the study period. We defined self-reported COVID-19 vaccination status as having ever received a COVID-19 vaccination. Confounding variables of interest included age, sex, race/ethnicity, country of birth, family income, family size, marital status, education, region, insurance status, occupation, industry of employment, and survey year; hours worked per week was considered a potential effect modifier.

We conducted all analyses in RStudio version 4.4.1.,[3] downloaded MEPS data using the RStudio package "MEPS,"[4] and adjusted all descriptive and inferential statistics for MEPS's complex survey design.

We calculated descriptive statistics both overall and by PSL status and measured the association between access to PSL and COVID-19 vaccination status, both unadjusted and adjusted for covariates of interest, using logistic regression with a logit link; we used a quasibinomial distribution to account for potential overdispersion. We also estimated overall associations stratified by hours worked per week (< 35, 35–40, > 40). We used marginal effects analysis to estimate the covariate-adjusted percentage of respondents who reported ever receiving a COVID-19 vaccine by PSL status and occupation or industry group, with unadjusted proportions calculated for comparison.

RESULTS

Our analytic sample (n = 15 089) represented approximately 114.5 million US individuals employed during 2021 or 2022 (Table A, available as a supplement to the online version of this article at https://ajph.org); 22.6% reported not having access to PSL. Compared with those without PSL, those with PSL were more frequently White (61.4%), born in the United States (82.7%), married (58.0%), and college-educated (73.6%); they also tended to be older (mean = 41.9 years), to have higher total family incomes ($92 515), and to have smaller families (2.89 members). Respondents with PSL were more frequently employed in professional and related occupations (31.3%) and education, health, and social services industries (29.4%), while those without PSL were more frequently employed in service occupations (24.6%) and construction (10.7%) or leisure and hospitality (15.0%) industries.

Respondents with access to PSL more frequently reported having ever received a COVID-19 vaccination than those without PSL (85.8% compared with 72.3%; Table B, available as a supplement to the online version of this article at https://ajph.org). This association was significant after controlling for confounders of interest (adjusted odds ratio [AOR] = 1.33; 95% confidence interval [CI] = 1.14, 1.55); stratified analyses indicated this association was significant in those working 35 to 40 (AOR = 1.53; 95% CI = 1.22, 1.93) and greater than 40 hours (AOR = 1.57; 95% CI = 1.13, 2.17) per week, but not less than 35 hours per week (AOR 1.02; 95% CI = 0.72, 1.43; Table C, available as a supplement to the online version of this article at https://ajph.org). Within all occupation and industry groups, both the unadjusted and covariate-adjusted proportion of respondents reporting ever receiving a COVID-19 vaccine was higher in those with PSL compared with those without (Figure 1; Table D, available as a supplement to the online version of this article at https://ajph.org). These differences were significant in all occupation and industry groups assessed apart from farming, fishing, and forestry occupations and information industries; other services industries; and natural resource and mining industries.

DISCUSSION

This study's findings, which represented more than 114 million employed US adults aged 18 to 64 years, suggest that workers with access to PSL are significantly more likely to report being vaccinated for COVID-19 than those without. This association was not significant in respondents working less than 35 hours per week, suggesting PSL gives full-time workers time to receive vaccines and recover from their side effects. Previous research has highlighted associations between PSL and vaccine uptake. For instance, many of the same occupations with low rates of PSL access early in the COVID-19 pandemic also had low rates of COVID-19 vaccination uptake (e.g., farming, fishing, and forestry occupations).[5,6] Moreover, prepandemic analyses suggest that PSL increases uptake of vaccines for other infectious diseases, such as influenza, in workers with PSL access.[7]

Interpretations of national-level associations between PSL and preventive health care uptake are complicated by the wide variation in PSL access in the United States. As the United States

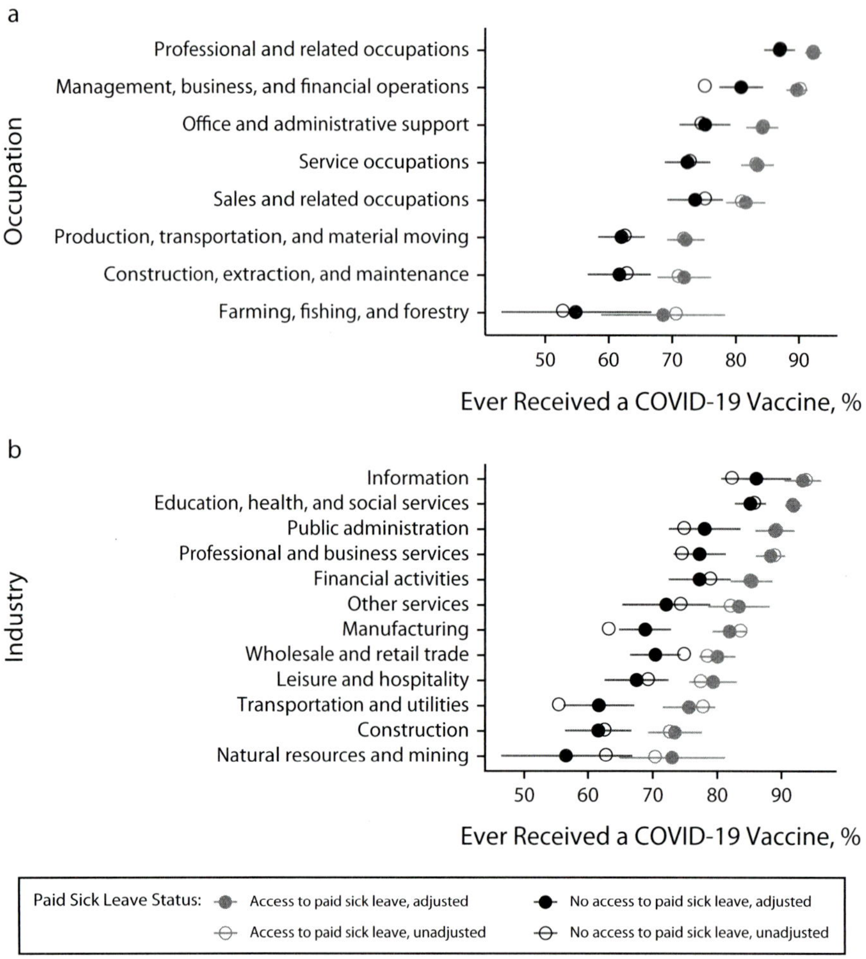

FIGURE 1— Percentage of Employed Adults Aged 18–64 Years Reporting Ever Receiving a COVID-19 Vaccine Stratified by Access to Paid Sick Leave Status and by (a) Occupation or (b) Industry of Employment: US Medical Expenditure Panel Survey (MEPS), 2021–2022

Note. Occupation and industry information in MEPS is coded using Census occupation and industry codes. Natural resources and mining industries are separate classifications but were combined here because of small cell sizes. "Other services" industries include establishments providing service not captured by other industry codes, including but not limited to equipment or machinery repair, religious services, and advocacy. The weighted sample size was n = 114 478 885. Results are presented both unadjusted and adjusted for respondent age, sex, race/ethnicity, country of birth (born in United States or not), family income, family size, marital status, education, region, insurance status, and survey year using marginal effects analysis of quasibinomial logistic regression models with a logit link.

does not have a national PSL policy, variation between state and local policies results in significant geographic and industrial variation in PSL access, potentially influencing the patterns observed in this study; some states exclude construction and agricultural workers from PSL laws,[8] both of which had low vaccination rates relative to other occupational or industrial groups in our study.

This study is subject to certain limitations. First, our analysis represents US adults employed by other persons and is not representative of those who lost employment during our study period. Second, although personal perspectives related to vaccine safety, effectiveness, and side effects have previously demonstrated associations with COVID-19 vaccination rates,[9] this information is not captured by MEPS. However, these personal perspectives likely do not influence an individual's access to PSL, and our findings are consistent with previous results measuring associations between PSL and preventive health care uptake.[1,7] Third, MEPS does not collect information related to workplace vaccination or PSL policies (e.g., if an employer requires their employees to receive a vaccine or voluntarily provides PSL), which may be associated with PSL access and COVID-19 vaccination status within our sample.

PUBLIC HEALTH IMPLICATIONS

These findings indicate that millions of US workers did not have access to PSL throughout 2021 to 2022. Expanding PSL access nationwide has the potential to reduce the spread of infectious diseases in the United States by increasing vaccine access among employed adults, helping working parents stay up to date with their children's vaccination schedule,[10] and preventing workplace spread of infectious diseases by allowing workers to stay home when sick.[11] Moreover, PSL has been noted to increase access to nonvaccine preventive health care resources (e.g., physician visits)[7] and is associated with decreases in occupational injuries in US workers,[12] potentially improving chronic disease outcomes in the United States. AJPH

ABOUT THE AUTHORS

Eric W. Lundstrom is with the Epidemic Intelligence Service, Centers for Disease Control and Prevention (CDC), and the Division of Field Studies and Engineering, National Institute for Occupational Safety and Health, Cincinnati, OH. Rebecca Tsai is with the Division of Field Studies and Engineering, National Institute for Occupational Safety and Health, Cincinnati. Abay Asfaw is with the Economic Research and Support Office, National Institute for Occupational Safety and Health, Washington, DC.

Note. The findings and conclusions in this report are those of the author(s) and do not necessarily represent the official position of the National Institute for Occupational Safety and Health, CDC.

CORRESPONDENCE

Correspondence should be sent to Eric W. Lundstrom, 1150 Tusculum Ave, Cincinnati, OH 45226 (e-mail: elundstrom@cdc.gov). Reprints can be ordered at https://www.ajph.org by clicking the "Reprints" link.

PUBLICATION INFORMATION

Full Citation: Lundstrom EW, Asfaw A, Tsai R. Access to paid sick leave and COVID-19 vaccination status among employed adults aged 18–64 years in the United States, 2021–2022. *Am J Public Health*. 2025;115(8):1308–1311.

Acceptance Date: February 24, 2025.

DOI: https://doi.org/10.2105/AJPH.2025.308095

ORCID iDs:

Eric W. Lundstrom https://orcid.org/0000-0001-9776-0134

Abay Asfaw https://orcid.org/0000-0002-4729-7302

Rebecca Tsai https://orcid.org/0000-0001-8656-9836

CONTRIBUTORS

E. W. Lundstrom downloaded all data, performed all analyses, and drafted the article for submission. All authors were involved in the conceptualization of the study and critical revision of the article and reviewed and approved the final article before submission.

ACKNOWLEDGMENTS

The authors would like to thank Anasua Bhattacharya (National Institute for Occupational Safety and Health) for providing valuable comments and suggestions on this article.

CONFLICTS OF INTEREST

The authors declare no conflicts of interest.

HUMAN PARTICIPANT PROTECTION

This activity was reviewed by the CDC, was deemed research not involving human participants, and was conducted consistent with applicable federal law and CDC policy.

REFERENCES

1. Schnake-Mahl AS, O'Leary G, Mullachery PH, et al. Higher COVID-19 vaccination and narrower disparities in US cities with paid sick leave compared to those without. *Health Aff (Millwood)*. 2022;41(11):1565–1574. https://doi.org/10.1377/hlthaff.2022.00779
2. US Department of Health and Human Services Agency for Healthcare Research and Quality. Medical Expenditure Panel Survey (MEPS). 2024. Available at: https://meps.ahrq.gov/mepsweb. Accessed September 2, 2024.
3. R Foundation for Statistical Computing. R: A language and environment for statistical computing. 2010. Available at: https://www.R-project.org. Accessed September 2, 2024.
4. Mitchell E. Package "MEPS." GitHub. 2021. Available at: https://github.com/e-mitchell/meps_r_pkg. Accessed September 2, 2024.
5. Hawkins D. Disparities in access to paid sick leave during the first year of the COVID-19 pandemic. *J Occup Environ Med*. 2023;65(5):370–377. https://doi.org/10.1097/JOM.0000000000002784
6. Henneberger PK, Cox-Ganser JM, Guthrie GM, Groth CP. Estimates of COVID-19 vaccine uptake in major occupational groups and detailed occupational categories in the United States, April–May 2021. *Am J Ind Med*. 2022;65(7):525–536. https://doi.org/10.1002/ajim.23370
7. Lamsal R, Napit K, Rosen AB, Wilson FA. Paid sick leave and healthcare utilization in adults: a systematic review and meta-analysis. *Am J Prev Med*. 2021;60(6):856–865. https://doi.org/10.1016/j.amepre.2021.01.009
8. Pomeranz JL, Silver D, Lieff SA, Pagan JA. State paid sick leave and paid sick-leave preemption laws across 50 U.S. states, 2009–2020. *Am J Prev Med*. 2022;62(5):688–695. https://doi.org/10.1016/j.amepre.2021.11.018
9. Baack BN, Abad N, Yankey D, et al. COVID-19 vaccination coverage and intent among adults aged 18–39 years—United States, March–May 2021. *MMWR Morb Mortal Wkly Rep*. 2021;70(25):928–933. https://doi.org/10.15585/mmwr.mm7025e2
10. Asfaw A, Colopy M. Association between parental access to paid sick leave and children's access to and use of healthcare services. *Am J Ind Med*. 2017;60(3):276–284. https://doi.org/10.1002/ajim.22692
11. Asfaw A, Rosa R, Pana-Cryan R. Potential economic benefits of paid sick leave in reducing absenteeism related to the spread of influenza-like illness. *J Occup Environ Med*. 2017;59(9):822–829. https://doi.org/10.1097/JOM.0000000000001076
12. Asfaw A, Pana-Cryan R, Rosa R. Paid sick leave and nonfatal occupational injuries. *Am J Public Health*. 2012;102(9):e59–e64. https://doi.org/10.2105/AJPH.2011.300482

Expiration of the Expanded Child Tax Credit and Energy Insecurity in US Households With Children, 2021–2022

Cecile Yama, MD, MSHPM, Jordan M. Rook, MD, Lauren E. Wisk, PhD, Rebecca Dudovitz, MD, MSHS, Diana Hernández, PhD, David P. Eisenman, MD, MSHS, and Kathryn M. Leifheit, PhD, MSPH

Objectives. To assess the relationship between the expiration of the expanded child tax credit (ECTC) and changes in energy insecurity among US households with children from 2021 to 2022.

Methods. We used nationally representative survey data to evaluate changes in energy insecurity among credit-eligible versus -ineligible households during and after the ECTC expansion. We performed difference-in-differences analyses to estimate changes in energy insecurity in the 2 groups and conducted stratified analyses by percentage of the federal poverty line.

Results. There was a 0.95 percentage point increase in inability to pay energy bills (95% confidence interval = 0.07, 1.85) among households with children but no difference in other measures of energy insecurity. Stratified analyses showed that households at 200% to 399% and 400% to 599% of the federal poverty line experienced increases in energy insecurity after expiration of the ECTC. We saw no differences in the lowest-income groups (< 200% federal poverty line).

Conclusions. The expiration of the ECTC was associated with increased inability to pay energy bills, suggesting that the credit prevented some forms of energy insecurity in households with children. Associations were limited to middle-income groups, indicating benefits were limited to this income stratum. (*Am J Public Health*. 2025;115(8):1312–1321. https://doi.org/10.2105/AJPH.2025.308105)

Energy insecurity, defined as the inability to adequately meet basic household energy needs, is a pervasive health-related social need in the United States.[1] Although more than 1 in 4 US households experience some form of energy insecurity,[2] only 22% of income-eligible households receive federal Low Income Home Energy Assistance Program (LIHEAP) assistance annually.[3,4] Increasingly extreme temperatures have created a context in which the share of households experiencing energy insecurity may continue to grow.[5] Energy insecurity is higher among households with children and lower-income households.[2,6,7]

Energy insecurity harms children's health and may contribute to health disparities. Its immediate effects are experienced as extreme home temperatures, heat- and cold-related illnesses, alternative and hazardous heating strategies, trade-offs between competing necessities, and parental stress.[1,8] When income is insufficient to cover the cost of living expenses, families are forced to choose between food and energy. This so-called "heat or eat" dilemma has dire consequences for children's health: children are more often diagnosed with failure to thrive in wintertime, and families with threatened utility shutoff are more likely to report that their children are hungry.[9,10] If families prioritize other needs over utilities, children are subjected to unsafe indoor temperatures; nationwide, 11% of households with children reported keeping the home at an unsafe temperature.[2] Infants and toddlers in energy-insecure homes are also at increased risk for developmental delays.[11] A child living in a cold home is twice as likely to have respiratory problems and up to 5 times more likely to have mental health problems.[12,13]

Tax credits may prevent energy insecurity and related adverse health effects. Tax credits are a form of non-directed cash benefit that gives families the autonomy to spend flexibly where their need is greatest. Under the American Rescue Plan Act of 2021 (Pub L No. 117–2), the child tax credit was expanded from $2000 to up to $3000 to $3600 per child annually (depending on household income and child age) and made fully refundable. Half the value of the credit was distributed in monthly advance payments from July to December 2021, with the remainder of the credit distributed upon tax filing.[14] All 2-parent households with incomes less than $150 000 and single-parent households with incomes less than $112 500 qualified to receive $300 per month for each child aged 5 years and younger and $250 per month for children aged 6 to 17 years during this 6-month period.

The expanded child tax credit (ECTC) lifted 2.1 million children above the poverty line, resulting in a historic low of 5.2% children in poverty at the end of 2021; its expiration increased child poverty to 12.4%.[15,16] Previous studies have found that, by supplementing families' budgets, implementation of the ECTC was associated with a 26% relative reduction in food insufficiency and a 1.9 percentage point (pp) absolute reduction in food insecurity.[17,18] Conversely, the expiration of the ECTC in December 2021 was associated with a 17% to 23% relative increase in food insufficiency.[19] We hypothesized that the ECTC may have similarly protected against energy insecurity, another form of material hardship.

Tax credits may benefit families who do not qualify for other benefit programs because of the "benefit cliff" phenomenon. Federal benefit programs such as the Supplemental Nutrition Assistance Program and LIHEAP, which helps families pay energy bills, are available only to families with incomes up to 130% and 150% of the federal poverty level (FPL; as determined by these respective programs), respectively.[20,21] Low-income families above these thresholds may not qualify for benefits despite household needs. Thus, the child tax credit presents an approach to addressing family health-related social needs that are above the benefit cliff threshold and may offset loss of benefits because of employment income exceeding a threshold.[22]

To our knowledge, there are no studies evaluating the impact of tax credit programs on energy insecurity. We aimed to (1) assess whether expiration of the ECTC was associated with changes in the prevalence of energy insecurity among those eligible for the credit, and (2) identify disparate consequences of ECTC expiration between income subgroups. Findings can inform future iterations of the child tax credit, in particular for households who may exceed income limits for existing benefit programs.

METHODS

We used nationally representative, cross-sectional data from the Household Pulse Survey (HPS). The HPS is an online survey conducted by the US Census Bureau to collect real-time data regarding the impact of COVID-19 on the US population that began in April 2020 and is continuing, with new collection cycles starting every 4 weeks. HPS wave 34 was the first to include items on energy insecurity. We used data from waves 34 to 48 of the HPS (July 2021–August 2022: response rate = 4.4%–7.9%), which included approximately 6 months during ECTC payments and 6.5 months after the ECTC expired. One adult (aged ≥ 18 years) per household responded to the HPS and provided responses for themselves and their household.

We applied several exclusions to the HPS to arrive at our final analytic sample. Survey waves 34 to 48 included 971 836 respondents. To increase comparability between eligibility groups by focusing our analysis on households with working-aged adults, we excluded respondents older than 65 years (n = 397 072; 40.8%). We additionally excluded individuals in the top 1% of income, as income eligibility for the credit was capped at $400 000 (~1500% of the FPL for a family of 4 in 2021) for joint tax filing (n = 3283; 3.3%).[23] Finally, we excluded respondents who did not have complete covariate or outcome data, apart from those missing income data (n = 9274; 1.0%). Our main analytic sample was made up of 562 207 participants (Table 1). We used a subsample of 88 864 participants who self-reported that they had received a monthly ECTC payment from survey waves 34 to 42 (during disbursement of the credit) to better understand spending patterns among those who received the ECTC.

Expanded Child Tax Credit Comparison Groups

We defined ECTC eligibility for the purpose of this study based on responses to "How many people under 18 years old currently live in your household?" Households with children were eligible for the ECTC (treatment group), and those without children were not eligible for the ECTC (control group). Previous studies of associations between the ECTC and social needs have compared

TABLE 1— Sample Characteristics by Expanded Child Tax Credit (ECTC) Eligibility: Household Pulse Survey, United States, July 2021–August 2022

Characteristic	Comparison Groups, No. (%) or Mean ±SD: ECTC Ineligible (Without Children; n = 337 055[a])	Comparison Groups, No. (%) or Mean ±SD: ECTC Eligible (With Children; n = 225 152)	P[b]
Age, y			<.001
18–24	15 340 (8.8)	4 723 (5.1)	
25–44	106 406 (38.0)	131 171 (63.4)	
45–64	215 309 (53.2)	89 258 (31.5)	
Mean age caregiver, y	44.5 ±0.05	40.2 ±0.04	
Sex at birth			<.001
Male	136 687 (51.5)	81 321 (44.2)	
Female	200 368 (48.5)	143 831 (55.8)	
Race/ethnicity			<.001
Non-Hispanic White	254 896 (67.7)	155 623 (57.7)	
Hispanic	25 932 (11.7)	23 643 (17.1)	
Non-Hispanic Black	23 160 (10.4)	18 527 (13.2)	
Non-Hispanic Asian	16 723 (4.8)	14 163 (5.8)	
Other[c]	16 344 (5.3)	13 196 (6.3)	
Education level			<.001
Less than high school graduate	4 868 (4.8)	5 469 (8.2)	
High school graduate or general equivalency diploma/ equivalent	36 295 (27.2)	23 127 (26.2)	
Some college or 2-yr degree	105 739 (31.1)	68 027 (30.5)	
College graduate	106 618 (21.7)	66 432 (18.4)	
Graduate degree	83 535 (15.3)	63 097 (16.8)	
Household income, % of the FPL			<.001
0–199	65 728 (19.5)	57 327 (25.5)	
200–399	80 699 (23.9)	54 045 (24.0)	
400–599	63 881 (19.0)	52 165 (23.2)	
≥600	116 131 (34.5)	52 413 (23.3)	
Missing	10 616 (3.2)	9 202 (4.1)	
Marital status			<.001
Married	167 429 (43.6)	167 521 (67.7)	
Not married	169 626 (56.4)	57 631(32.3)	
Number of people in household			<.001
1	86 623 (26.3)	0	
2	172 316 (48.6)	15 917 (7.3)	
≥3	78 116 (25.0)	209 235 (92.7)	
Housing ownership			<.001
Own	228 160 (60.1)	170 226 (66.2)	
Rent	104 354 (38.0)	52 207 (32.1)	
Occupied/nonrented	4 541 (1.9)	2 719 (1.7)	

Continued

AJPH August 2025, Vol. 115, No. 8

TABLE 1— Continued

Characteristic	Comparison Groups, No. (%) or Mean ±SD		P^b
	ECTC Ineligible (Without Children; n = 337 055[a])	ECTC Eligible (With Children; n = 225 152)	
Housing type			<.001
Apartment	86 252 (29.8)	27 744 (17.0)	
Single-family house	237 162 (64.9)	188 945 (77.4)	
Mobile home	11 528 (4.5)	7 815 (5.2)	
Other	2 113 (0.8)	648 (0.4)	
Public benefits: household receives SNAP/food stamps	22 358 (9.3)	26 871 (18.9)	<.001

Note. FPL = federal poverty level (determined by Health and Human Services for 2021 and 2022, matched with survey data collected in each of these years); SNAP = Supplemental Nutrition Assistance Program.
[a]Total weighted participants = 70 053 457. All percentages reflect weighted values.
[b]*P* values represent weighted χ^2 test.
[c]Other indicates respondent selected "any other race alone or race in combination."

these 2 groups, adjusting for potential confounders.[17–19] By comparing change over time (before vs after ECTC expiration) in outcomes between ECTC-eligible versus -ineligible groups (the treatment vs. control group, respectively), we were able to derive an intent-to-treat estimate of the ECTC's impact on families with children. The intent-to-treat approach is more valid and policy relevant than a per protocol analysis comparing outcomes between families who did versus did not receive the ECTC because (1) it does not rely on potentially biased self-report of ECTC receipt, and (2) it reflects a real-world scenario in which not all eligible families received the tax credit (i.e., noncompliance).

Outcome

We examined 3 measures representing distinct dimensions of energy insecurity: inability to pay energy bills, foregoing basic necessities to pay energy bills (henceforth referred to as "trade-offs"), and keeping the home at an unsafe temperature. The questions in the HPS that describe these components of energy insecurity are (1) "In the last 12 months, how many times was your household unable to pay an energy bill or unable to pay the full bill amount?"; (2) "In the last 12 months, how many months did your household reduce or forego expenses for basic household necessities, such as medicine or food, in order to pay an energy bill?"; and (3) "In the last 12 months, how many months did your household keep your home at a temperature that you felt was unsafe or unhealthy?" Response options were "almost every month," "some months," "1 or 2 months," and "never."

We dichotomized responses, assigning a value of 0 for "never" and 1 for all other responses. This was based on our understanding that any degree of energy insecurity could be detrimental to one's health and is consistent with the US Energy Information Administration's reporting approach.[2] The Cronbach's alpha indicated that these measures had low internal consistency, leading us to treat them as separate outcomes representing distinct, and possibly increasingly severe, forms of energy insecurity.

Statistical Analyses

In all analyses, we used HPS household survey weights to produce nationally representative estimates. First, we described characteristics of our ECTC-eligible and ECTC-ineligible groups, using χ^2 statistics to compare frequencies of sociodemographic characteristics between groups. Second, we conducted a difference-in-differences (DiD) analysis with repeated cross-sections to assess associations between ECTC eligibility and changes in energy insecurity following expiration of the ECTC. Those surveyed from July 21, 2021, through February 7, 2022 (survey waves 34–42), during the disbursement period of the ECTC, constituted the "preexpiration" group; those surveyed March 2, 2022, through August 8, 2022 (survey waves 43–48), after expiration of the ECTC, constituted the "postexpiration" group. Although the last monthly ECTC payment was reportedly sent in December 2021, we decided to conservatively group respondents in wave 42 (January 26, 2022–February 7, 2022) in the "preexpiration" period because many respondents to the HPS were still reporting receipt of the ECTC during that period (n = 7265, or 38.8% of eligible households, reported receiving ECTC during survey wave 42).

We adjusted our DiD models for covariates, including respondent age (18–24, 25–44, or 45–64 years), sex at birth (male or female), self-reported race and ethnicity, education level, income as a percentage of FPL, marital status, number of people in household, homeowner versus renter status, housing type, receipt of Supplemental Nutrition Assistance Program benefits, and state-level energy use and cost. We adjusted for race and ethnicity as proxies for experiences of structural racism, which decrease opportunities for wealth and homeownership and increase risk of energy insecurity.[1,24] We calculated percentage of FPL by assigning respondents the midpoint values of their reported income range, relative to household size–specific federal poverty guidelines (i.e., the FPL) from 2020 and 2021.[25]

We used percentage of the FPL as opposed to income brackets, as it better reflects household-level poverty and is more useful for understanding implications of the ECTC relative to other FPL-based federal benefit programs. Additionally, we used US Energy Information Administration data to create a measure of customer average energy costs by state–month (data in cents/kilowatt hours/month) to account for state-specific and seasonal variation in temperature and utility costs.[23] Additionally, our model included state fixed effects.

To better understand our overall estimates and identify subgroups particularly affected by ECTC expiration, we conducted stratified DiD analyses by income (using percentage of the FPL). To further understand the results of stratified analyses, we conducted post hoc analyses describing ECTC spending patterns by income in a subsample of respondents who were ECTC recipients (88 864 adults who reported receiving the ECTC during the preexpiration period, July 2021–February 2022).

Finally, we conducted several sensitivity analyses. First, we applied an event study specification to our main DiD models. An event study is a more flexible form of DiD approach that allows treatment effects to vary over time relative to treatment.[26] The model included dummy variables for HPS waves (with survey wave 42 set as the reference), interacted with the treatment indicator (i.e., ECTC eligibility). By graphing event study coefficients, we were able to check for potential violations to the parallel trends assumption underlying DiD analyses. We also performed event studies for all significant findings in the income subgroups.

We conducted 2 additional analyses to check our results' sensitivity to model specification. First, we ran a model that included controls for pandemic programs at the state–month level that might have a meaningful effect on energy insecurity. These included utility shutoff moratoria (1 = moratorium in place, 0 = no moratorium; coded based on dates in Benfer and Koehler's Eviction Moratoria & Housing Policy database)[27] and emergency rental assistance (cumulative dollars per capita distributed, based on data from US Treasury Department reports).[28] We chose not to include these controls in our main analysis because we did not expect them to affect energy insecurity differently between households with and households without children. In a second sensitivity analysis, we used HPS wave 41, fielded December 29, 2021, through January 10, 2022, as the reference wave.

We conducted a final sensitivity analysis to estimate "as treated" associations. Because we collected data on whether participants received the ECTC only during the preexpiration period (and not the postexpiration period), we could not use ECTC recipients as our intervention group; we instead used families with children as a proxy. To understand whether the experience of households that received the ECTC would have been comparable to the overall sample of households with children, we compared adjusted energy insecurity during the preexpiration period in (1) households without children, (2) those with children who received the ECTC, and (3) those with children who did not receive the ECTC. We used Stata/BE version 17.0 (StataCorp LP, College Station, TX) for all analyses.

RESULTS

Our sample of 562 207 adults represented 70 053 457 households nationally and 28 602 826 households with children. As seen in Table 1, compared with ECTC-ineligible adults, ECTC-eligible adults were younger (mean age 40.2 vs 44.5 years), were more likely to be women (55.8% vs 48.5%), were more often Hispanic (17.1% vs 11.7%) or non-Hispanic Black (13.2% vs 10.4%) individuals, and had lower incomes. ECTC-eligible individuals also reported lower educational attainment (e.g., 18.4% vs 21.7% with a college degree), were more likely to be married (67.7% vs 43.6%), and had a larger household size (i.e., households with 3 or more people; 92.7% vs 25.0%). They were more likely to be homeowners (66.2% vs 60.1%), live in a single-family home (77.4% vs 64.9%), and receive Supplemental Nutrition Assistance Program benefits (18.9% vs 9.3%).

Figure 1 shows marginal estimates, that is, the adjusted prevalence of each energy insecurity outcome, in ECTC-eligible and -ineligible groups before versus after expiration of the ECTC, as well as the pre–post change by eligibility group. Both households with and those without children experienced an increase in all 3 measures of energy insecurity when the ECTC expired. The magnitude of these increases differed by outcome: they were larger among ECTC-eligible versus -ineligible households for inability to pay energy bills and trade-offs but smaller for unsafe temperatures. Baseline inability to pay energy bills and trade-offs were more common among households with children (25.2% vs 21.4% and 33.1% vs 32.2%, respectively), whereas keeping the home at an unsafe temperature was more common among households without children (21.3% vs 17.9%).

Adjusted DiD analyses (Figure 2) demonstrated that ECTC expiration was associated with a 0.95 pp (95% confidence interval [CI] = 0.06, 1.85) increase in inability to pay energy bills among ECTC-eligible households compared to ECTC-ineligible households. Because the baseline prevalence of inability to pay bills was 22.9% in our sample, this 0.95 pp increase equates to a 4.2% relative increase associated with the expiration of ECTC. There was no significant overall difference in trade-offs or unsafe temperatures after expiration of the ECTC. There were mixed results in subgroup analyses by FPL. ECTC expiration was associated with an increase in inability to pay energy bills (1.94 pp; 95% CI = 0.11, 3.78) and an increase in trade-offs (2.82 pp; 95% CI = 0.85, 4.80) among households at 200% to 399% of the FPL. It was also associated with an increase in inability to pay bills of 2.34 pp (95% CI = 0.90, 3.80) among households at 400% to 599% of the FPL. There was a significant decrease of 1.9 pp (95% CI = −2.93, −0.86) in unsafe household temperatures among households at 600% or higher FPL. There was no change in any measure of energy insecurity for households at lower income levels.

Spending data (Figure 3) suggested that in each progressively lower stratum of the FPL, there was progressively higher spending on all competing necessities, including food, housing, utilities, and debt.

Visual inspection of event study coefficients (Figure A, available as a supplement to the online version of this article at http://www.ajph.org) showed a relatively flat pretreatment (i.e., during ECTC) trend, indicating that energy insecurity did not increase significantly among ECTC-eligible families relative to ineligible families before ECTC expiration and suggesting that the parallel trends assumption was satisfied. One notable exception to this was the event study for unsafe

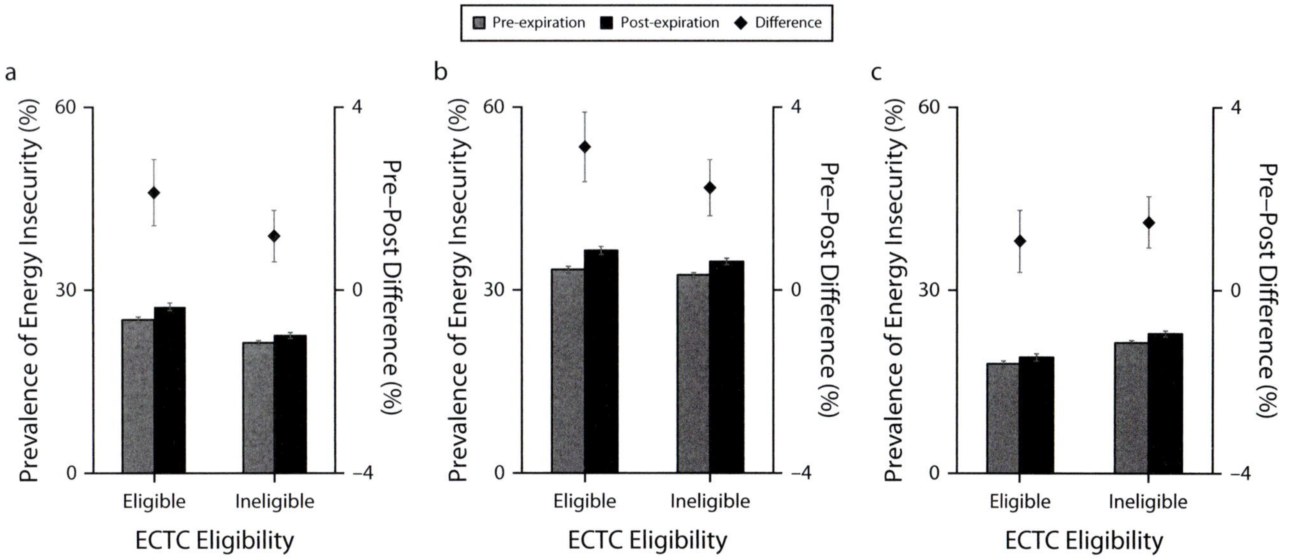

FIGURE 1— Adjusted Prevalence of Energy Insecurity Before and After the Expanded Child Tax Credit (ECTC) Expiration by (a) Inability to Pay Bills, (b) Trade-offs, and (c) Unsafe Household Temperatures: Household Pulse Survey, United States, July 2021–August 2022

Note. The graphs display marginal estimates (i.e., adjusted prevalence of energy insecurity before and after ECTC expiration based on ECTC eligibility). The left y-axis represents pre–post prevalence. The right y-axis and black diamonds reflect pre–post difference estimates. Whiskers indicate 95% confidence intervals. Analyses are adjusted and weighted.

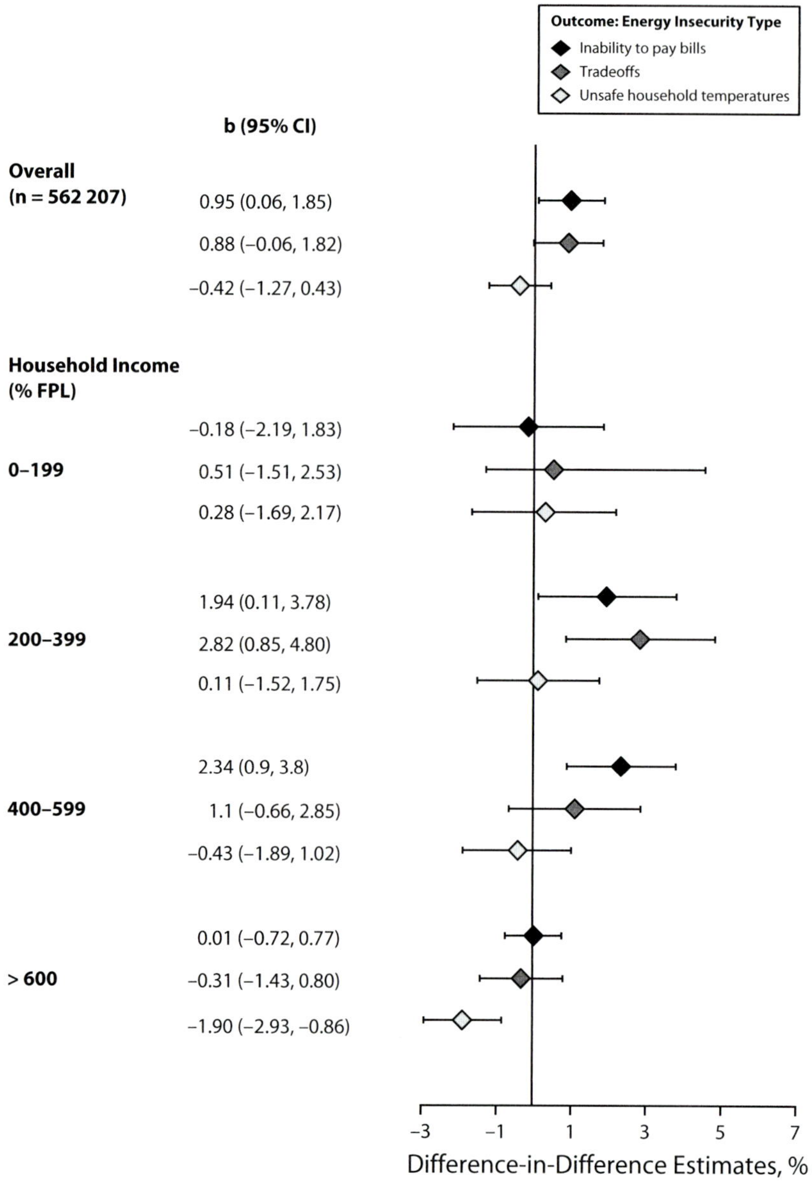

FIGURE 2— Difference-in-Difference Estimates of Energy Insecurity Among Households With Children After Expiration of the Expanded Child Tax Credit (ECTC): Household Pulse Survey, United States, July 2021–August 2022

Note. CI = confidence interval; FPL = federal poverty level (determined by Health and Human Services for 2021 and 2022, matched with survey data collected in each of these years). This figure represents difference-in-difference estimates of percentage point change in energy insecurity among ECTC-eligible households with children after expiration of the ECTC. Overall estimates are followed by stratified estimates by percentage of the federal poverty level (determined by Health and Human Services for 2021 and 2022, matched with survey data collected in each of these years). Error bars represent 95% confidence intervals.

temperatures among households at or above 600% of the FPL: in this group, report of unsafe temperatures was declining among ECTC-eligible households, relative to ineligible households, before expiration. Therefore, the DiD result showing a significant decrease associated with expiration may be spurious, possibly driven by preexpiration trends.

Our sensitivity analysis incorporating controls for state utility moratorium shutoffs and emergency rental assistance produced results that were qualitatively similar to our main results (Table A, available as a supplement to the online version of this article at http://www.ajph.org). Our analysis using wave 41 as a cutoff was broadly similar to our main results, although the coefficient for inability to pay energy bills was slightly attenuated (0.82 rather than 0.95; $P = .06$; Table A).

Comparison of adjusted energy insecurity in (1) households without

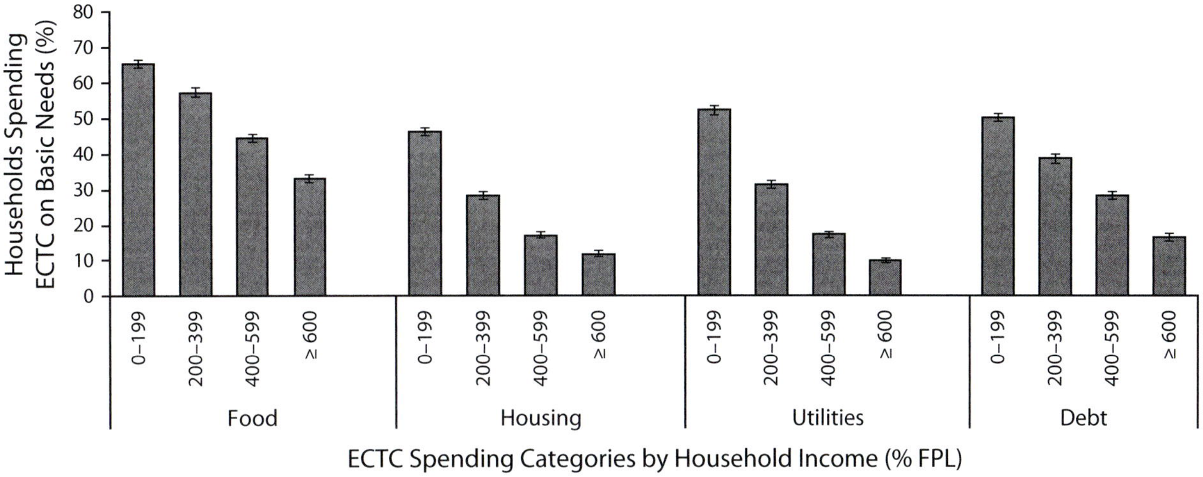

FIGURE 3— **Competing Expanded Child Tax Credit (ECTC) Spending Needs by Household Income: Household Pulse Survey, United States, July 2021–August 2022**

Note. FPL = federal poverty level (determined by Health and Human Services for 2021 and 2022, matched with survey data collected in each of these years). This figure depicts spending of ECTC recipients on competing basic necessities. It represents a subsample of 88 864 adults who reported receiving the ECTC during the disbursement period (survey waves 38–42; July 2021–February 2022). Respondents could select more than 1 category, so total spending does not equal 100%. The category of food includes groceries, eating out, and takeout. The category of utilities was specified to indicate both utilities and telecommunications, including natural gas, electricity, cable, internet, and cell phone. The category of housing includes spending on rent or mortgage. The category of debt indicates respondents who mostly spent their ECTC on debt. The categories of spending selected reflect categories commonly understood as basic necessities, but they do not encompass all possible spending categories.

children, (2) those that have children and reported receiving the ECTC, and (3) those that have children and did not report receiving the ECTC (Table B, available as a supplement to the online version of this article at http://www.ajph.org) revealed higher levels of inability to pay bills in both households that reported ECTC receipt and those that did not report receipt compared to ineligible households. Trade-offs were significantly higher in households that reported ECTC receipt compared to ineligible households. As stated in the "Methods" section, this was not our primary comparison for 2 reasons: (1) we find the intent-to-treat estimates more policy relevant, and (2) data on ECTC receipt were not available after ECTC expiration, making the DiD analysis unfeasible.

DISCUSSION

Ours is the first study, to our knowledge, to examine the association between expiration of the ECTC and household measures of energy insecurity. We found a statistically significant increase (0.95 pp) in inability to pay bills among ECTC-eligible households. Based on the 2022 estimates of households with children, this translates to an additional 308 560 households that have children and became energy insecure after ECTC payments ended.[29] We did not find statistically significant changes in overall measures of trade-offs or keeping households at unsafe temperatures. The latter is consistent with previous studies of energy insecurity, which have found low prevalence of unsafe temperatures[20]—either because it is a coping mechanism of last resort or owing to social desirability bias (parents of children may be hesitant to report "unhealthy" temperatures). These findings suggest that after ECTC expiration, households with children had greater difficulty paying energy bills, although we detected no difference in other, potentially more severe forms of energy insecurity.

Income-stratified results showed an increase in 2 measures of energy insecurity following expiration of the ECTC among eligible households at 200% to 399% of the FPL. We henceforth describe this group as "middle income," consistent with previous studies.[30] Respondents at 400% to 599% of the FPL had increased inability to pay energy bills after expiration but did not demonstrate any change in foregoing basic necessities. Taken together, these findings suggest that ECTC prevented milder forms of energy insecurity overall, in particular for middle-income families.

We propose 3 potential mechanisms through which the ECTC had the greatest impact on middle-income households. First, these households would not have been federally eligible for the LIHEAP or Supplemental Nutrition Assistance Program.[21] The protective association of the ECTC seen in the 200% to 399% of the

FPL group may reflect benefit cliff effects, whereby households who earn just above eligibility thresholds for benefit programs are ineligible despite existing needs.[22] Second, ECTC may not have affected energy insecurity among the lowest-income groups (0%–199% of the FPL) because of a greater number of competing needs, leading families to prioritize ECTC spending on necessities such as food. Third, lowest-income households may have had a lower uptake of the ECTC, as Karpman et al. have demonstrated,[31] which may explain the varying associations between ECTC expiration and energy insecurity by FPL.

Strengths and Limitations

Our study builds on previous work that examined the association between ECTC and other forms of material hardship. Shafer et al.,[17] Bovell-Ammon et al.,[32] and Rook et al.[18] have contributed to evidence of decreased food insecurity and insufficiency during the period of ECTC receipt. Our results are comparable to, albeit lower than, the 3.5 pp increase in food insufficiency identified by Bouchelle et al. in low-income households after ECTC withdrawal.[19] Our study demonstrates that the reduction in poverty may not be sufficient to address all forms of material hardship for the lowest-income households, given inequitable burdens of debt and competing necessities.

Our study had several limitations. Although we used nationally representative data from during and after ECTC disbursements, our data were limited by their serial cross-sectional nature. Additionally, although our sample size was large, stratified analyses may have been underpowered to make comparisons. Response rate for the HPS is low, and data are subject to nonresponse bias, although we partially accounted for this with survey weighting. Although we controlled for several potential confounders, households with and those without children and periods before and periods after ECTC expiration may differ in ways that are unmeasured. Our outcome variable asked participants to reflect back over 12 months and thus might not be sensitive to acute changes in household finances. Additionally, our intent-to-treat approach to measuring exposure based on presumed eligibility provided policy-relevant estimates of ECTC impact but likely biased results toward the null.

Public Health Implications

Our findings suggest that the ECTC may have prevented some forms of energy insecurity in households with children, particularly middle-income households; however, the ECTC did not address potentially more severe measures of energy insecurity or the experience of energy insecurity in the lowest-income households. Given the rise of energy insecurity, and with the knowledge that social needs lead to negative and costly health outcomes, federal and state governments should consider reinstating more generous child tax credit policies and distributing credits according to household need. AJPH

ABOUT THE AUTHORS

Cecile L. Yama and Jordan M. Rook are with the National Clinician Scholars Program, University of California, Los Angeles. Lauren E. Wisk, Rebecca Dudovitz, David P. Eisenman, and Kathryn M. Leifheit are with the David Geffen School of Medicine, University of California, Los Angeles. Diana Hernández is with the Mailman School of Public Health, Columbia University, New York, NY.

CORRESPONDENCE

Correspondence should be sent to Cecile Yama, 1100 Glendon Ave, Suite 900, Los Angeles, CA 90024 (e-mail: cecile.yama@gmail.com). Reprints can be ordered at https://www.ajph.org by clicking the "Reprints" link.

PUBLICATION INFORMATION

Full Citation: Yama C, Rook JM, Wisk LE, et al. Expiration of the expanded child tax credit and energy insecurity in US households with children, 2021–2022. *Am J Public Health*. 2025;115(8): 1312–1321.

Acceptance Date: March 1, 2025.

DOI: https://doi.org/10.2105/AJPH.2025.308105

ORCID iDs:

Cecile Yama https://orcid.org/0000-0002-7434-9497

Jordan M. Rook https://orcid.org/0000-0003-3579-4704

Rebecca Dudovitz https://orcid.org/0000-0001-9457-0562

Kathryn M. Leifheit https://orcid.org/0000-0003-3980-9715

CONTRIBUTORS

C. Yama performed the formal analyses and wrote the original draft of the article. C. Yama, J. M. Rook, L. E. Wisk, and K. M. Leifheit conceptualized the study and developed the methodology. R. Dudovitz provided guidance on study design. D. Hernández provided subject matter expertise on energy insecurity. D. P. Eisenman provided subject matter expertise on weather and energy insecurity. K. M. Leifheit guided statistical methodology and analysis and supervised the study. All authors wrote and edited the article and reviewed and approved the final version.

ACKNOWLEDGMENTS

This study was funded by the Los Angeles County Department of Health Services through the National Clinician Scholars Program Fellowship (to C. Y.); the VA Office of Academic Affiliations through the National Clinician Scholars Program Fellowship (to J. M. R.); the National Institute of Diabetes and Digestive and Kidney Diseases (grants K01 DK116932 and R03 DK132439 to L. E. W.); the Health Resources and Services Administration, US Department of Health and Human Services (award UA6MC32492 to R. D.); the Life Course Intervention Research Network (award U9DMC49250 to R. D.); the Life Course Translational Research Network (to R. D.); and the JPB Foundation (to D. H.).

Note. The contents of this article are solely the responsibility of the authors and do not necessarily represent the official views of the funders.

CONFLICTS OF INTEREST

The authors have no conflicts of interest relevant to this article to disclose.

HUMAN PARTICIPANT PROTECTION

The University of California Los Angeles institutional review board deemed our study to be nonhuman participants research.

REFERENCES

1. Hernández D. Understanding "energy insecurity" and why it matters to health. *Soc Sci Med.* 2016; 2016(167):1–10. https://doi.org/10.1016/j.socscimed.2016.08.029
2. US Energy Information Administration. Residential Energy Consumption Survey (RECS). Form EIA-457A. 2024 Household Questionnaire Specification. Available at: https://www.eia.gov/survey/form/eia_457/RECS%20457%20A_Questionnaire%20Content.pdf. Accessed May 16, 2025.
3. Martín C. Families need more help to keep the lights on and the water running during the pandemic. April 15, 2020. Available at: https://www.urban.org/urban-wire/families-need-more-help-keep-lights-and-water-running-during-pandemic. Accessed May 6, 2025.
4. Graff M, Carley S. COVID-19 assistance needs to target energy insecurity. *Nat Energy.* 2020;5(5):352–354. https://doi.org/10.1038/s41560-020-0620-y
5. Hernández D. Energy insecurity: a framework for understanding energy, the built environment, and health among vulnerable populations in the context of climate change. *Am J Public Health.* 2013;103(4):e32–e34. https://doi.org/10.2105/AJPH.2012.301179
6. Hernández D, Aratani Y, Jiang Y. Energy insecurity among families with children. January 2014. Available at: https://www.nccp.org/wp-content/uploads/2020/05/text_1086.pdf. Accessed May 11, 2025.
7. Hernández D. Energy insecurity and health: America's hidden hardship. Health Affairs Health Policy Brief. 2023. Available at: https://www.healthaffairs.org/do/10.1377/hpb20230518.472953. Accessed May 11, 2025.
8. Lane K, Ito K, Johnson S, Gibson EA, Tang A, Matte T. Burden and risk factors for cold-related illness and death in New York City. *Int J Environ Res Public Health.* 2018;15(4):632. https://doi.org/10.3390/ijerph15040632
9. Frank DA, Roos N, Meyers A, et al. Seasonal variation in weight-for-age in a pediatric emergency room. *Public Health Rep.* 1996;111(4):366–371.
10. Bhattacharya J, Deleire T, Haider S, Currie J. Heat or eat? Cold-weather shocks and nutrition in poor American families. *Am J Public Health.* 2003; 93(7):1149–1154. https://doi.org/10.2105/AJPH.93.7.1149
11. Cook JT, Frank DA, Casey PH, et al. A brief indicator of household energy security: associations with food security, child health, and child development in US infants and toddlers. *Pediatrics.* 2008;122(4):e867–e875. https://doi.org/10.1542/peds.2008-0286
12. Mohan G. Young, poor, and sick: the public health threat of energy poverty for children in Ireland. *Energy Res Soc Sci.* 2021;71:101822. https://doi.org/10.1016/j.erss.2020.101822
13. Institute of Health Equity. The health impacts of cold homes and fuel poverty. May 2011. Available at: https://www.instituteofhealthequity.org/resources-reports/the-health-impacts-of-cold-homes-and-fuel-poverty/the-health-impacts-of-cold-homes-and-fuel-poverty.pdf. Accessed May 11, 2025.
14. Internal Revenue Service. Advance child tax credit payments in 2021. Available at: https://www.irs.gov/credits-deductions/advance-child-tax-credit-payments-in-2021. Accessed May 6, 2025.
15. Burns K, Fox LE. The impact of the 2021 expanded child tax credit on child poverty. November 22, 2022. Available at: https://www.census.gov/library/working-papers/2022/demo/SEHSD-wp2022-24.html. Accessed May 6, 2025.
16. Parrott S. Record rise in poverty highlights importance of child tax credit; health coverage marks a high point before pandemic safeguards ended. September 12, 2023. Available at: https://www.cbpp.org/press/statements/record-rise-in-poverty-highlights-importance-of-child-tax-credit-health-coverage. Accessed May 6, 2025.
17. Shafer PR, Gutiérrez KM, Ettinger de Cuba S, Bovell-Ammon A, Raifman J. Association of the implementation of child tax credit advance payments with food insufficiency in US households. *JAMA Netw Open.* 2022;5(1):e2143296. https://doi.org/10.1001/jamanetworkopen.2021.43296
18. Rook JM, Yama CL, Schickedanz AB, Feuerbach AM, Lee SL, Wisk LE. Changes in self-reported adult health and household food security with the 2021 expanded child tax credit monthly payments. *JAMA Health Forum.* 2023;4(6):e231672. https://doi.org/10.1001/jamahealthforum.2023.1672
19. Bouchelle Z, Vasan A, Candon M, Kenyon CC. Food insufficiency following discontinuation of monthly child tax credit payments among lower-income US households. *JAMA Health Forum.* 2022;3(11):e224039. https://doi.org/10.1001/jamahealthforum.2022.4039
20. Hernández D, Laird J. Surviving a shut-off: US households at greatest risk of utility disconnections and how they cope. *Am Behav Sci.* 2022; 66(7):856–880. https://doi.org/10.1177/00027642211013401
21. Nikolla D. Are heat and eat policies affecting SNAP household participation? July 26, 2016. Available at: https://vtechworks.lib.vt.edu/server/api/core/bitstreams/a5a3dd48-3ab4-48c8-952a-88c9535649dc/content. Accessed May 11, 2025.
22. Anderson T, Coffey A, Daly H, Hahn H, Maag E, Werner K. Balancing at the edge of the cliff. January 11, 2022. Available at: https://www.urban.org/research/publication/balancing-edge-cliff. Accessed May 11, 2025.
23. US Energy Information Administration. Electric power monthly. February 2025. Available at: https://www.eia.gov/electricity/monthly. Accessed May 11, 2025.
24. Loya J. Ethno-racial and down payment disparities in mortgage credit access. *Race Soc Probl.* 2023;15(4):376–394. https://doi.org/10.1007/s12552-022-09378-z
25. Hest R. Four methods for calculating income as a percentage of the federal poverty guidelines (FPG) in the Behavioral Risk Factor Surveillance System (BRFSS). August 17, 2023. Available at: https://www.shadac.org/four-methods-calculating-income-percent-federal-poverty-guidelines-fpg-behavioral-risk-factor. Accessed May 11, 2025.
26. Goodman-Bacon A. Difference-in-differences with variation in treatment timing. *J Econom.* 2021;225(2):254–277. https://doi.org/10.1016/j.jeconom.2021.03.014
27. Benfer E, Koehler R. Eviction moratoria & housing policy: federal, state, commonwealth, and territory. February 6, 2023. Available at: https://www.openicpsr.org/openicpsr/project/157201/version/V2/view. Accessed May 11, 2025. https://doi.org/10.3886/E157201V2
28. US Department of the Treasury. Emergency rental assistance program. Available at: https://home.treasury.gov/policy-issues/coronavirus/assistance-for-state-local-and-tribal-governments/emergency-rental-assistance-program. Accessed May 6, 2025.
29. Hemez P, Washington CN, Kreider RM. America's families and living arrangements: 2022. May 2024. Available at: https://www.census.gov/library/publications/2024/demo/p20-587.html. Accessed May 6, 2025.
30. DeVoe JE, Tillotson CJ, Wallace LS. Insurance coverage gaps among US children with insured parents: are middle income children more likely to have longer gaps? *Matern Child Health J.* 2011; 15(3):342–351. https://doi.org/10.1007/s10995-010-0584-9
31. Karpman M, Maag E, Kenney G, Wissoker D. Who has received advance child tax credit payments, and how were the payments used? November 2021. Available at: https://taxpolicycenter.org/sites/default/files/publication/163132/who-has-received-advance-ctc-payments-and-how-were-the-payments-used_0.pdf. Accessed May 11, 2025.
32. Bovell-Ammon A, McCann NC, Mulugeta M, de Cuba SE, Raifman J, Shafer P. Association of the expiration of child tax credit advance payments with food insufficiency in US households. *JAMA Netw Open.* 2022;5(10):e2234438. https://doi.org/10.1001/jamanetworkopen.2022.34438

Preventing Real-World Pediatric Vehicular Heatstroke Events With Technology

Jalaj Maheshwari, MSE, Emma Sartin, PhD, MPH, Gregory Chingas, MS, and Kristy B. Arbogast, PhD

Objectives. To determine if currently available technologies can prevent real-world pediatric vehicular heatstroke cases.

Methods. We systematically reviewed cases of children dying in hot vehicles to identify "exemplar" scenarios. Exemplar events were defined as cases that were distinct from others based on characteristics of the child, caregiver, and the setting or context in which the event occurred. We then determined whether available detection, alerting, and intervention technologies would have functioned as intended in each scenario.

Results. We identified 10 exemplar cases. Technologies' effectiveness varied drastically; some would have functioned as intended in all exemplar cases, and others in only 1 or 2. No single technology by itself could have prevented all deaths.

Conclusions. A combination of vehicle technologies is needed to reduce cases of pediatric vehicular heatstroke.

Public Health Implications. The Hot Cars Act (2021) mandates that vehicles have child safety alert systems in 2025. However, it does not provide any specific guidelines to manufacturers about which technologies should be used. Our results highlight technologies that may be most effective in preventing pediatric vehicular heatstroke and underscore the importance of utilizing multiple features in tandem.
(*Am J Public Health*. 2025;115(8):1322–1326. https://doi.org/10.2105/AJPH.2025.308109)

AJPH August 2025, Vol. 115, No. 8

Since the late 1990s, there have been more than 950 pediatric vehicular heatstroke deaths (i.e., children dying in hot vehicles) in the United States.[1] These deaths occur in various ways: about 53% of children are forgotten, about 25% gain access to vehicles without their caregiver knowing, and the rest are knowingly left (usually with no intention of harm, 19.6%; 1.7% have unknown circumstances).[1] To address this public health problem, mitigating solutions must address all scenarios.

Notably, beginning in 2025, all new passenger vehicles less than 10 000 pounds must be equipped with a child safety alert system.[2] Available technologies function as detection, alert, and intervention systems.[3–5] Indirect detection technologies determine the presence of a child through logic-based algorithms; they do not actively scan for occupants inside the vehicle. For example, if a rear door has been opened and closed before a trip, the caregiver will be prompted to check for a child. Conversely, direct detection technologies scan for human activity inside the vehicle using varying sensors. For example, heartbeat sensors scan the vehicle environment to detect the presence of an occupant. If an occupant is detected, alerting technologies aim to notify a rescuer (e.g., the caregiver, bystanders, second-degree contact) through visual, auditory, or haptic alerts. Lastly, interventions prevent occupants from overheating once they are detected (e.g., the vehicle's air conditioner turning on).

Because of caregivers' low perceived threat, there has been a poor uptake of behavior-based solutions to vehicular heatstroke (e.g., checking the back seat of the vehicle for an occupant after every drive).[6] However, most US caregivers report positive attitudes toward having mitigating technologies in their vehicle.[6] Thus, incorporating these technologies into vehicles—particularly together in varying packages—may be a promising approach to reduce deaths from pediatric vehicular heatstroke.[3,5] With a goal of informing education, legislation, advocacy, and manufacturing efforts, the objective of this study was to determine if, and if so, which combination of, currently available technologies may prevent real-world pediatric vehicular heatstroke cases.

METHODS

Broadly, we reviewed pediatric vehicular heatstroke deaths to identify "exemplar" scenarios. Exemplar events were defined as cases that were distinct from others based on characteristics of the child, caregiver, and setting or context in which the event occurred. We then determined whether detection, alerting, and intervention technologies would have prevented the death in each scenario.

Figure A (available as a supplement to the online version of this article at https://ajph.org) provides an overview of our search process to identify and characterize exemplar cases. First, we identified and reviewed media reports and other documented information about deaths that occurred between 2011 and 2019 cataloged in NoHeatStroke.org.[1] Incidents where more than 1 pediatric victim was involved were classified as separate incidents (e.g., a pair of siblings resulted in 2 cases). This produced 354 cases. For cases that occurred between 2011 and 2013, or 130 of the 354 cases, we contacted sheriffs' offices, police departments, county records centers, and similar public record entities to request the detailed police records. Of the 130 requests, 48 were acquired (electronically or via regular mail), 51 were not responded to, and 31 were refused. Reasons for refusal included loss of records, active legal action pending in case, state refusal because of the victim being a juvenile, or state refusal because of laws limiting public access to police reports. Using all available or gathered sources of information, we created summative reports for each incident. Summative reports included information specific to the child (age, sex, race, ethnicity, underlying medical conditions), incident (date and location), vehicle (make, model, type, model year, and color), child's restraint status (if the child was seated in a child safety seat, the type of child safety seat, and if they were restrained into the child safety seat or into the vehicle by a seat belt), environment (interior and exterior temperatures, location of child in the vehicle, where the vehicle was located or parked, general incident circumstances), and caregiver (sex, race, ethnicity). For the 224 cases that occurred between 2014 and 2019, we thoroughly examined media reports to determine if scenarios differed from the 130 already classified. If they were suspected to be distinct from any of the 130 cases already reviewed, we requested full police reports following the process described previously.

For each of the exemplar cases, we explored whether an individual or a combination of technologies could have mitigated the child's death. Technologies—described in detail in Table A (available as a supplement to the online version of this article at https://ajph.org)—were identified from 2 previous studies.[3,5] Case reviews assessing and agreeing upon the technologies' effectiveness were conducted with a panel of subject-matter experts from academia and industry.

RESULTS

Overall, across the 354 cases, we identified 10 distinct scenarios in which a pediatric vehicular heatstroke fatality occurred, described in detail in Table B (available as a supplement to the online version of this article at https://ajph.org). These exemplar scenarios were deemed distinct based on the age of the child, the location inside the vehicle where the child was found, the immediate surroundings of the vehicle, and the caregiver's status.

Table 1 depicts each technology's effectiveness across exemplar cases. By themselves, no technologies would have prevented all events. Instead, we found that a combination of indirect detection, direct detection, alerting, and intervention features is needed. While effective in several cases, none of the indirect detection technologies were universally effective because of caregivers intentionally leaving children in vehicles. Notably, global positioning system–related reminders would not have mitigated or prevented any cases. Among direct detection–based technologies, heartbeat sensors were determined to be the most effective (detecting the child in each scenario) because they do not require a child to be in certain positions within the vehicle. Carbon dioxide, optical, pressure, ultrasonic, and radar/radio-frequency detection technologies were also found to be effective, successfully detecting children in 80% to 90% of cases. Conversely, chest restraint sensors would have only been able to detect 1 child. Among alerting technologies, notifying a second-degree contact was the only technology that would have effectively brought intervention to every

TABLE 1— Exemplar Cases of Pediatric Vehicular Heatstroke Events and Their Mitigating Solutions: United States, 2011–2019

	Exemplar Cases										
	Child in Rearward-Facing Child Restraint Seat	Child on Vehicle Floor	Trunk Entrapment	Child in Front Passenger Seat	Child in Booster Seat	Cellphone in Vehicle	Caregiver Indisposed and Aware	Caregiver Indisposed and Unaware	Vehicle Close to Adults	Vehicle Distant From Adults	Total Use
Indirect detection											
Bluetooth connection	1	0	0	1	0	0	1	1	1	1	6
Door logic	1	0	0	1	0	0	1	1	1	1	6
Global positioning system device	0	0	0	0	0	0	0	0	1	1	2
Direct detection											
Chest restraint sensor	1	0	0	0	0	0	1	0	1	1	4
Carbon dioxide sensor	1	1	0	1	1	1	0	1	1	1	8
Heartbeat sensor	1	1	1	1	1	1	1	1	1	1	10
Optical sensor	1	1	0	0	1	1	1	1	1	1	8
Pressure sensor	1	0	0	1	1	1	1	1	1	1	8
Ultrasonic sensor	1	1	0	1	1	1	1	1	1	1	9
RADAR/radio frequency sensor	1	1	0	1	1	1	1	1	1	1	9
Alerting											
Primary (1°) contact notified	1	1	1	0	1	0	1	0	1	1	7
Secondary (2°) contact notified	1	1	1	1	1	1	1	1	1	1	10
Chime warning noise	1	0	0	1	1	0	1	0	1	1	6
Corresponding app	1	1	1	0	1	0	1	0	1	1	7
C-pillar button alarm	1	0	0	1	0	0	1	0	1	1	5
Daycare mobile app	0	0	0	0	1	0	0	0	1	1	3
Headlights	0	0	0	1	0	1	0	0	0	0	2
Horn	1	1	1	1	1	1	1	1	1	0	9
Infotainment display	1	0	0	1	1	0	1	0	1	1	6
Subscription-based electronic security or communications service	1	1	1	1	1	1	1	1	1	1	10

Continued

TABLE 1— Continued

	Exemplar Cases										
	Child in Rearward-Facing Child Restraint Seat	Child on Vehicle Floor	Trunk Entrapment	Child in Front Passenger Seat	Child in Booster Seat	Cellphone in Vehicle	Caregiver Indisposed and Aware	Caregiver Indisposed and Unaware	Vehicle Close to Adults	Vehicle Distant From Adults	Total Use
Vehicle key fob	1	1	1	1	1	0	1	0	1	1	8
Wristband transmitter	1	0	0	0	0	0	1	0	0	0	2
Intervention											
Air conditioner on	1	1	0	1	1	1	0	1	1	1	8
Doors unlock	0	1	0	1	0	1	0	1	0	0	4
Trunk opens	0	1	1	0	0	1	0	1	0	0	4
Windows roll down	0	0	0	0	0	1	0	0	0	0	1

Note. For more information about each technology or intervention, refer to Table A (available as a supplement to the online version of this article at https://ajph.org).

child (assuming they were detected) from overheating, in both cases where children were left behind intentionally or unintentionally by caregivers. The most effective second-degree contacts would be emergency medical services or 911. The second-best alerting feature was the vehicle using its horn, which would have alerted individuals to 9 of the 10 children (1 child was not in proximity to anyone who could intervene). Turning the air conditioner on inside the vehicle was the most effective intervention strategy assessed, preventing about 80% of cases.

DISCUSSION

Ultimately, we did not identify any one solution to preventing pediatric vehicular heatstroke. Because of the array of scenarios, combinations of technologies are necessary. That said, within specific categories, some technologies were found to be more effective than others. Thus, moving forward, minimum technology requirements for vehicles should be established in tandem with novel education efforts. While we comprehensively reviewed pediatric vehicular heatstroke events to identify our exemplar cases, many of our requests for full reports were not fulfilled, and, of those that were obtained, many contained substantial amounts of redacted or missing information. This may have resulted in missing unique cases. Lastly, we focused on technologies described in previous research; novel technologies may have been developed since these studies, and some of the technologies described are no longer produced. Future work must identify how caregivers will interact with, use, and feel toward mitigating technologies. The findings of this study are critical to inform ongoing policy, manufacturing, and advocacy efforts. AJPH

ABOUT THE AUTHORS

Jalaj Maheshwari is with the Center for Injury Research and Prevention (CIRP) at the Children's Hospital of Philadelphia. Emma Sartin was with CIRP at the Children's Hospital of Philadelphia at the time of the study and with the Department of Health Policy and Organization at the University of Alabama at Birmingham at the time of writing the article. Gregory Chingas was at Drexel University, Philadelphia, at the time of the study. Kristy B. Arbogast is with CIRP at the Children's Hospital of Philadelphia and the Perelman School of Medicine at the University of Pennsylvania, Philadelphia.

CORRESPONDENCE

Correspondence should be sent to Jalaj Maheshwari, Roberts Center for Pediatric Research, 2716 South St, Floor 13, Philadelphia, PA 19146 (e-mail: maheshwarj@chop.edu). Reprints can be ordered at https://www.ajph.org by clicking the "Reprints" link.

PUBLICATION INFORMATION

Full Citation: Maheshwari J, Sartin E, Chingas G, Arbogast KB. Preventing real-world pediatric vehicular heatstroke events with technology. *Am J Public Health*. 2025;115(8):1322–1326.

Acceptance Date: March 4, 2025.

DOI: https://doi.org/10.2105/AJPH.2025.308109

ORCID iDs:

Jalaj Maheshwari https://orcid.org/0000-0003-2710-7521

Kristy B. Arbogast https://orcid.org/0000-0002-1694-4562

CONTRIBUTORS

J. Maheshwari conceptualized and designed the study, designed the data collection instruments, collected data, carried out initial analyses and case studies, supervised and coordinated data collection, drafted the initial article, and critically reviewed and revised the article. E. Sartin drafted the initial article and critically reviewed and revised the article. G. Chingas collected data and carried out initial analyses and case studies. K. Arbogast critically reviewed and revised the article.

ACKNOWLEDGMENTS

The authors would like to acknowledge the National Science Foundation (NSF) Center for Child Injury Prevention Studies Industry–University Cooperative Research Center at the Children's Hospital of Philadelphia (CHOP) and the Ohio State University (OSU) for sponsoring this study and its Industry Advisory Board (IAB) members for their support, valuable input, and advice.

Note. The views presented here are solely those of the authors and not necessarily the views of CHOP, CIRP, OSU, the NSF, or the IAB members.

CONFLICTS OF INTEREST

The authors have no conflicts of interest to disclose.

HUMAN PARTICIPANT PROTECTION

The CHOP institutional review board deemed this study exempt as the data analyzed are publicly available for anyone to access.

REFERENCES

1. Null J. Heatstroke Deaths of Children in Vehicles. No Heat Stroke. 2023. https://www.noheatstroke.org. Accessed February 2, 2025.
2. HR 3164, 117th Congress (2021-2022). Hot Cars Act of 2021 (2021, May 13). Available at: https://www.congress.gov/bill/117th-congress/house-bill/3164/text. Accessed February 2, 2025.
3. Glenn E, Glenn TL, Neurauter ML. Pediatric vehicular heatstroke: review of literature and preventative technologies. National Surface Transportation Safety Center for Excellence. 2019. Available at: https://vtechworks.lib.vt.edu/items/9a6097a4-2195-4b3c-941f-6c5e3da274d6. Accessed June 11, 2025.
4. Glenn T, Glenn E, Neurauter L. Pediatric vehicular heatstroke: evaluation of preventative technologies. National Surface Transportation Safety Center for Excellence. 2021. Available at: https://vtechworks.lib.vt.edu/items/2252f770-e8d4-477d-85ac-09dbb5b96f5e. Accessed June 11, 2025.
5. Arbogast KB, Belwadi A, Allison M. Reducing the potential for heat stroke to children in parked motor vehicles: evaluation of reminder technology. National Highway Traffic Safety Administration. 2012. Available at: https://www.nhtsa.gov/sites/nhtsa.gov/files/811632.pdf. Accessed June 11, 2025.
6. Sartin E, Metzger KB, Maheshwari J. US caregivers' attitudes and risk perceptions towards pediatric vehicular heatstroke: a national survey. *Accid Anal Prev*. 2023;190:107147. https://doi.org/10.1016/j.aap.2023.107147

Collecting Data Is Just the First Step: The Importance of Training Providers for Patient Encounters

Shine Chang, PhD, and Miria Kano, PhD

ABOUT THE AUTHORS

Shine Chang is with the Department of Health Disparities Research, University of Texas MD Anderson Cancer Center, Houston. Miria Kano is with the University of Colorado Cancer Center and the Colorado School of Public Health, Anschutz Medical Campus, Aurora.

The article by Tamí-Maury and Millett[1] makes a strong case for the regular and repeated collection of sexual orientation and gender identity (SOGI) information for health care patients and study participants, recognizing that an individual's sexual or gender identity, openness to change, and behaviors may change over time. Policies and practices that discount the potential of such changes and subsequent failure to collect updated identity information may have serious implications for a patient's feelings of safety and trust, the quality of health care delivered, and the accurate collection and interpretation of research findings. Addressing barriers to the collection of SOGI data and the incorporation of SOGI information into clinical care and research are crucial, as the proportion of individuals self-reporting as sexual or gender minorities (SGM) has increased significantly over time.[2]

Many hospital systems, including cancer centers, have only recently begun to implement routine SOGI data collection from patients, yet these undercollected and underused data are relevant to patient safety, trust in clinical care teams, and engagement in health recommendations intended to improve patient outcomes. Research reveals that creating fields in health records for the collection of SOGI data is not enough.[3] Training to increase staff competence and confidence in providing welcoming and culturally respectful care to their SGM patients and their caregivers is essential. Likewise, training for health care teams ensures that clinicians know how to best incorporate such information into clinical care, how to respond to SOGI disclosure during patient encounters, and how to relate such disclosures to clinical recommendations, treatment decisions, and treatment plans. These professional behaviors are key to good patient–clinician encounters, not only for SGM patients but for all patients.

Knowing that some clinicians will disregard patient SOGI information, incorrectly believing that treating everyone the same way is an acceptable approach, what can Tamí-Maury and Millett suggest as strategies for fostering conversations with clinicians to facilitate the understanding of how ignoring such patient information and patient identity may hinder personalized care and risk offending patients and their loved ones, in addition to damaging patient–clinician trust? What do the authors suggest as best practices for preparing clinicians for encounters with SGM patients and their caregivers? For researchers, what methods would be appropriate for analyzing data reported by individuals reporting fluid SOGI status or changes in SOGI status? And how might these fluid data best be used? AJPH

Letters to the editor referring to a recent *AJPH* article are encouraged up to 3 months after the article's appearance. By submitting a letter to the editor, the author gives permission for its publication in *AJPH*. Letters should not duplicate material being published or submitted elsewhere. The editors reserve the right to edit and abridge letters and to publish responses. Text is limited to 400 words and 7 references. Submit online at www.editorialmanager.com/ajph. Queries should be addressed to the Editor-in-Chief, Alfredo Morabia, MD, PhD, at editorajph@apha.org.

CORRESPONDENCE

Correspondence should be sent to Shine Chang, PhD, The University of Texas MD Anderson Cancer Center, Department of Health Disparities Research, 1155 Pressler St, Unit 732, Houston, TX 77030 (e-mail: ShineChang@MDAnderson.org). Reprints can be ordered at https://www.ajph.org by clicking the "Reprints" link.

PUBLICATION INFORMATION

Full Citation: Chang S, Kano M. Collecting data is just the first step: the importance of training providers for patient encounters. *Am J Public Health*. 2025;115(8):1327–1328.

Acceptance Date: March 1, 2025.

DOI: https://doi.org/10.2105/AJPH.2025.308106

ORCID iD:
Shine Chang https://orcid.org/0000-0003-3804-9697

CONTRIBUTORS

The authors contributed equally to and have agreed to be accountable for all aspects of this work.

ACKNOWLEDGMENTS

We are grateful for the thoughtful insights provided by Irene Tamí-Maury and Thomas Millett.

CONFLICTS OF INTEREST

The authors have no conflicts of interest to disclose.

REFERENCES

1. Tamí-Maury I, Millett TJ. Recommendations and implementation considerations for the routine collection of sexual orientation and gender identity data in research and practice. *Am J Public Health*. 2024;114(8):777–781. https://doi.org/10.2105/AJPH.2024.307695
2. Jones JM. LGBTQ+ identification in US now at 7.6%. *Gallup*. March 13, 2024. Available at: https://news.gallup.com/poll/611864/lgbtq-identification.aspx. Accessed December 30, 2024.
3. Kamen CS, Pratt-Chapman ML, Meersman SC, et al. Sexual orientation and gender identity data collection in oncology practice: findings of an ASCO survey. *JCO Oncol Pract*. 2022;18(8):e1297–e1305. https://doi.org/10.1200/OP.22.00084

Tamí-Maury and Millett Respond

Irene Tamí-Maury, DMD, DrPH, MSc, and Mary-Louise E. Millett, MPH

ABOUT THE AUTHORS

Irene Tamí-Maury is with the Department of Epidemiology, University of Texas Health Science Center at Houston (UTHealth Houston) School of Public Health, and the UTHealth Houston School of Public Health Center for Health Promotion and Prevention Research (CHPPR). Mary-Louise E. Millett is with the Department of Health Promotion and Behavioral Sciences, UTHealth Houston School of Public Health, CHPPR, and the UTHealth Houston Institute for Implementation Science.

We appreciate the thoughtful commentary on our article[1] and the recognition of the importance of routinely collecting and updating sexual orientation and gender identity (SOGI) data in health care and research settings. We fully agree that simply creating fields in health records and data collection research instruments is not enough: comprehensive training for clinicians and health care staff is essential to ensure that SOGI data are not only collected but meaningfully incorporated into clinical care and research.

To address the challenge of clinicians disregarding SOGI information under the premise of treating all patients the same, we advocate a combination of structural and educational interventions. Institutional policies should mandate SOGI data collection and emphasize its clinical relevance,[2] and training programs should equip providers with the skills to integrate this information into patient-centered care. Strategies such as case-based learning, standardized patient encounters, and implicit bias training can help clinicians understand how acknowledging and addressing SOGI identity foster trust and improve health outcomes.[3]

Regarding best practices for preparing clinicians to engage with sexual and gender minority patients and caregivers, we recommend ongoing education on culturally responsive communication, inclusive language, and the specific health needs of sexual and gender minority populations.[4] For example, the National LGBTQIA+ (lesbian, gay, bisexual, transgender, and queer plus) Health Education Center offers training initiatives, comprehensive resources, and expert consultation to help organizations enhance the quality and cost efficiency of care provided to sexual and gender minority individuals. Providing concrete examples of how SOGI information influences screening recommendations, risk assessments, and treatment decisions can further reinforce its value in clinical practice.

For researchers analyzing SOGI data, longitudinal approaches can capture changes over time while ensuring data integrity and confidentiality.[5] Mixed methods research (combining quantitative and qualitative approaches) can offer a more comprehensive understanding of how identity shifts relate to health behaviors and outcomes.[6] Furthermore, sensitivity analyses that account for variability in SOGI reporting can help refine statistical models and improve the accuracy of findings.[7]

Ultimately, using SOGI data requires a commitment to inclusivity, methodological rigor, and the ethical use of participant-reported information. By addressing these considerations, we can ensure that health care and research practices truly reflect and respond to individuals' experiences.

We appreciate the opportunity to continue this important discussion and look forward to ongoing dialogue on improving health equity through inclusive data collection and clinical practice. AJPH

CORRESPONDENCE

Correspondence should be sent to Irene Tamí-Maury, DMD, DrPH, MSc, Assistant Professor, Department of Epidemiology, University of Texas Health Science Center at Houston, School of Public Health, Department of Epidemiology, 1200 Pressler St, RAS Suite E-641, Houston, TX 77030-3900 (e-mail: Irene.Tami@uth.tmc.edu). Reprints can be ordered at http://www.ajph.org by clicking the "Reprints" link.

PUBLICATION INFORMATION

Full Citation: Tamí-Maury I, Millett MLE. Tamí-Maury and Millett respond. *Am J Public Health*. 2025;115(8):1328–1329.

Acceptance Date: April 9, 2025.

DOI: https://doi.org/10.2105/AJPH.2025.308155

ORCID iDs:
Irene Tamí-Maury https://orcid.org/0000-0002-1404-8641

Mary-Louise E. Millett https://orcid.org/0000-0002-6599-5622

CONTRIBUTORS

I. Tamí-Maury conceptualized and drafted the response. M. L. E. Millett critically revised it. Both authors approved the final version to be published.

CONFLICTS OF INTEREST

The authors declare that they have no conflicts of interest.

REFERENCES

1. Tamí-Maury I, Millett MLE. Recommendations and implementation considerations for the routine collection of sexual orientation and gender identity data in research and practice. *Am J Public Health.* 2024;114(8):777–781. https://doi.org/10.2105/ajph.2024.307695
2. Grasso C, McDowell MJ, Goldhammer H, Keuroghlian AS. Planning and implementing sexual orientation and gender identity data collection in electronic health records. *J Am Med Inform Assoc.* 2019;26(1):66–70. https://doi.org/10.1093/jamia/ocy137
3. Oda FS, Stiehl CM. Sexual orientation and gender identity (SOGI): a tutorial on ethical data practices. *Behav Anal Pract.* 2025;18(1):275–290. https://doi.org/10.1007/s40617-024-01014-z
4. Cheung CK, Lee H, Francis-Levin N, et al. Provider preparedness to care for sexual and gender minority adolescent and young adult cancer patients: a scoping review. *Pec Innov.* 2024;5:100343. https://doi.org/10.1016/j.pecinn.2024.100343
5. Taris TW. *A Primer in Longitudinal Data Analysis.* Thousand Oaks, CA: SAGE; 2000. Available at: https://methods.sagepub.com/book/mono/a-primer-in-longitudinal-data-analysis/toc. Accessed May 30, 2025.
6. Fetters MD, Curry LA, Creswell JW. Achieving integration in mixed methods designs—principles and practices. *Health Serv Res.* 2013;48(6 pt 2):2134–2156. https://doi.org/10.1111/1475-6773.12117
7. Saltelli A, Ratto M, Andres T, et al. *Global Sensitivity Analysis. The Primer.* Chichester, UK: Wiley; 2008. https://doi.org/10.1002/9780470725184

Erratum In: "Intersectional HIV Stigma Among Black Women: Regional Differences and Implications From the Black Women First Initiative"

In: Scott JC, Rocco M, Kitchen M, et al. Intersectional HIV stigma among Black women: regional differences and implications from the Black Women First initiative. *Am J Public Health*. 2025;115(S1):S75–S84.

When originally published, one of the institutional review boards was listed incorrectly in the Human Participant Protection section. The section should read:

The study was approved by the University of Massachusetts Lowell, and the Boston University Charles River and Medical Campus institutional review boards, protocols 20-147 and 5832X. AJPH

https://doi.org/10.2105/AJPH.2025.308037e

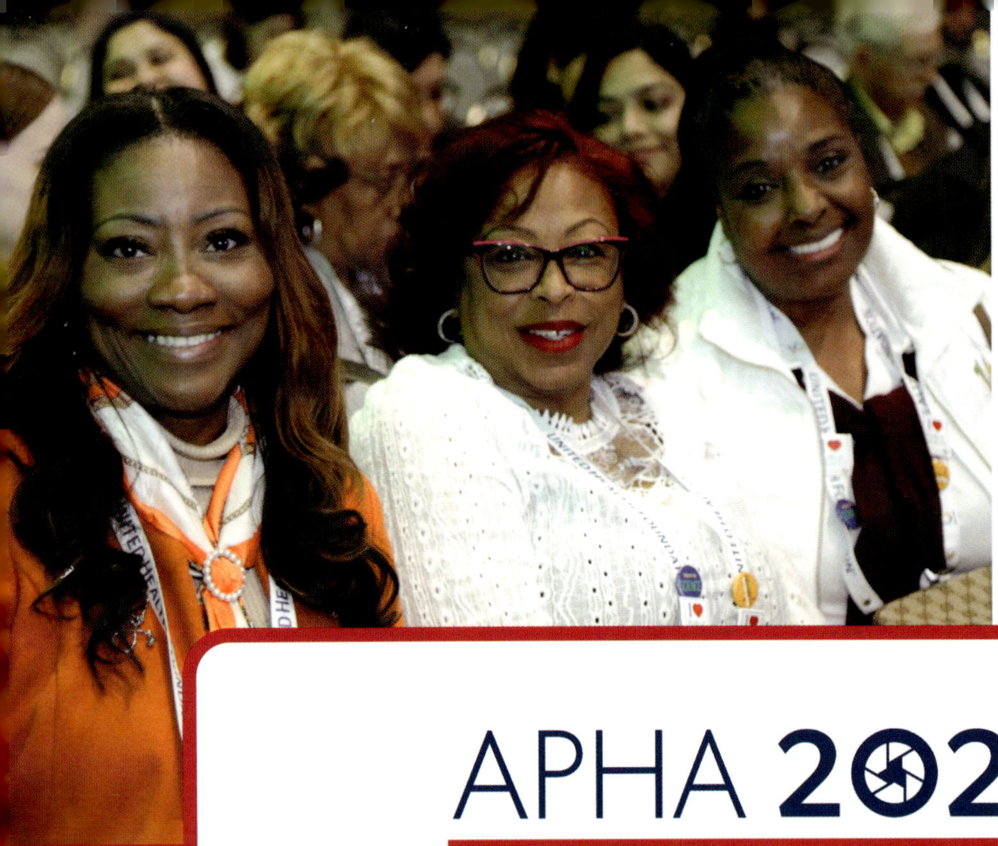
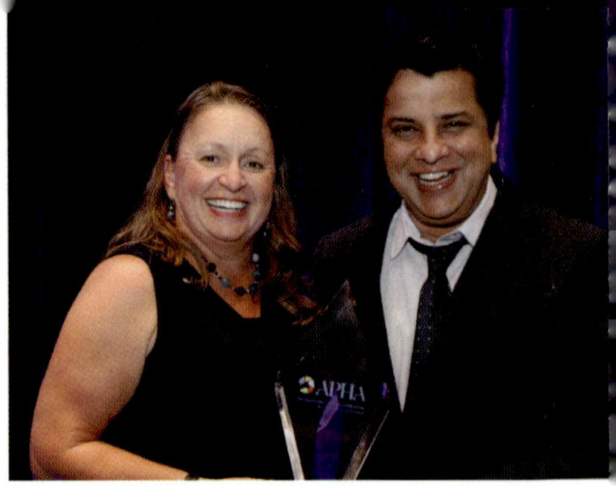
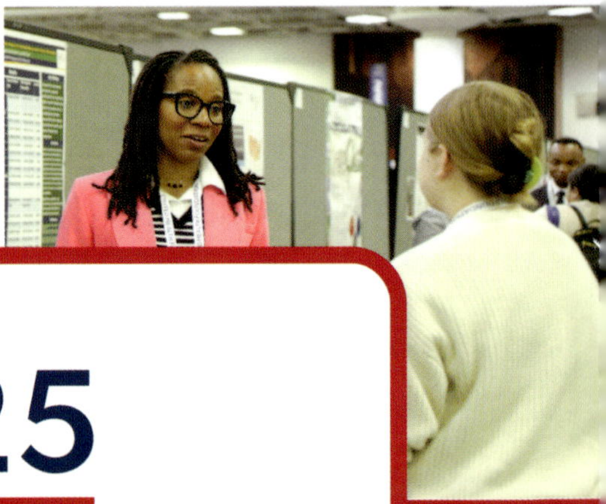